Sexuality

Other titles in *The Essential Glossary* series

FRENCH CULTURE AND SOCIETY Michael Kelly
SPANISH CULTURE AND SOCIETY Barry Jordan
GERMAN CULTURE AND SOCIETY Holger Briel
FRANCOPHONE STUDIES Margaret Majumdar
AMERICAN LITERATURE Stephen Matterson
IRISH STUDIES John Goodby, Alex Davis,
Andrew Hadfield, Eve Patten

VICTORIAN CULTURE AND SOCIETY Adam C. Roberts
POST-COLONIAL STUDIES John Thieme

Sexuality
The Essential Glossary

Edited by Jo Eadie

A member of the Hodder Headline Group
LONDON
Distributed in the United States of America by
Oxford University Press Inc., New York

First published in Great Britain in 2004 by
Arnold, a member of the Hodder Headline Group,
338 Euston Road, London NW1 3BH

http://www.arnoldpublishers.com

Distributed in the United States of America by
Oxford University Press Inc.,
198 Madison Avenue, New York, NY10016

© 2004 Arnold

The advice and information in this book are believed to be true and
accurate at the date of going to press, but neither the author nor the publisher
can accept any legal responsibility or liability for any errors or omissions.

British Library Cataloguing in Publication Data
A catalogue record for this book is available from the British Library

Library of Congress Cataloging-in-Publication Data
A catalog record for this book is available from the Library of Congress

ISBN 0 340 80675 3 (hb)
ISBN 0 340 80676 1 (pb)

1 2 3 4 5 6 7 8 9 10

Typeset in 10/13pt Minion by Phoenix Photosetting, Chatham, Kent
Printed and bound in Malta.

What do you think about this book? Or any other Arnold title?
Please send your comments to feedback.arnold@hodder.co.uk

Contents

Preface   vii

Contributors   xiii

Glossary   1

Bibliography   247

Preface

From the specialized vocabularies of the street to those of the classroom, sexuality finds itself anatomized and labelled by an intimidating array of concepts, argots, and phrases. Students working through academic material ask themselves why some writers describe marriage as 'heteronormative', some as 'heterosexist', and others as 'heteropatriarchal'; or what it means to speak of sex as variously 'scripted', 'performed' and 'commodified'. Those reading journalism, biographies, pamphlets and other primary materials might be wondering what the difference is between a 'butch bottom' and a 'lesbian boy'. Even the most commonplace features of our sexual landscape – 'honeymoon' or 'orgasm' – have acquired a history of analysis and argument. And everyone, of course, has heard of a few practical activities that they've never quite known the meaning of – maybe 'circle jerk' or 'rainbow kissing'.

As sexual cultures – and the study of them – blossom within what is, with differing degrees of inaccuracy, variously called the West, the First World, or the industrialized nations, it seems timely to offer a guide to the key terms. Although the phrase 'sexuality studies' has never quite taken off, courses, journals and publishers focusing on sexuality have. In all these sites, sexuality serves as the meeting point of a range of approaches – ethnography, textual studies, archival history, oral history, abstract theory; and it has therefore become a topic that is central to a number of disciplines, while also crossing and confusing the lines between them. This glossary is firmly located in this post-disciplinary tradition, with entries moving easily between history and social theory, philosophy and legal studies, literature and economics, psychology and social policy. It takes its lead from what we might call a postfoucauldian, post-queer – but emphatically *not* postfeminist – consensus across those disciplines: that gender inequality is still to be fought for; that desire and sexual practice are the variable products of culture; that sexual identity is unstable and surprising; that collective struggle and individual liberty can make strange bedfellows.

At the same time, this glossary comes very much out of a tradition of sexual politics. It is broadly an assertion of sexual pluralism, taking it as read that sexual freedoms have to be fought for, that sexual silences are harmful, and that sex is a contested area where our rights have yet to be made fully guaranteed. At the same time, it shows a suspicion that sexual liberation is not unproblematically a force for 'good': the last 40 years of sexual politics have generated their own problems – whether in terms of sectarianism within communities, the depoliticizing commodification of sexual styles by the market-place, or the unravelling of larger social gains by a retreat into the false security of biol-ogy and genetics.

Because sexuality is therefore a sort of 'war of ideas', I have elected to offer what is pri-marily a conceptual glossary, charting the ideas and arguments that circulate around almost 400 key terms – rather than merely the bare facts about each. Being as they are at the centre of these debates, my brief to the 50 contributors was to avoid being partisan – but also to avoid being dull. They succeeded in striking an admirable balance between covering the key arguments in each topic, while also suggesting their own particular lines of thought. I therefore hope that the glossary proves challenging and unexpected at times – as well as thorough and informative. For their unstinting work – and respon-siveness to my editorial demands – they have my deepest gratitude.

Making the most of the glossary

The initial remit of this glossary was to cover around 400 key words, but the field extends so much further beyond this that the reader will find the book best read if accompanied by other glossaries from the fields that overlap: terms such as 'hege-mony', 'surplus repression' and 'citationality' are much used around sexuality, but since they already have ample coverage in glossaries of sociology, Marxism and literary the-ory, you will not find them here. Also excluded were terms which require a definition, rather than a discussion – an old fashioned dictionary should define 'vulva' and 'pre-puce' for you. Inevitably, given the richness of sexual argot, we have not covered all the slang for all sexual practices, and readers may want to supplement this book with *The Deviants Dictionary* (http://public.diversity.org.uk/deviant/index.html), Pranzarone's *Glossary of Sexual Slang* (http://www.sexuality.org/l/sex/slang.html) or the *Dictionary of Sexology* (http://www.sexuality.org/l/sex/sexdict.html), when they find that 'gang bang' and 'spit roast' never made it into the final edition. And terms where there seemed relatively little academic or political material to discuss were also cut – hence, oddly, we have a glossary of sexuality without 'fuck' in it.

Presentation

Terms are arranged alphabetically, and set out the key arguments relating to their topic. Singling out individual terms such as these obviously leads to a fair amount of interconnection, and the glossary is heavily cross-referenced to encourage readers to build up a fuller picture of whatever topic they explore. When we have felt it would be useful to read other terms alongside, these have been put in small capitals. For instance, starting from AIDS will take you on to ACTIVISM, CONDOMS, DENTAL DAMS, HIV and SAFE(R) SEX, hence building up a far more detailed picture than any one entry could offer on its own. Equally, where an entry uses terms that may in themselves be unfamiliar for a new reader, they have been capitalized to alert you to a definition offered elsewhere. Unless particularly relevant, we have not capitalized the terms lesbian, gay, heterosexual, bisexual, transsexual, or feminism, since they occur so frequently.

The references within entries pick out the most important and interesting items of reading within the area – amounting to a bibliography of around 1,000 items. Where terms open up onto a much larger field of debate, a key item of further reading is suggested that can serve as a more in-depth exploration of the territory. For those terms which have not merited a full entry, but which readers are nevertheless likely to be looking up, there are cross-references to other relevant entries.

Structure

To offer readers a broad picture of what the book covers, the entries in the glossary can be grouped into five general areas: Theoretical Concepts; Identities, Acts and Orientations; Sexual Culture; Sexual Politics; and The Body. If a reader wants to work through a particular set or subset of entries in a certain area, these can be mapped out as follows (terms may be included in more than one section as appropriate).

1. Theoretical concepts

Key concepts: appropriation; assimilation; binary; classical sexuality; coital imperative; commodification; critical heterosexual studies; desexualization; desire; developmental narrative; deviance; early modern sexuality; erotophobia; essentialism; ethnic model; fantasy; flaneur/flaneuse; fluidity; gender capital; heteronormativity; homoerotocism; hybridity; hyperfemininity; hypermasculinity; hypersexual; identification; imitation; intimacy; *jouissance*; lesbian and gay studies; masquerade; medieval sexuality; modern sexuality; narrative; negotiation; normalization; objectification; obscenity; paraphilia; parody; phallocentrism; postmodern sexuality; premodern sexuality; public/private; queer theory; role; self-definition; sexual capital; sexual citizenship; sexual difference; sexual dimorphism; sexual orientation; sexual politics; sexual practice; sexual space; sexual stratification; sexualization; shame; situational homosexuality; social constructionism; sociobiology; stigma; trans studies; trans theory; voluntarism.

Terms coined by individual writers: abject; anti-gay; compulsory heterosexuality; confessional society; epistemology of the closet; epistemology of the fence; female masculinity; gender blending; heterosexual matrix; hom(m)osexual; homosocial; homoness; hydraulic model; lesbian continuum; lesbian gender; libidinal economy; male lesbian; minoritizing; non-heterosexual; performance; performativity; perverse dynamic; plastic sexuality; pleasure and danger; pomosexual; pure relationship; repressive hypothesis; *scientia sexualis*; script; sexual contract; straight mind; universalizing; zami.

Psychoanalysis: castration complex; cathexis; developmental narrative; disavowal; erogenous zones; fantasy; fetishism; hysteria; incest taboo; latency; libido; narcissism;

object-choice; Oedipus complex; penis envy; perversion; phallic mother; phallocentrism; phallus; polymorphous perversity; pre-oedipal; psychoanalysis; repression; sexual difference; *vagina dentata*; voyeurism.

Sexology: autoerotism; inversion; Kinsey scale; Klein sexual orientation grid; paraphilia; perversion; sexology; third sex.

2. Identities, acts and orientations

Sexual orientations: asexuality; bisexuality; heterosexuality; homosexuality; monosexuality; paedophilia; pansexual.

Sexual identities: berdache; bi; bicurious; bi-dyke; bottom; butch; femme; FtM; gay; genderqueer; hermaphrodite; heteroflexible; intersex; leathersex; lesbian; lesbian boy; men-who-have-sex-with-men; MtF; political lesbianism; post-gay; queer; SM; stone butch; straight; switch; tomboy; top; trans; transgender; transman; transwoman; transsexual; transvestite; two-spirit; whore; woman-identified woman; womyn; zami.

Sex acts: auto-erotic asphyxiation; barebacking; bestiality; bondage; buggery; circle jerk; coitus interruptus; coprophilia; daisy chain; douching; exhibitionism; feltching; fisting; foreplay; frottage; golden showers; group sex; incest; infantilism; intercourse; intergenerational sex; interracial sex; kissing; leathersex; masturbation; mummification; oral sex; orgasm; packing; pederasty; penetration; public sex; rainbow kissing; rimming; safe(r) sex; shaving; SM; sodomy; telephone sex; tribadism; virtual sex; voyeurism; watersports.

3. Sexual culture

Sex lives: adolescence; age of consent; AIDS; bed-death; divorce; family; fidelity; HIV; honeymoon; infidelity; marriage; *ménage-à-trois*; mistress; monogamy; pre-pubescence; romance; seduction; serial monogamy; sex education; sex manuals; sexual health; STDs; triad.

The sex industry: brothel; commodification; erotica; hard core; money shot; pimp; pornography; prostitution; red light district; sex industry; sex tourism; sex work; soft core; stripping

Subcultures: barebacking; bi-dyke; bottom; butch; butch/femme; camp; clone; closet; coming out; cottaging; cross-dressing; cruising; cuddle buddies; daddy; dominatrix; drag king; drag queen; dyke; fag/faggot; fag hag; femme; fetishism; FtM; fuck buddies; genderfuck; genderqueer; ghetto; leathersex; lesbian boy; lesbian chic; lesbians who have sex with men; lesbigay; LGBT; lipstick lesbian; MtF; non-monogamy; pansexual; passing; polyamory; polyfidelity; PWA/PLWA; queerbashing; recreational sex; rough trade; safeword; sapphism; scat; scene; sex parties; slash-fiction; SM; stone butch; straight acting; swinging; switch; top; triad; vanilla; womyn; zami.

Sexual props: cervical cap; condom; dental dam; dildo; IUD; packing; pill; rohypnol; sex toys; strap on; teledildonics; viagra; vibrator.

Sexual(ized) states: androgyny; asexuality; celibacy; effeminacy; frigidity; gender dysphoria; gender euphoria; impotence; innocence; intersex; masculinity; nudity; virginity; virility.

4. Sexual politics

Sexual politics: activism; age of consent; AIDS crisis; anti-gay; appropriation; assimilation; biphobia; body fascism; body politics; censorship; coalition politics; community; compulsory heterosexuality; compulsory monosexuality; consent; de-gaying; don't ask, don't tell; double standard; erotophobia; ethnic model; family values; feminism; free love; heteropatriarchy; heterophobia; heterosexism and homophobia; heterosexual privilege; homophile; homophobia; homosexual panic; interracial sex; internalized oppression; LGBT; liberation; lifestyle politics; outing; political lesbianism; pride; public/private; queer; re-gaying; reclaiming; separatism; sex positive / sex negative; sex radical; sex wars; social purity; transphobia; visibility.

Reproductive politics: abortion; artificial insemination; biological parent; coitus interruptus; condom; contraception; gay fathers; infertility; IUD; IVF; lesbian mothers; pregnancy; social parent; sperm donor; sterilization.

Gender politics: berdache; cross-dressing; female masculinity; femininity; gender blending; gender capital; gender euphoria; gender dysphoria; genderfuck; genderqueer; hermaphrodite; hyperfemininity; hypermasculinity; intersex; masculinity; sexual dimorphism; trans theory; transgender; transman; transwoman; transsexual; transvestite; two-spirit.

Sexual violence: date rape; FGM; male rape; rape; rohypnol; sexual abuse; sexual harassment; SM.

5. The body

Body modification: clitoridectomy; cosmetic surgery; FGM; HRT; male circumcision; piercing; sterilization.

Body parts: anus; breast; clitoris; erogenous zones; gay gene; gay brain; mouth; nipple; penis; pubic hair; semen; skin; testicles; vagina.

Bodily states and condition: AIDS; ejaculation; erection; female ejaculation; gender dysphoria; HIV; impotence; intersex; *jouissance*; menopause; menstruation; nudity; orgasm; polymorphous perversity; pregnancy; STDs; virginity.

Body politics: abortion; body fascism; body politics; essentialism; FGM; hermaphrodite; intersex; sexual difference; sexual health; SM; transgender; transsexual; viagra.

Why read?

And finally, no-one should overlook that most primal of childhood pleasures: leafing through a dictionary to look up dirty words.

Jo Eadie
November 2003

Contributors

Dan Allman, HIV Social, Behavioural and Epidemiological Studies Unit, Department of Public Health Sciences, University of Toronto, Canada.

Serena Anderlini-D'Onofrio, Department of Humanities, University of Puerto Rico at Mayaguez.

Caroline Bainbridge, Psychosocial Studies, University of East London, UK.

Paul Baker, Department of Linguistics and Modern English Language, Lancaster University, UK.

David Bell, Media, Journalism and Cultural Studies, Staffordshire University, Stoke-on-Trent, UK.

Mary K. Bloodsworth-Lugo, Department of Philosophy, Washington State University, Pullman, USA.

Josephine Brain, Gender Institute, London School of Economics, London, UK.

Chris Brickell, Gender and Women's Studies Programme, University of Otago, Dunedin, New Zealand/Aotearoa.

Rebecca Chalker, Department of Women's and Gender Studies, Pace University, New York, USA.

Melinda Yuen-ching Chen, Department of Linguistics, University of California at Berkeley, USA.

Ta-wei Chi, Department of Comparative Literature, UCLA, USA.

Tamarah Cohen, EFL Instructor, Kansai Gaidai University, Japan.

Andrew W Cranmer, independent scholar, Lake Echo, Canada.

Ivan Crozier, Science Studies Unit, University of Edinburgh, UK.

Jo Eadie, Social Sciences, The Open University in the East Midlands, Nottingham, UK.

Alex Evans, Graduate Research Centre for the Humanities, University of Sussex, UK.

David T. Evans, Educational consultant in sexual health (freelance), London, UK.

Natalia Gerodetti, Institut d'Études Politiques et Internationales (IEPI), University of Lausanne, Switzerland.

Rachael Groner, English Department, Temple University, Philadelphia, PA, USA.

Clare Hemmings, Gender Institute, London School of Economics, London, UK.

Liz Highleyman, journalist and health educator, San Francisco, USA.

Sally Hines, Centre for Interdisciplinary Gender Studies, University of Leeds, UK.

Myra J. Hird, School of Sociology and Social Policy, Queen's University, Belfast, UK.

Linda Kiernan, Combined Departments of History, University College, Dublin, Republic of Ireland.

Marc Lafrance, Faculty of Medieval and Modern Languages, University of Oxford, UK.

Ana Lopes, International Union of Sex Workers, London, UK.

Karen E. Lovaas, Department of Speech and Communication Studies, San Francisco State University, USA.

Sara MacBride-Stewart, Department of Gender Studies, University of Canterbury, Christchurch, New Zealand/Aotearoa.

Caroline J. McKenzie, Women's and Gender Studies Department, University of Toledo, Ohio, USA.

Mark McLelland, Centre for Critical and Cultural Studies, University of Queensland, Brisbane, Australia.

Kelly McWilliam, School of English, Media Studies, and Art History, University of Queensland, Brisbane, Australia.

Susan Mooney, Department of English, University of South Florida, Tampa, USA.

Amy Mullin, Department of Philosophy, University of Toronto, Canada.

Sylvia Posocco, Gender Institute, London School of Economics, London, UK.

Annie Potts, Department of American Studies, University of Canterbury, New Zealand/Aotearoa.

Nicholas Rees-Roberts, Department of English, University of Nancy, France.

Paul Reynolds, Centre for Studies in the Social Sciences, Edge Hill College, Ormskirk, UK.

Stefanie S. Rixecker, Environment, Society and Design Division, Lincoln University, New Zealand/Aotearoa.

Gary Schmidt, Department of Modern Languages, Luther College, Decorah, Iowa, USA.

Alison Smith, English Department, University of Central Florida, Orlando, USA.

Linnea A. Stenson, Program Director, Steven J. Schochet Center for GLBT Studies, University of Minnesota, USA.

Karen Throsby, Gender Institute, London School of Economics, London, UK.

Jill Weiss, School of Social Science and Human Services, Ramapo, NJ, USA.

Christopher West, independent scholar, Brighton, UK.

Iain Williamson, School of Behavioural Studies, University College Northampton, UK.

Julie Wuthnow, Department of American Studies, University of Canterbury, New Zealand/Aotearoa.

Abject　From a PSYCHOANALYTIC perspective Kristeva (1982) proposes that humans must perform an imaginary separation from our innate biological elements. In order to define ourselves as self-contained beings we must REPRESS the fact of our biological origins in the womb, and in order to define ourselves as rational beings we must forget the messy, biological components of our bodies. Having repressed the memory of this PRE-OEDIPAL connection, substances that remind us of it, such as blood, mucus, pus, and excrement, become 'abject': revolting, and in need of cleaning away. However, since these substances are an appealing reminder of a time that we have been forced to forget, their messiness also remains strangely attractive. For Kristeva, abjection is a necessary psychic process, which all human societies must face, while Stallybrass and White (1986: 200–1) suggest that abjection is a historically specific obsession, produced by the social regulations of MODERN SEXUALITY.

Various SEXUAL PRACTICES are often imagined as dangerous due to their association with abject bodily fluids. Grosz (1994: 198–202) argues that SEMEN is unsettling for men, since it reminds them of the FLUIDITY of their own bodies. Some bodily processes are also more powerfully abjected than others, such as sex acts involving menstrual blood or excrement – RIMMING and RAINBOW KISSING. SEXUAL HEALTH education must therefore take account of irrational fears in enabling people to feel comfortable with their own bodily processes. Furthermore, whole groups may be declared abject when represented in terms that associate them with reviled bodily substances. For instance, in the AIDS CRISIS, imagery of disease was affixed to both gay men and PROSTITUTES by politicians and the mass media (Gilman 1993). (**Jo Eadie**)

Abortion　Abortion is the deliberate termination of a PREGNANCY. Women may choose to abort an unplanned pregnancy, or a planned pregnancy where the foetus is unviable or has been diagnosed with a serious disability. Abortion may be used to terminate a pregnancy resulting from a RAPE, or women may decide to end a pregnancy following a change of personal circumstances such as job loss or relationship breakdown. Women may also find themselves coerced into undergoing abortions in some countries as a result of strict population control policies, or where a foetus is of the 'wrong' sex (Hartmann 1995; Hadley 1997). Abortion is legal in most, but not all, Western nations.

Abortion is a highly contested arena. 'Pro-life' campaigners argue that life begins at conception, and therefore, that abortion is murder. From this perspective, the line between CONTRACEPTION and abortion becomes blurred, since both the PILL and the IUD work by preventing the implantation of a fertilized egg (Clarke 2000). In the United

States, anti-abortion campaigns have led to the killings of doctors who perform abortions and the bombing of abortion clinics. A quarter of the world's population lives in countries where abortions are completely or almost completely prohibited, leading to the deaths worldwide of over 500 women daily as a result of unsafe terminations (Hadley 1997). Concerns about the use of abortion to terminate foetuses with disabilities have also been raised by disability activists who argue that this devalues the lives of those who are disabled. These concerns highlight the links between abortion and other routinely used reproductive technologies such as amniocentesis and ultrasound, which are used to detect foetal abnormalities. The 'pro-choice' lobby shifts the focus of the debate from the foetus to the woman, arguing that she has a right to choose or refuse an abortion. Feminists argue that without a 100 per cent reliable form of reversible CONTRACEPTION, the denial of access to abortion constitutes a restriction on women's sexual freedom (Petchesky 1984). (**Karen Throsby**)

Further reading

Hadley (1997); Riddle (1997).

Activism   Activism is the process of attempting political influence by individual or collective action. It has played a pivotal role in the lives of sexual minorities in the twentieth century, taking place across a broad spectrum of sexual issues, from lesbian, bisexual, gay and transgender rights, to HIV treatment funding, and the freedom to practise SM, and has resulted in many of the rights sexual minorities enjoy today. Perhaps the inspiration for most sexual activism, lesbian and gay activism has taken many forms, and was initially ushered in by the early twentieth-century rise of PSYCHO-ANALYSIS and the work of SEXOLOGISTS such as Havelock Ellis and Magnus Hirschfeld, who formed the earliest official gay activist organization, the German 'Institute for Sexual Science', later destroyed by the rise of Nazism. The 1950s saw the medical arguments of a few benevolent scientists slowly giving way to gay-run, HOMOPHILE groups such as the US 'Mattachine Society', who engaged in some political demonstration, albeit limited by fear of adverse consequences (Miller 1995: 333–57).

A new open-ness for lesbian and gay activism, and for sexual activism in general, was begun after a 1969 raid on the Stonewall Inn, a Manhattan gay bar, during which the occupants, led by DRAG QUEENS, rioted, resulting in days of protest (see Miller 1995). Galvanized by British law reform and the tide of social and sexual change in the 1960s, particularly the strengthening of FEMINIST activism, the 1970s saw British gay activism burgeoning, with the rise of the comparatively conservative CHE (Campaign for Homosexual Equality), alongside the more radical Gay Liberation Front, who staged 'Zaps' (disruptive theatrical stunts designed to gain press coverage) on targets such as religious conferences and the Miss World competition (Lucas 1994: 141–57). In the late 1980s, after a period of comparative quiet, gay activists rose to the challenge of the AIDS crisis, with ACT-UP (the 'AIDS Coalition To Unleash Power') advocating civil disobedience zaps on apathetic government agencies (see Miller 1995: 439–61). This new wave of radicalism led to the creation of 1990s groups such as Queer Nation, Outrage, and the Lesbian Avengers, among whom some advocated 'OUTING' (the exposure of CLOSETED people in power) (see Signorile 1994); more 'respectable' legal and parliamentary 'rights' campaigns continued alongside. Such co-existence demonstrates something of the central methodological question for twentieth- (and twenty-first-) century political action: should activists *demand* or *persuade*? (**Alex Evans**)

Further reading

Miller (1995).

Adolescence   Adolescence is generally used to refer to a discrete stage of human lifespan development which is perceived as a transitional phase between childhood and adulthood, and which involves qualitative changes of a biological, cognitive and socio-emotional nature. Adolescents are often represented in a negative manner (Lesko 1996) although widely accepted beliefs about adolescence being an invariably turbulent time are not supported by the academic literature in this area (Offer and Schonert-Reichl 1992). Certain difficulties in delineating adolescence arise because typically within capitalist societies there is no agreement on when an individual enters the period of adolescence or when s/he achieves adult status. In many non-capitalist cultures there are clear rites of passage where a youth experiences certain rituals or is set certain tasks. Typically these mark the transition from childhood to adulthood and within many of these societies 'adolescence' as such is therefore an essentially meaningless concept. Adolescence should therefore be viewed as a socio-historical construct.

Puberty is generally taken to indicate the onset of adolescence. It has been estimated that the average duration of pubertal development is approximately four years, typically between the ages of 10–15 for girls and 11–16 for boys. Pubertal development involves primary sexual changes such as ovulation and spermatogenesis (the production of eggs and SEMEN in females and males respectively) and secondary sexual characteristics such as the growth of body hair. The timing of puberty varies significantly across individuals and being an early or late developer may influence body image and sexual behaviour including MASTURBATION.

It has been demonstrated that adolescence may be a period of vulnerability for many lesbian and gay young people who violate HETEROSEXIST assumptions and who are likely to experience significant prejudice as they COME OUT and aim to construct a stigmatized SEXUAL IDENTITY (D'Augelli and Patterson 2001). The AGE OF CONSENT varies significantly across countries for both same-sex and heterosexual partners and may criminalize sexually active adolescents in different ways. (**Iain Williamson**)

Further reading

Coleman and Roker (1998).

Age of consent   The age of consent refers to the legal age, as defined in legislation, at which an individual is considered sufficiently mature to agree to engage in sexual acts with another person. Modern age of consent laws derive from Victorian attempts to curb child prostitution and were aimed at preserving the chastity of young girls (Kinkaid 1993) but the law has proven a blunt instrument for regulating human desire. For instance, acts considered 'sexual' as well as the ages considered appropriate for performing them differ cross-culturally (between nations) and within different subcultures (between various immigrant and religious groups within one nation). Also, some jurisdictions apply different ages (always higher) to homosexual sex (which is sometimes illegal) or apply different ages to males and females. In some American states, for instance, male–male SODOMY is always illegal, irrespective of age, whereas in Japan homosexuality is not mentioned in the criminal code, meaning there is no age of consent for male–male sex (McLelland 2000: 38). 'Statutory rape' refers to situations in which an older male has sex with a female or male below the legal age of consent and is prosecuted irrespective of whether the younger partner agreed to the act. Some civil rights' groups have argued that this denial of agency on the part of youths under the official age of consent disregards their basic human right to control the use of their own bodies whereas others insist that these regulations are essential to prevent child SEXUAL ABUSE. Some countries, such as the Netherlands, have attempted to deal with this complex situation by introducing a two-tier age of consent of 12 and 16 respectively (for both heterosexual and homosexual acts) with the higher age being deemed to apply in situations where there is a complaint by the minor or other evidence supplied that the sex act was coerced. (See also CONSENT.) (**Mark McLelland**)

AIDS   The progressive breakdown of the immune system in Acquired Immune-Deficiency Syndrome (AIDS) is the result of the destruction of the body's protective T-Cells by HIV (the Human Immunodeficiency Virus). HIV infection may initially be largely asymptomatic; however, stripped of its natural defences, the body becomes susceptible to diseases uncommon in otherwise healthy persons (such as Kaposi's Sarcoma, a rare skin cancer). The sudden preponderance of these illnesses in US urban gay men led to eventual identification of the syndrome in 1981, initially (inaccurately) known as GRID (Gay Related Immune-Deficiency). In 1982, US health agencies coined the term 'AIDS' as a more neutral label for an illness already gaining widespread notoriety – and which is largely heterosexually transmitted in the non-Western world.

Initially combated preventatively by campaigns to promote SAFE(R) SEX, the late 1990s saw the arrival of 'combination therapies', *cocktails* of drugs which have dramatically improved the health of many PWAs (Persons With AIDS), although debilitating side effects, complex dosage procedures, and concerns about the long-term efficacy of treatments (which do not work for everyone), mean that HIV remains an extremely serious illness. The potential for the slowing or reversal of 'seroconversion' (the replication of the virus) in patients has made terms like 'ARC' (AIDS-Related Complex), and indeed, 'AIDS', less common. Health professionals now tend to refer instead to stages of HIV infection.

AIDS' perceived associations with certain groups and activities have made it a nexus of social/ cultural abjections. Critics have noted the prevalence in AIDS discourse of such socially unacceptable signifiers as homosexuality, death, and anal intercourse; IV drug-use, prostitution and promiscuity; and the so-called 'dark continent' of Africa (see Crimp (ed.) 1988). Such associations have facilitated a mobilization of racist, homophobic, misogynistic, socially conservative forces against groups affected by the disease. Treichler (1988) has declared an 'epidemic of signification', in which AIDS has produced countless ideological significations, apparent in the moralism of much medical and biological AIDS discourse, and in religious conservative characterizations of AIDS as *the wages of sin*, which have compared gay sexuality to 'shak[ing] your fist in God's face' (Jerry Falwell in Shilts 1987: 347). Further, media images of the physical suffering of AIDS have acted as 'confirmation' of popular myths: of the 'homosexual body' as physically distinct from that of the sexually 'normal', and homosexuality itself imagined as a sickness (Watney 1988).

Alongside the burgeoning of cultural ACTIVISM tackling mass media AIDS representations, political activists such as ACT-UP ('AIDS Coalition To Unleash Power') have responded vigorously to the AIDS CRISIS, labelled by playwright Larry Kramer a new 'holocaust', caused by 'genocid[al]' political inaction (Kramer 1994: 163). This new, firebrand, demeanour in the gay movement produced the in-your-face politics of the QUEER movement. (**Alex Evans**)

Further reading

Crimp (ed.) (1988); Shilts (1988).

AIDS crisis   The grim period in the history of the Western AIDS epidemic, from the late 1980s into the mid-1990s, which saw rapid increases in HIV infection, death, and illness. The onset of the AIDS crisis was met with frantic ACTIVISM in the gay COMMUNITY, later formalized and funded as a vigorous voluntary sector, but this action was coupled with a dearth of resources and interest, from governments and statutory health providers (Kramer 1995; Watney 2001). Slowly, governments were persuaded to undertake prevention work, largely by the promotion of the idea of a potential heterosexual epidemic (Kramer 1995; Watney 2001). This may have been attained at a significant cost: a 'de-gaying' of AIDS which resulted in the misdistribution of resources in the fight against AIDS (King 1993: 169; see MEN-WHO-HAVE-SEX-WITH-MEN). The Western AIDS crisis is now often referred to in the past tense – the arrival of new treatments has significantly slowed the progress of the disease and the days in which gay communities experienced 'serial bereavements' seem, for the moment at least, in the past. And yet, a kind of AIDS apathy has been widely noted by sexual health workers as a consequence of the proliferation of AIDS information during the 1990s – part of a 'Post-AIDS' identity among gay men (Watney 2001). Likewise, mainstream media panic has given way to a two-pronged complacency – that AIDS in the West is after all, 'just a gay disease', and that the foreseen heterosexual holocaust is taking place only, at a convenient arm's length, in the 'Third World'. Yet infection rates continue to rise in the West – in both gay and straight communities. (See also SAFE(R) SEX.) (**Alex Evans**)

Androgyny   A combining of MASCULINITY and FEMININITY in gender PERFORMANCE and/or gender identity, from the Greek *andro* (male) and *gyne* (female). The term may imply gender duality, that is, a simultaneous expression of both culturally prevalent genders, or it may imply gender neutrality and/or transcendence of conventional gender constraints. As Halberstam argues, androgyny should not be confused with cross-gender identification or presentation (PASSING) (1998: 57, 284 note 19), but it is sometimes used to refer to the (transient) gender identity of TRANSSEXUALS in the process of sex-change. Androgyny is not specific to any sexual orientation: it is, for example, variously applied to queer styles like the lesbian 'andro-dyke' and to the mainstream 1990s youth culture of unisex clothing.

Until the end of the eighteenth century, the woman who displayed signs of masculinity, especially if accompanied by same-sex desire, was often assumed to be a physical HERMAPHRODITE (Trumbach 1994). By the end of the nineteenth century, gender variance was likely to be read as sexual DEVIANCE: 'the homosexual' was identified by SEXOLOGISTS in terms of an INVERSION of gender, 'a kind of interior androgyny' (Foucault 1990: 43). As a symbol for transcending the bipolarity of gender, androgyny became a topic of feminist debate in the mid-1970s, seeming to promise 'the elimination of obligatory sexualities and sex roles' (Rubin 1975: 204), and was also embraced by the anti-sexist men's movement as an alternative to traditional oppressive masculinity. More recent political attention has shifted to a multiplicity of gender variations – beyond the implicit BINARISM of androgyny – analysed for their relative potential to disrupt HETERONORMATIVITY (see GENDERQUEER and GENDERFUCK). Meanwhile a burgeoning body of anthropological and historical literature on cross-dressing and ritual forms of androgyny (see BERDACHE and TWO-SPIRIT) has highlighted the cultural and historical specificity of the modern West's biological model of SEXUAL DIMORPHISM (see, for example, Herdt 1994). (**Josephine Brain**)

Anti-gay   More commonly a synonym for HOMOPHOBIA, the term was redeployed as a book edited by Mark Simpson (1996) and a burgeoning political (or anti-political movement) which aims to rattle the bars of the cage that is mainstream gay culture. The anti-gay movement turns upon the ASSIMILATION of DEVIANCY within gay culture – an assimilationist tendency which renders the rich diversity of sexual and political expression within the LGBT COMMUNITY to a palatable bland and seemingly beautiful mirror image of a heterosexual norm. As a philosophy, anti-gay challenges gay cultural discourses which reproduce the mainstream dialectic of conceiving the world as either normal or deviant. At its purest, anti-gay rallies against the self-righteousness of the supposedly deviant or alternative yet surprisingly mainstream philosophy of gay community norms which assume, for example, that CAMP is the height of wit and intrinsic to a gay sensibility (Simpson 1996). Contrary to the HETERONORMATIVITY of gay norms that envision a shared sensibility or a uniform gay identity, and one which has little room for expressions of alternative viewpoints or lifestyles, an anti-gay philosophy sets out to embrace the most marginal of the marginal such as queercore, punks and DRAG QUEENS and KINGS without necessarily rendering them all one happy family. For a proponent of this philosophy, at fault is a mainstream culture and mantra that good, clean gayness is honourable and deserving, and other 'transgressive' cultural movements are less so. For Simpson and others, the blame lies within gay political organizations, media and commerce which tend to gentrify gay identity through the unanalytical and unobjective manipulation of emotional response buttons such as the trauma of COMING OUT, QUEERBASHING, legal equality, or AIDS. In essence an anti-gay philosophy asks us to celebrate diversity without APPROPRIATION or CENSORSHIP. At its core, then, is a critique against the uniformity, mediocrity and manner in which mainstream gay culture tends to serve the interests of the institutions that propagate it. (See also POST-GAY.) (**Dan Allman**)

Anus   Cats lick them, dogs sniff them, but many humans treat the anus as one of the most maligned parts of the body. Many erotic practices can be performed with the anus, including oro-anal licking (RIMMING/analingus), pleasure-pain stimulation e.g. tickling and spanking (see SM), defecatory procedures such as douching, enemas or colonic irrigation, and penetrative forms of sex. The latter includes penetration with, or encirclement of, penises (see BUGGERY and FELTCHING), DILDOS and SEX TOYS or substitutes such as food or large objects including fists / arms (brachio-colonic penetration, also called FISTING or 'fist-fucking'). For some people, the anus is also a highly sexualized bodily zone for AUTOEROTIC stimulation. Whilst historical references bear witness to the phenomenon of anal eroticization, many cultures proscribe and STIGMATIZE all forms of anal sex, essentially because of the ABJECT relations to defecation (see COPROPHILIA), its lack of procreative ability (Davenport-Hines 1990), and the supposed loss of MASCULINITY of the recipient (Bersani 1988). In English, reference to anal sex is also used to insinuate 'creeping up to' a person in authority (e.g. 'brown-nosing', 'arse-licking the boss'), or as derogatory terms of abuse towards gay men ('arse-bandit', 'turd-burglar', etc.). Its almost universal association with male homosexuality hides two key facts: that not all homosexual males participate in anal sex, and that non-homosexuals, both male and female, can and do enjoy it too. Various anal sexual practices are illegal in different states throughout the world. However, epidemiological evidence from international sexual health studies witnesses that neither laws, condemnation nor fear of infection can stop this human activity: they only serve to invisibilize its occurrence, and put the participants outside the reach of effective health promotion initiatives. As with all forms of unprotected sex, many anal sex practices can carry health risks, such as transmitting pathogens or damaging the anal mucosa or rectal canal, which can be diminished or avoided completely by adopting appropriate SAFE(R) SEX practices. (**David Evans**)

Appropriation   Appropriation features in a broad range of disciplines and practices, from law and economics to graphic design and post-colonial studies. Across these fields appropriation typically refers to seizing and using something – for example, a word, language, biological or cultural practice – that expressly belongs to someone else, usually without the owner's consent (see, for example, Gill 2001). For example, leading designers such as Versace have appropriated SM accessories in their designs and fashion shows (Raphael 1998: 1). There is a power dynamic inherent in appropriation, 'a relationship between cultural unequals – a dominant culture that appropriates and a weaker culture that has no control over its representations or products' (Ashley and Plesch 2002: 3). Above all else, the concept stresses the motivating idea of 'gain[ing] power over' the appropriated (ibid.). However, marginalized cultures can also (re)appropriate various cultural artefacts back from the dominant culture as part of a collective resistance to their oppression (see Healey 1996). For instance, in the early 1990s gays and lesbians (re)appropriated the term QUEER. Previously a term of insult it was reclaimed as the fashionable term for all people who identify as non-HETERO-NORMATIVE. This is part of a broader shift in scholarship that has begun to acknowledge that appropriation is not necessarily a one-way process of dominator over dominated. It is 'potentially a two-way process, one in which exchange and creative response may take place' (Ashley and Plesch 2002: 6). (**Kelly McWilliam**)

Artificial insemination   Artificial insemination (AI) is delivery of sperm into the vagina by means of a syringe. AI allows women to become PREGNANT without sexual contact with the sperm provider, and is used by heterosexual women whose male partners are infertile or who are unable to have penetrative sex (Mason 1993); lesbian and single women (Saffron 1994); and in surrogacy arrangements contracted by homosexual and heterosexual couples. Where donor sperm is obtained through a clinic or sperm bank, the donor usually remains anonymous, although the purchasing woman will usually be able to select a donor based on particular characteristics such as IQ or physical appearance (Schmidt and Moore 1998). Sperm donors can also be recruited privately, either through advertisements (Hogben and Coupland 2000) or through personal acquaintances. This is particularly common among lesbians using AI, who go on to negotiate varying degrees of contact and co-parenting between the mother, the child and the biological father (Saffron 1994). These novel parenting arrangements constitute a significant challenge to the model of the heterosexual FAMILY. In contrast, where AI is used by heterosexual couples to circumvent the male partner's infertility, the donor almost always remains anonymous, and the vast majority of couples keep the fact that the social father is not the biological father secret from the child (Mason 1993; see BIOLOGICAL PARENT and SOCIAL PARENT). Differing legal systems may or may not allow anonymous sperm donors to be traced by their biological children, and legal changes in this area can impact upon the availability of sperm donors. Relative to the more sophisticated reproductive technologies such as IVF, AI is cheap, low risk and within the woman's control, although prior testing for HIV and other STDs cannot be guaranteed when sperm is obtained through unregulated sources such as the Internet or mail order companies. (**Karen Throsby**)

Further reading

Saffron (1994).

Asexuality   An absence of desire and/or sexual signals. Asexuality may be an actual lack of interest in sexual engagement or a description (sometimes derogatory) applied to behaviours which do not appear conventionally sexual. It is not to be confused with abstinence or CELIBACY which imply a wilful refusal of sex, and differs from the sexual unresponsiveness implied by frigidity and IMPOTENCE in that it suggests a fundamental indifference to sex. Since PSYCHOANALYSIS posits sexuality as the central force in shaping subjectivity, asexuality is usually seen as a consequence of REPRESSION or of bio-chemical or mechanical 'abnormality'. However, asexuality may be thought of more positively as a (conscious) cultural rejection of sexual identities.

The representation of certain subjects as 'asexual' is deeply embedded within dominant power relations. As lesbian historians have pointed out, same-sex relations between women during the eighteenth and nineteenth centuries were often constructed as asexual (Faderman 1981; Trumbach 1994). While this is part of a wider tendency to render lesbianism invisible, it is also intricately related to hierarchies of gender, 'race' and class. In the early nineteenth-century Woods and Pirie libel case for example (Faderman 1981: 147–56), two Edinburgh schoolmistresses accused of lesbianism were awarded damages for defamation of character because it was inconceivable to the judges that 'decent' (read: white, Western, middle-class) women were capable of willingly engaging in sexual activity beyond the dutiful gratification of their husbands. This was in a context when homosexual acts between men were severely punished and in which working-class and black women were often represented as debauched. Some theorists have criticized a tendency within lesbian scholarship to assume the asexuality of relations between women, in a focus on 'romantic friendships', for example (Halberstam 1998: 55–6). (**Josephine Brain**)

Assimilation   To assimilate is when a minority group changes to fit into mainstream culture, such as when emigrants learn the customs and practices of their new homeland in order to fit in. There are times when assimilation is a valuable skill, such as in

PASSING, when an FtM person, for example, successfully passes for male in a public bathroom. In other cases, such as in some mainstream gay, lesbian, bisexual, and transgender activist groups, assimilation is a stated or implied goal – such as the 1950s HOMOPHILE movement. To assimilate, in these cases, is to NORMALIZE the variety of sexualities that are presently considered in the minority. Such normalization might include toning down CAMP behaviour or changing verbal cues that might identify members of a sexual minority group. A more extreme form of assimilation can be illustrated by Chandler Burr, a gay writer who considers himself an 'ardent assimilationist', and who says that he would 'not be opposed to considering genetic surgery' to cure himself of homosexuality (quoted in Warner 1999: 19). In Burr's case, to normalize homosexuality may include erasing it altogether. Other LGBT activist groups may not define assimilation as literally as Burr, but to normalize all forms of sexuality that are not heterosexual may result, preferably or not, in the eradication of 'homosexuality' in its present form. QUEER politics critiques mainstream ACTIVIST groups for not going far enough in their redefinition of 'normal' sexual identities and practices. The goal of queer politics is to eradicate 'homosexuality' and 'heterosexuality' in favour of a more fluid definition and practice of sexuality. Definitions of SEXUAL CITIZENSHIP vary and the debate continues about to what extent society should require assimilation and/or should validate a wider range of visible forms of sexuality (see PUBLIC/PRIVATE). (**Rachael Groner**)

Autoerotic asphyxiation   Known also as asphyxophilia, breath control play, terminal sex or 'scarfing', this highly STIGMATIZED practice is potentially lethal, factors which make it impossible to be sure how widespread it is. While breath control performed by others is part of the repertoire of some BDSM participants, auto-erotic asphyxiation, or AeA, involves the participant – characteristically young (e.g. 12–25) white males – using various forms of breath control on themselves and in isolation. Gags, restraints or a hanging neck-noose, can all serve to restrict the flow of oxygen in an attempt to heighten sexual excitement. The goal is to achieve orgasm and escape without passing out or dying (markc63 1996). Sometimes associated with other high risk-taking practices, AeA is frequently not suspected until death has occurred. The participants are often private, solitary characters, despite a few being public figures. They tend to be high achievers and not suspected of having any unusual (sexual) tendencies. Participants are overwhelmingly heterosexual, and some CROSS DRESS during the event. The motivation can be a purely physical/emotional one of heightened sexual pleasure, but some theorists situate the psychogenic motivation in a need to be punished, or to assuage guilt in an extreme masochistic manner. People who suffer excessive guilt at masturbation and other sexual practices, typically members of religiously conservative families, are prime candidates for AeA. Participants are not considered to have suicidal ideations, rather a SEXUAL PREFERENCE that predisposes them to danger (Allram 2000). Even in those who do not die, detrimental physiological changes in the body, and the instantaneous danger of a no-return hypoxic collapse, mean that this practice is never free from danger in life, or to life itself (Wiseman 2002). It is usually family members who discover the tragic death, and at that same moment, realize fully what has happened. Many try to 'sanitize' the scene before calling for emergency aid; thus, statistical evidence is more likely to record death by accident or suicide than a sexual practice gone wrong. (**David Evans**)

Autoerotism   Also called 'autoeroticism', or desire directed at oneself, this is most commonly thought of as MASTURBATION, although the originator of the term, Havelock Ellis (1898), tried to expand the term to include other sexual phenomena involving the self, such as NARCISSISM, dancing, HYSTERIA, and day dreaming. In doing so, Ellis was trying to break down the powerful negative stereotypes of the masturbator that had become widely dispersed in the nineteenth century, relying as they did on the thin, pasty individual who was suffering from spermatorrhoea (see SEMEN). Sigmund Freud, although strenuous in his efforts to limit Ellis's broad scope, essentially agreed with Ellis's schema. Autoerotism was an important theoretical development in the field of sexual psychology, as it posited the viewpoint that all individuals were inherently and naturally sexual. Feminism has encouraged women to find liberation in the autonomy of autoerotism (Haraway 1990: 150), which challenges the dominant construction of the female body as primarily a vehicle for male pleasure, using this as a starting point to discovering their own bodies and rejecting the SHAME and STIGMA often culturally attached to the female body. As such, it forms a central component of the feminist philosophy of Irigaray (1985b) who sees in the image of the two lips of the VAGINA touching each other, an image of female power and wholeness (see Whitford 1991:149–91). (**Ivan Crozier** and **Jo Eadie**)

B

Barebacking   Derived from horse-riding without a saddle, this is a term used to account for a culture of unprotected sex among gay men. Whereas the term 'relapse' signifies occasional unsafe sex practices (Warner 1995), barebacking is more precisely the ideology of risk-taking by seropositive men who are prepared to turn a blind eye to mutations of the HIV virus, or who are tired of being policed by AIDS; and by seronegative men who deny the real threat of contamination or who are ignorant of the inevitable mutant strains of the virus and unknown long-term effects of the existing drugs. Many young gay men are left, through lack of any government initiative, to believe that AIDS is old hat since the introduction of second-generation anti-retroviral drugs in the mid-1990s (Lestrade 2000). Barebacking is the logical evolution of the 'relapse' into the public sphere, feeding into common fantasies gay men harbour of returning to a pre-AIDS sexual LIBERATION. The bareback ideology is about rejecting the perceived emasculation of gay men by AIDS, about marketing contamination and illness as titillating transgression, co-opting the idea of Gay Liberation as mere hedonistic LIFESTYLE POLITICS. Mainstreaming unsafe sex neutralizes the shame and transforms the risk of contamination into a seemingly ethically acceptable lifestyle choice. Out goes collective responsibility; in comes individual freedom. Lately, prevention activists have been discussing 'risk/harm reduction' strategies to target gay men according to sero-status: positive, negative or unknown. Such strategies prove effective when dealing with the complexity of sexual relations – how psychological vulnerability and unconscious fantasy are vectors in seroconversion (Odets 1995). The danger is that the maximalist discourse (a CONDOM every time) is positioned as out of step with the supposed reality of contemporary gay sex lives. Prevention risks being abandoned in favour of damage limitation, which invariably takes unprotected sex as a starting block. (See also SAFE(R) SEX). (**Nicholas Rees-Roberts**)

BDSM   See SM.

Bed death   This term refers to the belief that as the length of a relationship increases, the frequency of sex between partners decreases, until the relationship becomes completely sexless. Most therapists and advice columnists agree that 'bed death' occurs when illness, work-related stress, family crises, children, and other stressors negatively impact on a relationship. As well, inevitable shifts in sexual desires will affect long-term relationships. While 'Lesbian bed death' is the most commonly heard term, 'gay bed death' and 'straight bed death' also occur: while the straight mainstream may not admit to bed death, 'you do see – quite often – women's magazines touting "Six Ways to Spice Up Your Love Life"'; this is also true among gay males, although gay culture is more equipped to deal with NON-MONOGAMY' (Bayrd 2002:30). Well-known clinicians such as JoAnn Loulan have documented inhibited sexual desires between women in long-term relationships, but others do not believe 'lesbian bed death' exists as a clinical entity. More radical understandings suggest that 'it is not useful to count the number of sex acts per week without knowing what we are counting' (Johnson 2002: 5). The question itself may be problematic when sex between women may not be defined by distinct genital acts in the same way that sex is when a PENIS is involved. This can further work to pathologize what is actually a wide-ranging collection of intimate activities that exist in lesbian relationships. (**Linnea Stenson**)

Berdache   A term originally used by European colonizers of North America to refer to indigenous peoples who exhibited aspects of behaviour or appearance not normally associated with their biological sex. It refers most often to males who take on the social ROLE of women, but sometimes refers to females who take on male roles as well. Individuals became berdache either through childhood preferences for activities associated with the other gender, or through vision quests in early adolescence. In both cases, berdache were then socialized and dressed as members of that gender, and often married members of the same sex (who were not themselves berdache). These relationships were sometimes sexual, but how often this was the case is a matter of dispute. In addition, some claim that berdache status was associated with enhanced spiritual powers or standing within the community. Given its specific cultural context, it should *not* be equated in a simple way with Western concepts of either HOMOSEXUALITY or CROSS-DRESSING.

The figure of the berdache has become significant in the context of contemporary gay IDENTITY politics. Some have argued that the apparent acceptance of berdache within North American indigenous communities can provide a model of tolerance and respect for diversity and also serve as a source of pride for indigenous LGBT people of today (Roscoe 1998; Williams 1986). Others argue that this interpretation romanticizes the experiences of the berdache, and obscures differences between the varied traditions of different North American cultures. They also contend that the term itself, as a pejorative relic of the colonial period, should be abandoned in favour TWO-SPIRIT, a name coined by QUEER indigenous North Americans themselves in the early 1990s (e.g. Jacobs *et al.* 1997). (**Julie Wuthnow**)

Further reading

Roscoe (1998).

Bestiality   Sometimes referred to as zoophilia, bestiality means human sexual interaction with non-human animals. Sex with animals is fiercely taboo in most human cultures, yet somewhat sketchy evidence suggests that it is not too uncommon a practice. It is also a thriving subgenre of PORNOGRAPHY. Assembling information from sex surveys, court records and media reports, Dekkers (1994) offers the most insightful overview of this SEXUAL PRACTICE. As he notes, bestiality is associated today with childhood experimentation with sex, and with two distinct groups of animals: farm animals and domestic pets. In the case of the former the carnal eroticism of breeding animals is combined with an unromantic and similarly animalistic human sexuality and a possible naivety concerning sexual taboos (Bell 2000). Indeed, Dekkers goes as far as to suggest that in some rural communities ADOLESCENT sex with animals is seen as preferable to sex between adolescents. In the case of pets, sex can be seen as an extension of the love and intimacy shared between animals and their owners (Franklin 1999). In both cases, of course, the animals are seen as pre-culturally, naturally sexual – and this in part accounts for their erotic appeal. Gathering empirical material on human–animal sex is tricky, for obvious reasons. Nevertheless, the Kinsey Reports

13

managed to procure fairly detailed information about what they coyly labelled 'animal contacts'. The researchers found bestiality to be a minority practice, usually confined to rural childhood and adolescence, and list the variety of practices they uncovered with clinical precision. Perhaps the most problematic issue raised by bestiality concerns CONSENT and exploitation, cornerstones of human sexual practice. Can a pet dog or a farmer's goat be said to consent to sex with its owner? Is bestiality just one more dimension to human abuse of animals? (**David Bell**)

Bi   Bi is short for bisexual or bisexuality. The term came into use during the bisexual movement, in the 1990s, when bisexuals claimed their own identity and the gay and lesbian community reconfigured itself to include bisexuals and bisexuality. Persons who refer to themselves as bisexuals, as in 'I'm bi', often use the term. It is also used in inclusive acronyms and/or abbreviations, such as LESBIGAY. More interestingly, the term has been used in a diacritical fashion, as a stand-in for the English preposition 'by', which, spelled as 'bi', alluded to the intermediate nature of bisexual orientations, and to the ubiquitous, if sometimes unacknowledged, presence of bisexuals in the master narrative of the sexual liberation movement. Some such titles are *Bi Any Other Name* (Ka'ahumanu and Hutchins (eds) 1990), and *Blessed Bi Spirit* (Kolodny 2000). (**Serena Anderlini-D'Onofrio**)

Bicurious   A recently coined term used by people who are interested in exploring sexual contact beyond that which they have been living so far. Although the term can be used by people whose primary orientation is towards their own sex, it is largely a term used by STRAIGHT people (see also HETEROFLEXIBLE). George (2001) suggests that it is particularly associated with RECREATIONAL SEX, as opposed to sexual practices organized around a strong identity or community. The term frustrates the certainties of DEVELOPMENTAL NARRATIVES of sexuality by leaving it open whether its user is making a transition to bisexuality, merely exploring some sexual alternatives – or indeed may be on their way to a gay or lesbian lifestyle, either temporarily or permanently. Its opponents see the term as demeaning BISEXUALITY by making it into no more than an act of temporary titillation. But more positively it can be seen as one of a number of new POSTMODERN identities which are open about their own provisionality and complexity, in the face of a sexual culture which expects sexuality to stay within BINARY classifications (see also LESBIANS WHO HAVE SEX WITH MEN). (**Jo Eadie**)

Bi-dyke   A subcultural slang term for a self-identified bisexual woman who either predominantly (or only) has sex with women, or who most strongly locates herself within the lesbian COMMUNITY. It is a term used by bisexuals, rather than one that is necessarily widely recognized within LESBIAN communities, making use of the QUEER convention of shortening (BI) or appropriating (DYKE) terms for political or cultural ends. Similar terms in a descriptive sense are 'bisexual lesbian' (Dajenya 1995) and 'lesbian-identified bisexual' (Hutchins and Ka'ahumanu 1990: 370). Similar terms in a politically performative sense would include 'bi-fag', 'butch queen', 'dyke daddy' and so on, where the function is to bring together queer terms in a challenging way.

The term bi-dyke is interesting insofar as it emerges from and signals the particular way in which bisexual women's community has developed and been theorized in the last three decades in English-speaking urban contexts. In both community and theoretical contexts, bisexual feminists have argued that BISEXUALITY and FEMINISM are linked in their mutual concern with women's independent sexuality, and in posing a direct challenge to that sexuality being externally defined. In this vein, Weise argues that 'we see bisexuality calling into question many of the fundamental assumptions of our culture: the duality of gender; the necessity of bipolar relationships . . . [and] the demand for either/or sexualities' (Weise 1992: ix). In addition, women-only bisexual groups form a large part of the US and UK bisexual support networks and political movements. This work has not been matched by a corresponding focus on bisexual men *qua* bisexual men: male bisexuality has tended to be addressed in mixed-sex volumes, through psychological or sociological structural vectors, or in relation to HIV and AIDS (although more recently, see Beemyn and Steinman 2001 and 2002). (**Clare Hemmings**)

Binary   Binaries are intrinsically linked with modernity and the ideals of the Enlightenment whereby meaning is constructed as either/or through the difference between the terms A and B. Examples are: mind/body, nature/culture, rational/emotional, or man/woman, white/black, heterosexual/homosexual. Binarism is a system which relies on these either/or definitions. What is problematic about binaries is that they are not internally equal but display violent hierarchy whereby one term governs the other. Meaning and definition work by exclusion and lie in the difference between the terms; meaning is therefore not intrinsic but constituted by boundaries. However, this formula universalizes and fails to recognize differences within categories as well as maintaining them as binary oppositions (Weedon 1997).

Within binarizing sexual politics differences are often perceived to be threatening and those who appear to be 'in-between' sexualities or genders are required to 'take sides' or are scapegoated – for instance, expecting bisexuals to 'come off the fence' (Eadie 1994) and TRANS people to PASS as a given gender (Bornstein 1994). Some sexual subcultures reiterate binaries, such as the insistence by some lesbians that one is either BUTCH or FEMME or the SM insistence that one is either TOP or BOTTOM. However, these binaries can also be positively eroticized within SM and BUTCH/FEMME culture. Furthermore, rather than being static, new identities are always being generated which seek to interrogate the reigning binaries within sexual subcultures, such as 'SWITCH' in SM. Thus being a continuous performance, sexual identities can both maintain binaries as well as advocate their blurring, for example, through the enactment of ANDROGYNY or through bisexuality as an ideal within sexual LIBERATIONIST thinking. In particular, both feminism and QUEER THEORISTS seek to expose and undo the constitution of binaries both theoretically and through activism. (**Natalia Gerodetti**)

Further reading

Herdt (1994); Wilchins (2002).

Biological parent   A biological parent is a person whose eggs or sperm were used to conceive a child, whether through vaginal intercourse, or through other conceptive technologies such as ARTIFICIAL INSEMINATION or IVF. Whilst parenthood is conventionally understood as a unitary concept to which biological relatedness between parent and child is fundamental, the new reproductive technologies highlight the extent to which parenthood can easily be fragmented into biological and social categories. A lesbian couple, for instance, might wish to distinguish between the child's biological mother and her/his other mother – or might wish to efface the distinction. The case of surrogacy offers an additional category of gestational motherhood, since IVF techniques enable contracting couples to use their own gametes, or those of donors, to create embryos which will be gestated by another woman on their behalf (Ragone 1998).

Outside of the use of reproductive technology or donor gametes, gestational motherhood is inseparable from biological motherhood. However, for men, biological parenthood is less certain, and there has been a rise in the availability of simple and discrete genetic tests to prove or disprove biological parenthood. Social and cultural assumptions of the primacy of biological relationships means that the discovery of non-paternity in this context is understood as producing a fundamental change in the relationship between the father and the child. It is also the case that a man might be a biological parent but be unaware of it, either because he donated sperm anonymously, or because he has no contact with the mother. In the context of reproductive technology, the certainties of biological parenthood have also been destablized, and there have been a number of mix-ups in IVF clinics, where the wrong embryos have been implanted. These errors have generally only become visible where the subsequent children have been racially different from their presumed biological parents and, as is also the case with gestational surrogacy cases, can produce competing parenthood claims (Hartouni 1997; Andrews 1999). (**Karen Throsby**)

Biphobia   Biphobia is a form of EROTOPHOBIA especially directed against BISEXUAL people. Like HOMOPHOBIA, biphobia exists both within and outside of the gay, lesbian, bisexual and transgender community. For many heterosexuals, biphobia can be the fear of not being completely straight, or of being near people who are not completely straight. For gay and lesbian people, biphobia can be the fear of not being completely gay or lesbian, of having desires that do not correspond to one's IDENTITY. Both within and outside of the queer community, biphobia became rampant during the AIDS scare, when, in the late 1980s, it was found that many queers had been behaving bisexually all the time, even as they had passed as gay or straight depending on what was necessary. This awareness was enhanced by the spread of AIDS outside of the traditional risk group of gay men. Straight people were biphobic due to the fear that bisexual behaviour would spread the infection beyond the gay community. Gays and lesbians were biphobic due to the fear that the practice of bisexuality, once uncovered, would destabilize their sense of identity, and the cultural notion the gay liberation movement had established, that one was 'born that way'. Bisexuality was understood as a phase, and not as an identity or form of desire in itself. Moreover, the idea that homosexuality was mentally healthy had recently been established, based on the new edition of the Diagnostic and Statistical Manual (DSM), of 1974, the first not to list homosexuality as a mental illness. As a result, gays and lesbians feared that fundamentalist social impulses would use the concept of bisexuality to claim once again that homosexuality could be cured. (**Serena Anderlini-D'Onofrio**)

Further reading

Ka'ahumanu and Hutchins (eds)(1990).

Bisexuality   The attraction to members of both sexes. Three common mistaken assumptions pervade thinking about bisexuality: that it entails *simultaneous* attraction to men and women; that it entails *equal* attraction to men and women; and that it entails sexual *activity* with both men and women. While these may be true for some bisexuals, others may be: attracted to different sexes at different times in their lives; more strongly attracted to one sex; sexually active with only one – or neither – sex. The KLEIN SEXUAL ORIENTATION GRID has been developed as a tool to illustrate the diversity of forms of attraction towards both sexes.

Sexual theory has offered a series of explanations for bisexuality. For early SEXOLOGY, bisexuality was seen as deriving from the fact that human biology contains both male and female components – a position that Freud rejected. Instead, he proposed that bisexuality was a result of the child's IDENTIFICATION with both parents: the psyche contains both what he refers to as active, masculine components, resulting from identification with the father (the desire to possess a woman) and passive, feminine elements, resulting from identification with the mother (the desire to be possessed by a man). As Butler (1990: 61) observes, in the Freudian model bisexuality is thus no more than 'the coincidence of two heterosexual desires within a single psyche'. Working from this assumption, Freud argued that this double desire would usually be REPRESSED as one or other identification became stronger, but that in some cases psychoanalysis might be able to restore a patient's 'full bisexual functions' (1991b: 375). Garber extends this Freudian approach by arguing that 'bisexuality is that upon the repression of which society depends for its laws, codes, boundaries, social organization – everything that defines "civilization" as we know it' (1995: 206). For Garber, such ABJECT desire may return to unsettle adult identities which are based on excluding some part of this desire as a result of COMPULSORY MONOSEXUALITY, a position supported by Hall and Pramaggiore (1996). But this stress on the subversive qualities of bisexuality should not make us overlook the ways in which it also occurs as an accepted part of conventional sexual practice in many cultures (Fox 1996: 9–13). The Bi Academic Intervention collective (1997), argue for bisexuality as following culturally determined paths, which may result in its being a licit expression of existing social structures: for instance, its apparent transgressions may model themselves on dominant models of racial supremacy or on the economic imperatives of capitalism.

Psychological work has shown how bisexuality plays an important part in the emotional and sexual lives of many people (see George 1993; Klein and Wolf 1985). Some may choose to organize a bisexual IDENTITY around their double desires, but others may also identify as lesbian, as heterosexual, or as gay. The unwillingness to name oneself as bisexual has been an important catalyst to activists, who have made bisexuality more credible and more visible through political action and the documenting of life histories (Hutchins and Ka'ahumanu (eds) 1990; Tucker 1995). These writers have coined a term for the hostility that they face: BIPHOBIA. Such writings challenge the primacy given to homosexuality in recent thinking about SEXUAL POLITICS, and instead argue that we must recognize a wider range of non-conformist sexualities. Against this some lesbian and gay theorists have seen bisexuality as an attempt to retain HETEROSEXUAL PRIVILEGE while enjoying the political cachet of an alternative sexuality (Wilkinson 1996) – leading to experimental identities such as BICURIOUS and HETEROFLEXIBLE. But in many organizations and events, the term LESBIGAY has developed as a shorthand way of indicating that lesbians, gay men, and bisexuals can – and want to – all be seen as part of a shared community. (**Jo Eadie**)

Further reading

Angelides (2001).

Body fascism   Body fascism is the enforcing of cultural ideals and norms of physicality through the persecution or exclusion of those whose bodies are not perceived to conform. Modern Western cultures stigmatize those who are perceived to be old, physically disabled, improperly sized, shaped, or raced, and who fail therefore to live up to certain models of physical desirability. Such perceptions tend to be 'explained' and 'naturalized' – overweight people are unhealthy or lazy; disabled people are sexually incapable – and yet the contingency of definitions of attractiveness is demonstrated by the mutability of representations of desirable bodies across history and cultures. Lesbian and gay cultures have had an ambiguous relationship with body fascism. Lesbian culture's FEMINIST outlook has encouraged the opposition of male-dominated models of beauty, although the rise of a more commercial lesbian culture has seen this stance become somewhat eroded in recent years. Gay male culture's body fascism has continued to escalate in the most hegemonic, COMMODIFIED streams of the scene, although some (sub-) subcultural strands have FETISHIZED bodies seen by the gay hegemony as undesirable (e.g. the 'Bear' and SM scene – the latter leading to some debate over the potential for SM to function as INTERNALIZED OPPRESSION, punishing unacceptable bodies). TELEPHONE SEX and other new technologies may have permitted those excluded by body fascism to engage in sexual interaction without the aesthetic constraints of the body (see also SEXUAL SPACE). In the partial deprofessionalization of PORNOGRAPHY and the exchange of 'amateur' images, 'imperfect' bodies may be becoming re-eroticized – although *perfect* amateur bodies may still be in high demand. The pornography industry has often fetishized bodies elsewhere considered undesirable; however, whether this is *liberation* or simple *exploitation* is a question for ongoing debate. (**Alex Evans**)

Further reading

Wolf (1993).

Body politics   A term developed within sociology and cultural studies to explore the link between the body and IDENTITY construction. Within body politics, practices such as diet, exercise and bodily adornment and modification are examined in relation both to the individual self and in terms of wider social and cultural interaction. The body is seen as central to the ways in which identity is constructed individually and collectively.

Foucault (1977) argued that distinct discourses were constructed around particular bodies in relation to institutional settings, such as hospitals, schools, prisons and armies. From a Foucauldian perspective, power is *inscribed* upon the body. Others read the body as a cultural *text,* by examining the ways in which bodies are represented in specific ways within certain societies and cultures. Feminist work has in this way explored eating disorders amongst women in terms of the relationship within Western society between normative FEMININITY and slenderness, emphasizing the links between eating disorders and notions of desirability (Bordo 1993). Similarly, a link has been made between the construction of normative MASCULINITY and fitness training programmes. Work on body politics also emphasizes the ways in which individuals employ agency to transform their bodies, and thus the meanings around identity, through *bodywork* practices; for example, PIERCING may be used to enhance sexual pleasure and/or to represent membership of a sexual subculture. Additionally body politics has explored representations of the body in relation to disability and HIV and AIDS. Here the emphasis is upon the ways in which dominant representations construct society's attitudes to the 'healthy' versus the 'sick' body. Writers have emphasized how representations, and their constructed meanings, produce value judgements around issues such as lifestyle choice, morality and risk behaviour. The body politics for the disability movement and HIV and AIDS movements have thus been concerned with subverting dominant representations to create alternative meanings of disability and experiences of HIV and AIDS. (**Sally Hines**)

Further reading

Bordo (1993).

Bondage   The act/art of restraining through the use of rope, scarves, cuffs, handcuffs, latex/leather, hoods, etc. Bondage might entail restraining the arms and/or legs, but may also involve complete immobilization. There is much debate as to the motivations for and pleasures of bondage, which include the NARCISSISM in being tied up and adored; the regression to childhood involved in being rendered passive; and the love/adoration expressed in taking time to bind a partner. Benjamin (1983) suggests that the desire to be controlled returns the participants to a parent–child relationship, in which the 'victim' is affirmed as needed and wanted, while the desire to bind another serves as a realization of the fantasies of power and independence which haunt us from our first childhood efforts to become separate and autonomous individuals – 'an attempt to relive an original differentiation which failed' (292). In particular, she suggests that the desire to be restrained serves as a compensation for the extreme levels of control and regulation over time, activity, and other people that we are all obliged to exercise within the rationalization of the modern social order (296). Conversely, McClintock (1993: 112) documents the particular pleasures in taking control enjoyed by social groups who normally have little access to power. In more sexual terms Adams (1996: 27–48) suggests that bondage multiplies the pleasures of the body, disrupting the hold over it normally exercised by genital sexuality. (**Caroline J. McKenzie**)

Bottom   Many gay men use this term to refer to the receptive partner in anal sex. For some men this is a reliable sexual choice which may become a self-label (Wegesin, Elwood and Bowen 2000) whilst for others it is a sexual position which may vary within and across sexual encounters (Underwood 2003). Cross-cultural research by Herdt (1997) suggests that in many (patriarchal) cultures men who identify as 'bottoms' are more widely stigmatized than men who adopt a TOP identity because of the association with being penetrated equating with femininity and weakness. The term is also used in relation to SADOMASOCHISM to refer to an individual who adopts a submissive role and allows him or herself to be dominated sexually by at least one other individual. Whilst such behaviour has tended to be pathologized, most encounters are scripted and rely heavily on ritual with little physical danger to the 'bottom'. Indeed, it is often argued within SM communities that bottoms hold the power in a SCENE, since they regulate sexual activities with the use of SAFEWORDS. (**Iain Williamson**)

Breast   Breasts are the fleshy appendages on the chest of the adult female. They are composed primarily of fatty tissue and mammary (milk-producing) glands. The tips of the breast are the NIPPLES and the areas of darker tissue surrounding the nipples are the areolae. Beyond their purpose of providing food for infants, breasts have acquired great cultural significance as symbols of nurturance and eroticism. Social notions of the ideal breast have varied greatly over time (Angier 1999; Latteier 1998; Yalom 1997). Stone-Age cultures left female figurines with immense breasts, thought to be fertility icons. Wall paintings from Minoan Crete showed women wearing tight bodices with exposed large breasts. In the Victorian era the hourglass figure with a full bosom and small waist – often achieved with a corset – signified health and wealth. In 1914 Mary Phelps Jacobs patented the first modern brassiere. In the early 1920s a slender boyish figure was the rage, but by the 1940s and 1950s Hollywood glamour queens and suburban housewives alike had adopted the pointed bullet bra. In the late 1960s and 1970s the small-breasted 'natural' look became popular, and many women abandoned their bras. It is widely (although spuriously) believed that feminists of this era burnt their bras to express their rejection of patriarchal notions of feminine beauty. In the 1980s and 1990s larger breasts were once again 'in', coupled with a slender, gym-toned body. Many women achieved this look with the padded push-up Wonderbra, while others opted for surgical breast enhancement (see COSMETIC SURGERY). Silicone gel breast implants were banned by the US Food and Drug Administration in 1992 due to health concerns, yet breast augmentation with saline implants remains a popular cosmetic procedure (Love and Lindsey 2000: 60–6). In recent years interest in the breast has focused on the growing epidemic of breast cancer, which has spawned a wave of activism similar to that pioneered by people with AIDS (Love and Lindsey 2000). Although breasts are used to sell everything from beauty products to beer – and much pornography is heavily breast-focused – Western women have typically been told they must cover their breasts, leading to controversies over the legality of toplessness and breast-feeding in public. (**Liz Highleyman**)

Brothel   From the Old English *brothen* (ruined) or *bréothan* (to go to ruin), a fixed or mobile establishment in which PROSTITUTES reside and offer their services, either as employees or on a commission basis. These businesses are usually managed by a Madam, who was or still may be a prostitute herself. Employees within a brothel, which can include men, must be prepared to meet varied sexual desires. Brothels may contain a 'torture-chamber', a 'dungeon' and other such themed rooms, catering for BONDAGE, SADOMASOCHISM and other FETISHES. Particular brothel employees may be assigned to certain clients, especially if they are regulars. The brothel can be traced back to the sixth century BC in Greece and 650 BC in China, however the term 'brothel' did not appear until 1593, being preceded by 'bawdy-house' (1552) and earlier by 'stew' (1362). Attempts were made in medieval Europe to abolish them totally, however they continued to gain in popularity. The brothel has featured in art and literature most famously in John Cleland's *Fanny Hill* (1748–1749). In nineteenth-century Paris mass brothels operated, leading to the term *tôles d'abattage* (demolition tables, slaughter tables) where tables were used instead of beds. In the 1970s it was reported that state-controlled brothels operated in West Germany, Spain, Holland and Belgium (Simons 1975). While it is currently illegal in the United Kingdom to operate a brothel they are common elsewhere in Europe and Asia, and in some US states, which has led in places to a vibrant SEX TOURISM industry. (**Linda Kiernan**)

Further reading

Jones (2000).

Buggery This derogatory term for anal intercourse is still widely used in legal statutes; for instance, the Sexual Offences (Amendment) Act (United Kingdom: 2000) reduced the minimum age 'at which a person, male or female, may lawfully consent to buggery from 18 to 16'. Buggery and SODOMY have many interchangeable representational meanings, but also profound differences in origins and legal understanding. Initially referring to a heretical eleventh-century Bulgarian sect, it was expanded to cover a wider range of heretical peoples, and later sexual dimensions were embellished denoting sacrilegious profanities, which led to state-sponsored brutalities and criminal sanctions (Dynes 1990a). Buggery pre-eminently represents anal intercourse, and other male same-sex activities and identities. Yet in the legal framework of the EARLY MODERN period it was also used to refer to so-called 'deviant' sex – anal and oral – between men and women, masturbation and BESTIALITY (Tomlinson 1999), suggesting that all non-procreative activities outside heterosexual marriage were seen as equally suspect. It is only in more recent centuries that the term has acquired its more specific meaning, as the modern figure of 'the homosexual' emerged. Despite this flexibility of meaning, there is little evidence that buggery was used as a term for lesbianism, indicating a general invisibilization of female sexuality. Different historical times and places portray a variety of approaches to anal intercourse, situating it anywhere from a cultural identifier of SEXUAL ORIENTATION, through to a conduit for consensual pleasure, from forced domination (MALE RAPE), to a mode of contraception and protector of vaginal VIRGINITY. Female-to-male anal intercourse using a STRAP-ON or DILDO signifies a rebellious abandonment of customary HETERONORMATIVE gender roles, and a performative translocation of sex from procreation to erotophilic emancipation.

Unprotected anal intercourse, referred to in certain gay circles as BAREBACKING, is unparalleled in means for transmitting sexual infections, and the primary mode for HIV transmission amongst male–male infections. (**David Evans**)

Butch A category of IDENTITY that refers to those overtly masculine in appearance or demeanour. Commonly deployed in gay and lesbian communities to refer to masculine lesbians, butch may be understood as 'a category of LESBIAN GENDER that is constituted through the deployment and manipulation of masculine gender codes and sym-bols' (Rubin 1992: 467). With reference to Anglo-American contexts, Halberstam (1998: 120) argues that butch amounts to 'a receptacle for all lesbian masculinity' and an important marker of FEMALE MASCULINITY. A polysemic and multi-dimensional cate-gory, butch is also implicated in understandings of DESIRE and SEXUAL PRACTICE. Thus, his-torically butches in BUTCH/FEMME communities were not only defined by masculine dress, demeanour and style, but often did, or were expected to, desire FEMMES (Rubin 1992). Butch may comprise a spectrum of identities often qualified in terms of rigid-ity and/or permeability, with 'soft' butch embodying porous and partial masculine IDENTIFICATIONS, and 'hard' and STONE BUTCH referring to progressively more male-identi-fied positions that are less sexually reciprocal and permeable (Halberstam 1998: 123).

Butch is in fact not exclusively lesbian, and rather often represents complex articu-lations of understandings of gender and sexuality which are context-specific and cul-turally nuanced. In gay male sexual culture in the United States, for instance, butch identities are linked the hyper-masculinity of the CLONE (Levine 1998). Further, ethno-graphic research points to the complex deployment of the term in gay, lesbian and transgender communities in New York City. In the context of DRAG balls, butches are 'female-bodied masculine persons' (Valentine 2002: 228) who adopt masculine names and may take testosterone injections when available. Butches here may take femme queens who 'walk the balls' as girlfriends. In turn, femme queens are 'male-bodied feminine persons' who feminize their bodies and at the balls parade alongside butch queens, i.e. 'masculine-identified gay men' (Valentine 2002: 228–9). On the ball scene, both butches and butch queens embody non-normative, masculine-inflected genders.
(**Silvia Posocco**)

Further reading

Halberstam (1998); Nestle (1992).

Butch/femme　　LESBIAN identities articulated in terms of masculine and feminine ROLES and styles. Butch/femme refers to the deployment of masculine and feminine demeanour, the articulation of specific forms of lesbian erotic identity (Nestle 1992: 14), and the creation of lesbian eroticized gender difference. As argued by Rubin (1992: 477), BUTCH and FEMME are 'ways of coding identities that are both connected and distinct from societal roles for men and women'.

Butch/femme historically pertains to gender and sexual identities and practices characteristic of working-class Anglo-American lesbian communities in the mid-twentieth century (Faderman 1991). Through oral history projects and historical research, Kennedy and Davis (1993) document butch and femme life and style in Buffalo, New York, from the 1940s to the 1960s. Here butch/femme roles drew unequivocally on contemporary heterosexual models of gender BINARISM and mostly structured erotic relations accordingly. However, they were foundational in the development of forms of public lesbian interaction and the inception of lesbian bar culture. Butch/femme communities therefore engaged in pioneering efforts at carving a space for public lesbian existence in pre-Stonewall times (Kennedy and Davis 1993: 6).

In the 1970s, lesbian feminists argued that butch/femme, as gendered articulations of lesbian identities, relations and DESIRE, amounted to a form of mimicry of heterosexuality (Jeffreys 1989). Grounded in stereotypes of SEXOLOGY, butch/femme are said to reproduce hierarchical gender relations, thus reinstating patriarchal arrangements and abetting the devaluation of the feminine, and of women. It is argued that these inherently derivative, asymmetrical and HETERONORMATIVE identities and relations should be replaced by reciprocal, non-hierarchical arrangements and consonant sexual conduct.

Despite the implication of butch/femme in SEX WARS controversies, the 1980s and 1990s witnessed a renaissance of lesbian gender-coded identities, or 'neo-butch/femme' (Faderman 1992: 579). Munt (1998b) cogently expresses the renewed interest in butch/femme identities and relations and argues that two distinctive and yet interrelated modes of articulation of butch/femme may be discerned. The 'epistemological mode' refers to lesbian knowledge practices that hinge on the PERFORMATIVE inscription of gender characteristics onto a female body, and result in the creation of 'LESBIAN GENDERS'. The 'ontological mode' corresponds to deployments of butch/femme that lay the ground for claims to a 'true' self. These analyses unsettle charges of uncritical dependence on heterosexuality and patriarchal power. Following Butler (1990: 123), they contend that butch/femme identities and desire may be predicated on 'dissonant juxtaposition' of gender signifiers, rather than gender conformity. Hence, 'the idea that butch and femme are in some sense "replicas" or "copies" of heterosexual exchange underestimates the erotic significance of these identities as internally dissonant and complex in their resignification of the hegemonic categories by which they are enabled' (Butler 1990: 123). The premise that COMPULSORY HETEROSEXUALITY is 'natural', 'original' and foundational is thus thrown into question (ibid. 124). (**Silvia Posocco**)

Further reading

Kennedy and Davis (1993); Nestle (1992).

Camp   A sensibility characterized by glamorous aesthetic excess and ironic humour, and connected with questions of gender and SEXUALITY. Camp artefacts or practices tend to demonstrate an inappropriate aesthetic excess, often expressed, or at least, 'read', in terms of gender confusion – from an excessive Art Nouveau lamp to a 'camping' gay man who calls his duffel coat 'my mink'. Historically, Sinfield (1994) claims that camp's defining moment was in the cultural constructions of sexuality, gender, and class, associated with Oscar Wilde's trial and the declining social power of the aristocratic leisured class in the nineteenth century. Discourse on camp, however, has ballooned since the publication of Susan Sontag's seminal 'Against interpretation: notes on camp' (1964), which concludes that camp is 'a form of aestheticism' (1964: 54), often relying on a contrast between 'silly or extravagant content and rich [usually 'glamorous'] form', and a sense of 'being-as-playing-a-role', that is, 'life as theater' (1964: 56). Gay criticism has often seen Sontag as an interloper in gay cultural practice, however. Gay left critics in the late 1970s and early 1980s sought to reconnect camp specifically to gay identity, suggesting that camp is 'a lie that tells the truth' originating in the duality of the CLOSETED queer's desire to both conceal and exploit his or her sexuality (Core 1984: 81). Camp's portent as gay cultural-*political* activity has generated extensive debate – as Richard Dyer points out, despite its 'radical/progressive potential', gay camp's often self-critical nature may reveal well-learned gay self-loathing (1999: 111).

QUEER THEORY again revitalized debate around camp in the 1990s. For the first time, scholars began explorations of lesbian camp (see DRAG KING). Continuing criticisms of Sontag's marginalization of camp's lesbian and gay heritage, Meyer (1994: 11) suggests that the confusing appearance of camp in the popular mainstream can be attributed to a 'queer trace' bleeding into a culture which re-appropriates items already APPROPRIATED and redirected by queer camp practice. Queer's unapologetic political stance also favoured camp as progressive political practice due to its potential for the disruption of hegemonic social values such as the worthiness of authenticity (Dollimore 1991: 307–25). Such attempts to indelibly ground camp in queer identity have been criticized, however, for their paradoxical absolutism on a subject which may hold the rejection of absolutes at its core (Cleto 1999b: 18–19). (**Alex Evans**)

Further reading

Cleto (ed.) (1999a).

Castration complex   A fear of castration which is the central mechanism in the psychoanalytic account of the OEDIPUS COMPLEX (Freud 1908: 1909). It is said to occur in both boys and girls, that is, in both the positive and negative forms of the Oedipus complex. In boys it marks the resolution of the Oedipus complex, while in girls it marks its beginning. Several factors influence the emergence of the castration complex in boys. There is usually a marked threat of punishment by the father for the boy's illicit DESIRE for the mother. This coincides with a visual reminder of the possibility of castration – this may result from the sight of the female genitalia or from the apparent disappearance of the PENIS during the act of coitus. The threat of castration thus takes on a heightened significance for the little boy. For Freud, entry into the castration complex signifies an entry into culture for the little boy insofar as the symbolic acceptance of the FANTASY of castration enables the REPRESSION of the boy's PRE-OEDIPAL attachment to the mother and encourages him to adhere to the law of the father. In boys, the castration complex marks the resolution of the Oedipus complex and the formation of the superego, the agency of the mind that regulates behaviour and morals.

By contrast, in girls, the castration complex marks the entry into Oedipal conflict. On witnessing the presence of the penis in males, the girl assumes that she has already been castrated by the mother, and she begins to seek compensation for this (see PENIS ENVY). There is a crucial difference between the male and female castration complexes in that, for the boy, the castration complex is a fantasy of what will happen to him if he fails to adhere to the social mores, while, for the girl, it seems as though castration is a lived fact. Paradoxically, however, it is difficult to see how the girl can be threatened by the loss of something she has never possessed. This is a fundamental flaw in Freud's articulation of the development of femininity and has been a key factor in feminist rejections of PHALLOCENTRIC Freudian ideas about female sexuality in particular (see Mitchell 1974: Chapter 8). (**Caroline Bainbridge**)

Cathexis Cathexis is a term coined by the translator of Freud's writings, James Strachey, to refer to the way in which psychical energy is invested in ideas or memories, body parts and objects, when we become powerfully attached to them. The original German term (*die Besetzung*) implies that something is being filled up or occupied. In PSYCHOANALYSIS, cathexis is associated with the instinctual (organic) drives of the unconscious. Cathexes are immensely powerful and are associated with the affective value of ideas and objects. It is interesting to consider the ways in which LIBIDO is bound up with cathexis. For example, FETISHISM can be seen as a cathexis, but so can being in love or the act of masturbation. The aim of the cathexis is to maintain balance in relation to libidinal energy. An excess of energy can lead to pain, whereas the release of energy leads to pleasure. (**Caroline Bainbridge**)

Celibacy From the Latin *caelebs*, unmarried; sometimes refers to 'no sexual relations', the purity of chastity, or mistakenly to ASEXUALITY, rather than a redirected way of sexual being (Goergen 1976). It is practised for numerous reasons, including asceticism, EROTOPHOBIA, voluntary choice or compulsory restraint. Ascetic celibacy is predominantly motivated by religious belief, as in parts of Hinduism (*bramacarya*), Buddhism and Christianity. In early Christianity, the VIRGIN replaced the martyr as the pinnacle of holiness, erroneously creating a dualist dichotomy between sexuality and spirituality; witness the 'Immaculate Conception', which sites the virginity of Mary at the zenith of transcended sexuality. For some, celibacy emanates out of a fear of sex or intimacy, or from a moral rejection of (certain) sexual activities e.g. due to internalized HOMOPHO-BIA. It may also include fear of infection, such as HIV, as well as rejection of sex through a zealous religious or moral conversion and internalized guilt (Connell and Dowsett 1999). A classic example of sexual revulsion is St Augustine's *Confessions*. Much of post-Augustinian Christianity has built its sexual 'theology' on a complete, Stoic, rejection of physical and sexual pleasures, called 'concupiscence' (Boswell 1995), for which Foucault (1990) asked why we continually burden ourselves with so much guilt from having once made sex a sin. Criminal, aberrant or uncharacteristic sexual activities of some 'celibate' people may be attributed to unhappiness with self-imposed celibacy, or to the fact that celibacy was 'chosen' by way of sublimating the undesirable inclination, which has now surfaced in its practice or actualization. Voluntary celibacy may be adopted prior to marriage, or as a requirement of a specific way of life. Some feminists have argued that since HETEROPATRIARCHAL society oppresses women by expecting them to organize their lives around being sexually desirable and available for men, celibacy should be considered as a feminist choice, by which women might direct their energies away from men and towards their own social, political and creative development (Densmore 1968). Enforced celibacy, particularly for women, has a long history in many cultures ranging from physical incarceration (e.g. in a nunnery or convent), through to the imposition of 'chastity belts' and FEMALE GENITAL MUTILATION. (**David Evans**)

Censorship   In its most extreme form the complete suppression of a speech act by an authoritative body; other forms include limiting distribution of a text, withdrawing financial support, ostracizing the writers, publishers, and distributors, and self-censoring. In countries in which speech is constitutionally protected, sexual speech has been subject to censorship under the regulatory category of OBSCENITY. In the eighteenth and nineteenth centuries, with the advent of PORNOGRAPHY as a distinct category of literature, governments passed laws aimed at preventing the dissemination of 'obscene' or 'immoral' materials, that were considered harmful to young people and undermining of community values (Heins 2001: 26–34). Such laws were used to forbid the general distribution of materials related to birth control, ABORTION, and sexual education; periodicals directed towards sexual minorities; pornography; as well as important literary works and scientific scholarship. The proliferation of sexual speech in recent decades following the relaxation of obscenity standards has led to calls for new restrictions on such speech. Anti-pornography feminists have argued that laws against pornography do not constitute censorship because pornography is an act that subordinates women, not pure speech that expresses an idea (Cornell 2000b: 19–165). SEX-POSITIVE feminists argue, however, that the suppression of female sexuality through censorship of sexual speech has historically been linked to women's inequality (Strossen 1995). An important question related to these debates is whether one can draw a line between speech as the communication of ideas and speech as an action that directly inflicts harm, as in SEXUAL HARASSMENT. Concerns central to censorship laws in the nineteenth century have resurfaced in discussions of the Internet. In 1997, The United States Supreme Court struck down the Communications Decency Act, which had attempted to ban all 'indecent' or 'patently offensive' speech on the Internet (Heins 2001: 157ff.). (**Gary Schmidt**)

Further reading

Wolfson (1997).

Cervical cap   A barrier method of CONTRACEPTION that blocks the entry of sperm and pathogens into the uterus. When used correctly and consistently, the cap is about 93 per cent effective; and 82 per cent with inconsistent use (Chalker 1987: 102–12). The cap has significant advantages over the diaphragm: it can be left in place for several days, thus providing greater spontaneity than other barriers and it cannot generally be felt by either partner. Unlike the condom and the diaphragm, the cap does not interfere with sexual sensation. Aside from lifelong abstinence, barrier contraception is the best preventative for most SEXUALLY TRANSMITTED DISEASES (STDs), but compliance, especially with condoms, has been disappointing. In the 1980s, cap providers reported good compliance with the cap among educated women, but recent research on this and other populations is lacking. While acknowledging the importance of developing contraceptives that can be used without male consent, some feminists contend that focusing research on female contraception de-emphasizes male responsibility in PREGNANCY and STD prevention. Yet, as long as women lack agency and equity in sexuality, and intercourse remains the centrepiece of most sexual activity, research on non-intrusive, woman-controlled contraception, such as the cervical cap, seems essential. Indeed, since the cervix is the chief vector of transmission of the human immunodeficiency virus (HIV) in women, with the availability of a vaginal virucide, the cap could also play a significant role in the prevention of AIDS and other STDs (Moench *et al.* 2001: 1–8). (**Rebecca Chalker**)

Child abuse   See AGE OF CONSENT; INTERGENERATIONAL SEX; PAEDOPHILIA; SEXUAL ABUSE.

Circle jerk   A term for GROUP SEX in which several men MASTURBATE together, either solo or, more usually, masturbating each other (cf. DAISY CHAIN). Circle jerks are not an uncommon feature of male ADOLESCENCE, when boys may masturbate in the same space, either with or without touching. To displace accusations of homosexuality, this can take the form of competitions to EJACULATE the most or the furthest, or games like 'toss the cookie' where boys race to ejaculate over a biscuit, and the loser eats it. Although nominally heterosexual boys are more likely to masturbate themselves than one another, there may be some touching – either by boys who know they are gay and for whom the circle jerk provides an alibi, or more casually for boys who see this particular context as allowing for same-sex interaction without their heterosexuality being compromised, for as Jenkins (1996) suggests, context plays a crucial role in defining the circumstances under which STRAIGHT young men may share sexual space comfortably (see SITUATIONAL HOMOSEXUALITY). Jerk Off or Jack Off (JO) clubs organized by the gay community in the 1970s provided opportunities for men to meet for mutual masturbation, and in turn gave rise to mixed 'Jack-and-Jill-Off parties' for bisexuals. During the AIDS CRISIS Jack Off clubs formed a crucial means of keeping SAFE(R) SEX sexy. Safe by definition, they ensured the survival of a sexual atmosphere which retained the key connotations of 1970s gay male culture – positively promiscuous, unconventional, casual – while showing that such an atmosphere was not incompatible with safe sex. They also demonstrate that public discourse can reconfigure SEXUAL PRACTICE in response to COMMUNITY needs (Altman 1986: 157–8). (**Jo Eadie**)

Circumcision   See FGM (FEMALE GENITAL MUTILATION); MALE CIRCUMCISION.

Classical sexuality   While periodization varies from culture to culture, for the Mediterranean world, the Classical period roughly runs from 400 BCE to 500 CE. The different cultures of the Mediterranean world – Greek, Roman, and Jewish – greatly influenced later MEDIEVAL European society politically, economically, and of course, sexually. Indeed, sexual language of the twenty-first century – terms such as ANDROGYNY, PORNOGRAPHY, and SODOMY as well as concepts such as the OEDIPUS COMPLEX – have their origin in Classical cultures.

In his influential series *The History of Sexuality* Michel Foucault provided the last 20 years with the impetus for re-examining the accepted notions of Western (European) sexuality. In the second volume Foucault considers sexual pleasure in the Classical past. Greek moralists, he argues, were concerned not with the nature of sexual behaviour but rather with the amount of sexual activity; was the individual sexually moderate or excessive (1985: 44–5)? While Christian writers wanted to determine and proscribe the very form of sexual relations, Greek sexual culture and behaviour accommodated the individual rather than a universal principle (ibid., 38–9, 62). That said, Greek culture did maintain laws addressing marriage and sexuality. While VIRGINITY upon marriage was valued, though not required, in Athenian brides (Cohen, 1991: 103), marriage was an important social institution. Marital fidelity was not simply a legal norm; as Cohen points out, adultery was an offence that compromised the '*philia* (love, friendship, attachment) between husband and wife' (ibid., 168). Classical Greek culture had great influence on both Roman civilization and early Christianity.

Roman sexual behaviour appears in at least two different though overlapping historical contexts: pagan and Christian. Both pre- and post-Christian Roman sexual culture were based on clear divisions between men and women, masculine and feminine, and superior and inferior. For men, Bullough points out, sex was regarded as a leisure activity and could appear within or without the marriage bed. Women, on the other hand, were to remain virtuous and faithful (1976: 129). Sexual ambiguity then was a great concern to Romans. Male sexuality was regarded as virile, thus positions or behaviour in which a man played a passive role was shunned; the majority of ancient Romans accepted HOMOSEXUALITY, but not sexually passive behaviour in men. Sexual roles were clearly laid out in the Roman and later Christian tradition. Masculinity, the virile male, was regarded as both the physical and moral superior of the femininity, the soft female. Male sexual aggressiveness, marked by the penetration and active role in impregnating women, was contrasted by the female passivity and role as receptacle to the male seed (Kuefler 2001: 19–21). While many of these ideas passed on to Christian Europe, Jewish thought also had an impact on early Christian behaviour.

Many of the Jewish and early Christian attitudes towards sexuality passed down through patristics such as Sts Augustine, Ambrose, and Jerome, to the MEDIEVAL world. Jewish tradition, like later Christian law, held that sexual relations must be confined to the marriage bed, though at times the Jewish culture embraced sexuality more readily than Christianity. Indeed in the Jewish tradition sexual relations between husband and wife on Friday nights could be regarded as a 'religious duty' (Bullough 1976: 74–8). Some sexual acts, such as male MASTURBATION and the subsequent loss of SEMEN, were abhorred as acts that denied the possibility of procreation. As in the MEDIEVAL view, sexual intercourse did not have to lead to pregnancy, but must be open to the possibility. Jewish scripture, much of which became scripture for Christians as well, often portrayed sexual and marital behaviour that would later become unacceptable. The great King Solomon, for instance, was reputed to have 700 wives and 300 concubines.

These Classical cultures, whether Greek, Roman, or Jewish, undoubtedly influenced later Christian ideals and attitudes. The ideals that were passed on to Medieval Europe, however, filtered through Christian commentators. In his essential study, *The Body and Society*, Peter Brown explored the idea of sexual renunciation in the early Christian world. Sexual renunciation was not simply a lifestyle choice; in an era of high mortality rates and low life expectancy, sexual renunciation could severely damage the growth and survival of a family. Indeed, Brown suggests that for the Roman population to remain stable, women must have had to bear at least five children (1988: 6). Sexual renunciation itself was not a Christian creation; Jewish groups such as the Essenes viewed sexuality suspiciously. While some groups attempted to reinforce the marriage bond as a central aspect of Jewish society, others abandoned sexuality altogether (Brown 1988: 39–40). Early Christian writers, including Augustine, Ambrose, and Jerome, prove the best starting point for understanding later Christian, Medieval, as well as a few twentieth-century sexual ideals.

Sexual cultures and traditions during the Classical period are not limited to either European or Mediterranean cultures. The flourishing sexual culture of India, for instance, provided the world with the well-known SEX MANUAL, the *Kama Sutra* of Vatsyayana. The *Kama Sutra*, however, is not simply a guide to sexual positions.

Rather this third-century text is a guide to living, finding a partner, committing adultery, and using drugs, as well as to sexual positions. (**Andrew Cranmer**)

Further reading

McClure (2002).

Clitoridectomy   See FGM (Female Genital Mutilation).

Clitoris   The genital organ of female sexual pleasure and ORGASM. The tip or *glans* of the clitoris is erroneously referred to as 'the' clitoris; in fact, the clitoris is an extensive organ system composed of erectile tissue, nerves, muscles and blood vessels, and is, hence, equivalent to the PENIS in extent and function. Anatomists and physicians in ancient Greece understood that the male and female genitals were equivalent and this concept was affirmed by Renaissance anatomists. But Enlightenment philosophers and physicians defined MENSTRUATION and PREGNANCY as pathologies that disabled women from public life and passionate sexuality (Laqueur 1990: 149–63). Gradually, essential clitoral structures were deleted from medical illustrations, or ascribed to the reproductive or urinary tracts. In 1904, Freud declared the VAGINA to be the focus of the mature woman's sexuality, and due to the prodigious influence of psychoanalysis, the concept of the clitoris as a powerful complex organ disappeared from medical texts and public consciousness in the twentieth century (Laqueur 1990: 233–7). Masters and Johnson (1966: 45–67) described the clitoral system and Sherfey (1972: 146–65) embellished and clarified their concept. The Federation of Feminist Women's Health Centers (1981: 33–57) produced a detailed description and illustrations of the clitoris, including all of the genital structures that interact to produce orgasm. Subsequently, anatomy texts have described an increasingly complex clitoris.

Heterosexual, intercourse-centred sex directly favours male orgasm, and the tiny female *glans* is often seen as a nuisance or as an impediment to its efficient achievement. In this regard, the knowledge that the clitoris is equal to the penis in size and potency may be threatening to many men (see also FGM). Yet some feminists argue that an understanding of the true extent and power of the clitoris has the potential to boost women's sexual self-image and interest in sex, promote the exploration of pleasure, and greatly enhance both partner sex and MASTURBATION. (**Rebecca Chalker**)

Clone   'Clone' is used to denote a particular, masculine gay male style or aesthetic: clones traditionally sport cropped hair, checked shirts and/or tightly fitting T-shirts, denim jeans (most often blue), and neatly trimmed moustaches; the hair and moustache are the most invariable elements of the look, but the parts may be arranged in various combinations without disqualifying individuals from the appellation. At various stages of his career Freddie Mercury dressed as a clone; for an amusing if somewhat acid vignette, see Pickles's description in his *Queens* (1986: 17–18). The clone look is often associated with post-Stonewall gay subcultures and interpreted as part of the 'masculinization of the gay man' (see Levine 1998) – that is, the large-scale repudiation of ways of understanding male homosexuality as essentially feminine (see EFFEMINACY) that took place in this period (although there has been some debate as to whether, in adopting the look, gay men are embracing or PARODYING dominant codes of masculinity). However in his introduction to Rodney Garland's *The Heart in Exile* (1995), Neil Bartlett observes the style well-established in 1950s Britain, and other commentators have argued that Tom of Finland's art – which appeared in American magazines from 1956 onwards – was in large part responsible for inspiring this look in gay male subcultures. Both these things suggest that gay men's affinity for such masculine accoutrements has enjoyed a rather longer history than the term itself; on this point see also Healy (1996: esp. 59–64). (**Chris West**)

Closet   The key metaphor of the gay liberation movement of the 1960s and onwards, 'COMING OUT of the closet' denoted an acceptance of one's own homosexuality or bisexuality, and an unembarrassed public disclosure of it. The closet is thus a silence imposed upon gays, lesbians, and bisexuals by a HETERONORMATIVE society, but which QUEER people maintain by staying hidden – and which they therefore have the power to overthrow. Sedgwick (1994: 11) suggests that the closet is therefore a PERFORMATIVE site: we are ordered into it, but can force our way out of it by uttering the magic words. However, this simple formula has its own complications: having admitted to homosexuality, one might still be closeted about certain desires or SEXUAL PRACTICES, such as SM or PAEDOPHILIA. Equally, to be 'out' in one environment does not preclude being closeted in others: work, family, church, and different friendship groups each have their own risks, and the calculation of whether to be in or out of the closet is taken in different ways with each group. Sedgwick (1991) argues that much Western culture is structured around a paranoid EPISTEMOLOGY OF THE CLOSET: a mode of inquiry in which knowing the truth is paramount, having secrets is taken as proof of weakness or corruption, and the state and its institutions assume that they must regulate what is known, and what may be made public. Indeed, she argues that the social meanings of secrecy and disclosure, and many of the terms dependent upon them – truth, sincerity, authenticity – 'are quite indelibly marked with the historical specificity of homosocial/homosexual definition' (ibid., 72), such that all forms of concealment attract the homophobic connotations of homosexuality (sickness, guilt, shame). Sedgwick's claim seems borne out by the fact that 'closet' has become the dominant metaphor for *any* embarrassing secret – we speak routinely now of a 'closet Catholic' or a 'closet soap addict'. However, in doing so the relative power and danger of certain closets over others has become overlooked. (**Jo Eadie**)

Coalition politics   Coalition politics is a form of ACTIVISM by which diverse COMMUNITIES join together to address a common concern. In the words of Young, 'In traditional coalitions diverse groups work together for specific ends which they agree interest or affect them all in a similar way' (1990: 188). By coming together, coalitions are thought to gain greater political leverage than if their members had worked as individuals or groups in isolation. In some instances, the formation of coalitions may be regarded as strategic since groups may come together for a specific purpose and not continue after the end has been achieved. Coalition politics have been contrasted to a politics of IDENTITY which base group formation on the common *identity* of members rather than on members' common *aims*. It has been said that Harvey Milk ushered into the gay LIBERATION struggle a politics of coalition by connecting 'typical' gay and lesbian concerns with those of other constituencies. In *The Hope Speech* (1978), Milk stated, 'I can't forget the faces of people who've lost hope. Be they gay, be they seniors, be they blacks looking for an almost impossible job, be they Latins trying to explain their problems and aspirations in a tongue that's foreign to them' (1997: 453). While the possible benefits of coalition politics are noted above, there has been debate concerning the role that majority communities should play vis-à-vis minority ones. One point of contention has been the possible loss of minority 'voice' when members of minority communities ally themselves with more mainstream groups and interests. In fact, the sort of group formed can, in turn, inform the very structure of public debate. As Jakobsen remarks: 'whether civil rights struggle is articulated as "minority protections" or "social justice for all" depends on whether civil rights is articulated with capitalist individualism or other struggles for social justice' (1998: 157–8). (**Mary Bloodsworth-Lugo**)

Further reading

Phelan (1994) Chapter 8.

Coital imperative   The coital imperative refers to the normative injunction to define sexual relations in terms of the PENILE penetration of a VAGINA. This injunction underlies HETERONORMATIVE sexual relations insofar as it requires that male and female anatomy undergird 'legitimate' sexual relations. That is, in heteronormative society, 'having sex' is *a priori* defined as necessarily entailing penile penetration of a vagina. This imperative excludes most forms of sexual expression. For instance, by definition, the coital imperative excludes all lesbian and gay sex (the use of DILDOS is considered by this imperative to be an attempt to replicate 'real' sex). More generally, the coital imperative excludes all sexual acts *other than* penile penetration of vagina (ORAL and ANAL sex, touching, petting, FELTCHING, FETISHISM, KISSING and so on). Lesbian feminists have theorized the implications of the coital imperative for lesbian IDENTITY: whilst Rich (1986) has argued against the coital imperative through a 'LESBIAN CONTINUUM' which involves a much broader and more inclusive definition of sexual relations, Wittig (1992) argues that because the category 'woman' is utterly dependent upon heternormativity for its existence, lesbians are not women. Frye (1983) has taken the point further by arguing that the specificity of lesbian sexuality, when sexual activity is normatively defined as requiring a penis, renders lesbianism impossible. As Ginzberg similarly argues, 'analytically, indeed tautologically, "lesbian" is self-referentially meaningless' when sexual relations are defined by the activity of a penis, and women are, by definition, excluded from having penises (1994: 83). Finally, the coital imperative constitutes an example of what Foucault (1990) terms a 'disciplinary technique' because of the way in which it regulates the ways in which people perform their identities (heterosexual, lesbian, homosexual and so on) and the ways in which pleasures become defined (legitimate, illegitimate, impossible and so on). (**Myra Hird**)

Coitus interruptus   Also known as 'pulling out', this is the interruption of penis–vagina intercourse before male EJACULATION. It is the oldest recorded form of CONTRACEPTION (reference may be found in Genesis 38: 8–9 in the story of Onan, leading onanism to be used as a term for both coitus interruptus and MASTURBATION) (Tannahill 1989: 64–6). It is also a very unreliable method of birth control with a failure rate of 19 per cent, due to either late withdrawal or the presence of sperm in the 'dew drop' of fluid produced by the man while aroused but before ejaculation. This form of contraception can be equally frustrating to both parties and should be rejected as an option considering its failure rate. In addition it does not protect against SEXUALLY TRANSMITTED DISEASES presenting further complications if a PREGNANCY does result. There are no side effects from using this method in itself, however it has been suggested that long-term practice can result in sexual dysfunction such as premature ejaculation in men (Hyde and DeLamater 1997: 198). (**Linda Kiernan**)

Coming out   The act of disclosing some truth about oneself to others, especially but not exclusively when this truth concerns SEXUAL ORIENTATION (one might come out as a lesbian; but one might equally well come out as an HIV positive person; or even as a fan of, say, trashy novels). However, Delany writes that earlier in the twentieth century 'coming out' referred to 'having one's first major homosexual experience' (1997: 20). It thus referenced the process of emerging *into* homosexual culture. This older usage was derived through analogy with the coming out of a debutante; it was superseded in the 18 months following the Stonewall riots in June 1969, during which time proponents of Gay Liberation exhorted their brothers and sisters to 'come out of the CLOSET'. Coming out in this later sense was central to the politics of Gay Liberation. It involved 'the acceptance, and *public demonstration*, of the validity of one's own homosexuality' (Weeks 1990: vii, my emphasis) and was seen as essential in the fight to combat HOMOPHOBIA in all its forms. Gay Liberationists therefore tended to see failure to come out as a sign of political cowardice, general conservatism, and/or INTERNALIZED OPPRESSION. In Britain the Committee for Homosexual Equality 'was sneered at for holding its meetings under an assumed name … and for its declining to "come out"' (ibid., 190).

There is not, however, a simple polarization between radical and conservative positions on coming out, in which the former equates with advocacy of it as a political strategy and the latter with rejection of it as such. Although Carl Wittman in his 'Gay Manifesto' urges gays to 'come out everywhere' (1992: 341), he recognizes that the cost may be very dear in terms of victimization at work, loss of friends, and exclusion from family (1992: 334–5). In more recent years this perspective has been differently inflected by non-white gay activists. Gupta argues that the family can be a tremendously important resource for black and brown gays, especially for immigrant peoples who live in 'a hostile white environment' (1989: 176). Injunctions to come out may implicitly enact a racism which must be challenged.

Such perspectives pose significant problems, therefore, for the practice of 'OUTING'. Outing people as gay relies on and assumes a clear identification of them as such; but *this* assumes a unified, unchanging, self-knowing subject, fully cognisant of their desires and in absolute control of the self they present to others. 'Coming out' construed as a kind of foolproof moment of self-construction ignores what is for many people a lived fluidity in identity. Conceived in this way, 'coming out' elides the situation of, for instance, someone who having come out as gay subsequently finds themselves needing to come out again as bisexual, or vice versa. It is perhaps best, then, to regard coming out as something that can rarely if ever be a completed event. It involves in this view a process of repeated, potentially diverse disclosures – since encounters with anyone or anything new may necessitate repetition of disclosure of (sexual) truths about oneself; and in addition, in the course of living we might find that we are not who we once thought we were. (**Chris West**)

Commodification   The process by which sexual acts and identities become transformed into marketable goods and services. The term covers both the sale of sex itself through PROSTITUTION and PORNOGRAPHY, and the ways in which financial transactions become a crucial part of sexual identities, such as the leather and torture SEX TOYS of SM practitioners, or the HONEYMOON holiday. Sex is heavily commodified, while at the same time it is held out to us as a place of romance and freedom (Singer 1993). The hostility often directed towards the commodification of sex can therefore be seen as a reaction to its contradictory position: commodification is seen as a debasement of an act whose ideological role within capitalism is to be an antidote to wage labour. Ironically, while wedding dresses, Valentine's Day cards, SEX MANUALS, romantic fiction, and even pornography, all promote a concept of sexuality as an escape from everyday commercial routines, they are the means by which it is turned into a marketable product.

Such public consumption of sexuality comes with its own limits on who is allowed to purchase, and what items are deemed suitable, which delimit appropriate sexual PERFORMANCE – the PREGNANT body is made unwelcome in lingerie departments since only certain types of sexuality are entitled to find their desire reflected in the market (Longhurst 1998). At the same time, marginal and illegal sexual markets have enabled dissident sexualities to acquire marketable forms, a process which has transformed the modern sexual landscape. For sexual subcultures, commodfication is a mixed blessing. It has enabled the purchase of places that are safe – yet in doing so may restrict access to the affluent (Field 1995), for 'where the state will not subsidize the formation and self-promotion of sexual minorities, little or nothing can be done ... without substantial private financial resources' (Califia 1994: 211). Even where the state supports sexual subcultures, this may involve conditions regarding acceptable types of behaviour. Furthermore, as a subculture becomes bound up with saleable objects, members may find their props and styles distributed to new markets – such as the use of traditions of gay photography in fashion magazines aimed primarily at heterosexual men (Mort 1996). Marxist critics object that the diversity of sexual possibilities is narrowed as commodification 'freezes' DESIRE, replacing its flux with fixed, repetitive, identical activities (Evans 1993).

Commodification has also been accused of inhibiting social justice, since it encourages sexual subjects to see themselves as individual consumers, who satisfy their needs through LIFESTYLE POLITICS, rather than as part of a collective social group who can demand large-scale social change (Chasin 2000). Yet this commercial model also brings with it new forms of collective organizing. The arguments by PROSTITUTES that they have the right to safe and sanitary working conditions like any other labourer (Cornell 2000a: 8–11), shows how the capitalist model can facilitate a demand for equal rights. (**Jo Eadie**)

Further reading

Evans (1993).

Community A group of people, connected by common cause or interest. Communities based on sexuality have flourished in the twentieth century – including those based around FETISHISM, SEX WORK, and POLYAMORY – facilitated by hard-fought legal changes, often building on longer historical traditions. In Britain, for example, Molly houses, where men would meet to enjoy social, and sexual interaction were recorded as far back as the seventeenth century (see Lucas 1994: 51–3). Although the term suggests that a community is accessible, homogenous, and welcoming, these are only ever partially the case. For instance, geographical lesbian and gay communities (or 'gay villages') have tended to appear primarily in metropolitan areas; however, developing communications technologies have permitted those who are geographically isolated to feel part of a sexual community (see SEXUAL SPACE). In terms of lesbian and gay politics, the supposed inclusiveness of 'the' community has sometimes elided differences between its various constituent groups, and many have argued for a plurality of 'communities' rather than a singular, monolithic entity. Lesbians have often been sidelined in what is solely a *gay* community, catering largely to the needs of gay men. The homogenization which was perceived to have taken hold of gay communities was a major motivating factor in the creation of QUEER culture (Seidman 1993), which aimed to reinscribe diversity (for instance, by expanding to include bisexuals and transsexuals – see LGBT). Communities also become crucial at times of crisis – such as an increase in political repression (see ACTIVISM): lesbian and gay communities have been vital in the AIDS CRISIS, acting as a prime network for the distribution of SAFE(R) SEX information and the provision of services for those affected by AIDS. (**Alex Evans**)

Compulsory heterosexuality   Compulsory heterosexuality refers to the range of practices and ideologies that naturalize, NORMALIZE and idealize heterosexual relations. Rubin (1975) first used the term to elucidate how the taboo on INCEST is preceded by a more basic taboo on homosexuality. Rich (1986) expanded Rubin's argument, theorizing that far from being a naturally occurring arrangement, heterosexuality is in fact a political institution: it is a SOCIAL CONSTRUCT bound up in and sustained through a variety of both positive and negative sanctions. Rich posits that the heterosexual imperative is inextricably tied to a sexist gender order – one that enables men to consolidate their power and control while simultaneously isolating women from one another and curtailing their potential. To counter the oppressive effects of HETEROPATRIARCHY, Rich proposes that women position themselves on what she calls the LESBIAN CONTINUUM. Despite its major contributions to the study of sexuality, Rich's work has been criticized for an 'anti-sex' attitude (Rubin 1984) and an inability to account for the intimate lives of men – be they gay, straight or bisexual. Aside from regulating the way in which men and women organize themselves erotically, Wittig (1992) asserts that compulsory heterosexuality produces a mythic and ostensibly 'essential' FEMININITY. Wittig's well-known phrase 'lesbians are not women' conveys the fact that – for this author – the category of woman is thoroughly conditioned by and made intelligible through its relationship to conventional heterosexual roles. Drawing on the insights of Rubin, Rich and Wittig, Butler (1990) insists on the need to complicate conceptions of heterosexuality in order to expose its multiple and indeed variable forms. For Butler, this process of complication will expose the utter contingency of sex, gender and sexuality, thus demystifying the HETEROSEXUAL MATRIX. (See also HETEROSEXISM.) (**Marc Lafrance**)

Compulsory monosexuality   This is a term used by bisexuals and PANSEXUALS to describe MONOSEXUALITY (lesbian, gay *and* heterosexual desire for only one sex) as an institution. It can usefully be seen as borrowing from and replying to Rich's (1986) often cited essay 'Compulsory Heterosexuality and Lesbian Existence', in which she argues that heterosexuality is not a choice but a socially and institutionally sanctioned set of practices that deny the validity of women's relationships to one another. Discussions of compulsory monosexuality, then, highlight the ways in which *desire for more than one sex* is similarly socially and legally prohibited through the institutionalized practices of marriage and domestic partnership, child rearing, inheritance, welfare benefits, media representations and narratives and so on. The term is frequently used to emphasize the social and cultural privileges afforded both homosexuals and heterosexuals through their singular desires.

For the SEXOLOGIST Stekel (1950), monosexuality is merely a surface act covering over the real bisexuality of an individual, while in the context of contemporary English-speaking bisexual communities, monosexuality is established as the opposite of bisexuality and includes both heterosexual and homosexual desire for a single sex. In the latter context, monosexuality is the privileged term, in relation to which bisexuality is pathologized or undermined (Highleyman 1992). The strategic importance of the term 'compulsory monosexuality' for the development of bisexual COMMUNITY is that it allows for the creation of a sense of common bisexual ground and struggle. Several writers have been critical of the use of the term however, arguing that to term all non-bisexuals 'monosexuals' erases the differences among lesbians, gay men and heterosexuals in terms of gender and sexual oppression (Blumenfeld and Hemmings, 1996). (**Claire Hemmings**)

Condom   Usually rubber or latex, but also made of other materials such as linen, gourds, tortoiseshell, leather, silk, oiled paper and sheep-gut. Condoms have traditionally been used for CONTRACEPTION and to act as barriers to STDs, including their use on shared DILDOS. Parisot (1987) reports acts of condom use during penetrative sex as early as 15,000 years ago. It was the Italian anatomist Gabriello Fallopio (1523–62) who recommended the wearing of a 'penis sheath' as a protection against disease. Most of us will know condoms for their modern sexual and public health importance. It was during the First World War that condoms were popularly exploited as a technique to control infection and disease among those enlisted. They became less public during the 1960s and 1970s, with the popularization of other forms of birth control, such as the PILL but took on a critical and worldwide importance with the advent of HIV and AIDS. Condoms offer reasonable protection against most sexually transmitted bacterial and viral infections because they can prevent the exchange of body fluids but condoms can fail. They can break, leak and slide off, but it should be noted that most reports of condom failure are the result of inconsistent or incorrect use, and not inappropriate construction or materials (Macaluso 1999). Condoms can be cut to open flat for use as an effective barrier for a variety of erotic activities such as RIMMING (see DENTAL DAMS). Condoms make excellent water balloons. (**Dan Allman**)

Further reading

Mindel (2000).

Confessional society   Arising from French philosopher Foucault (1990), the confessional society is posited on the practice of confession to regulate and determine sexuality. Thus, the EARLY-MODERN and MODERN subject's experience of sexuality is built on the relation of confession of sexuality; in the act of speech, the subject takes the inferior position, while the confessor occupies the silent, listening position of authority. Foucault explains how this basic eroticized relation has produced a SCIENTIA SEXUALIS (as opposed to the *ars erotica* practised by the ancients as well as in China, Japan, and Asia). Confessional practices came to permeate and determine many social practices: law, medicine, education, literature and other arts, psychotherapy, media communications (from journalism to the talk show to BLOGS, i.e. web logs or personal, online journals). Foucault explains: 'the confession became one of the West's most highly valued techniques for producing truth. We have since become a singularly confessing society' (59). The power dynamic of the confession has contributed to the formation of the modern sciences focusing on sex (medicine, psychiatry, pedagogy) in order to analyse and codify sex, further enhancing regulation. Especially since the 1960s, the intensified analysis and confession of sexuality, combined with relaxation of CENSOR-SHIP, has ostensibly produced more diverse expressions of sexuality in the public sphere, which in turn have assisted the successful promotion of tolerance, human and civil rights. The dynamic of the 'confessional society' informs the act of COMING OUT. While Foucault admits that confession can have a liberating effect for the subject, it also opens the subject to investigation and categorization by the social order. (**Susan Mooney**)

Consent   Consent refers to the notion that all sexual acts should be entered into freely, without coercion and with the informed agreement of all parties concerned. Where consent is not freely given, sex is defined as SEXUAL ASSAULT or RAPE. In practice, though, the notion of consent is problematic, particularly from a legal perspective since the AGE OF CONSENT differs widely across cultures. For instance, in some jurisdictions, the law does not recognize an individual's right to consent to same-sex sex. Similarly, individuals below the recognized age of consent are not considered sufficiently mature to agree to sexual acts which can lead to their partners being charged with statutory rape. Consent is, however, most problematic in BDSM subcultures (an overlapping abbreviation for BONDAGE and discipline, dominance and submission, and SADISM and MASOCHISM) which can involve the trading of pain resulting in physical harm. Despite the fact that participants in this subculture are generally very aware of the importance of consent, in some jurisdictions the law does not recognize an individual's right to consent to harm and so the 'dominant' or pain-inflicting partner is liable to charges of battery or assault. (**Mark McLelland**)

Further reading

Archard (1998).

Contraception   Contraception constitutes a range of techniques and technologies which aim to prevent conception, facilitating the separation of sex from reproduction.

There is nothing new about attempts to control fertility, with the use of herbs, amulets, pessaries and other folkloric methods dating back for centuries (Riddle 1997). Modern methods include: periodic abstinence; withdrawal before ejaculation (COITUS INTERRUPTUS); barrier methods such as CONDOMS, or the CERVICAL CAP; the use of spermicides; inter-uterine devices (IUD); oral, injectible or implantable hormones (e.g. Norplant, THE PILL); and surgical sterilization. Most contraceptive interventions focus on the female body, although several male hormonal contraceptives are currently in development (Clarke 2000; Oudshoorn 2000). Several of the contraceptive technologies also have non-contraceptive applications: the pill is used in the medical management of a range of menstrual disorders, and the condom is used to protect against the transmission of HIV and STDs.

Contraception is a highly contested area. The Catholic Church opposes the separation of sex from reproduction, and resists all contraceptive intervention; 'pro-life' activists oppose contraceptive technologies such as the pill and the IUD, which prevent implantation rather than conception, likening them to ABORTION. Feminists continue to campaign for contraceptive methods which are safe, reliable and woman-controlled. They have highlighted the risks of contraceptive technologies, such as the possibility of infection or pelvic inflammatory disease (PID) from IUDs and the potentially serious side effects associated with hormonal interventions, including increased vulnerability to HIV and other STDs (Clarke 2000). Other feminists have drawn attention to the use of women in developing countries for the testing of contraceptives which have later proved to be harmful (Rowland 1992), and the coercive use of contraception in population control programmes (Hartmann 1995). (**Karen Throsby**)

Further reading

Hartmann (1995).

Coprophilia　From the Greek compound *kopros* for dung or excrement, plus *philia*, a love of something or someone. Coprophilia, or the more popular term, SCAT refers to using excrement in sex. This may include defecating on a partner (including during anal intercourse), smearing or playing with fæces, defecating in clothing, using douches or enemas, manual (hand) evacuation, or eating shit. The latter is properly called *coprophagia*. Scat is frequently related to SM or bondage/domination SM (BDSM) sex; it may also be accompanied by WATERSPORTS. In sexual circles where colour-coded hankies denote a person's SEXUAL PREFERENCES, the colours would be beige or brown. Like many other more acceptable practices – say, heterosexual intercourse – there are a range of potential health risks, but appropriate SAFE(R) SEX choices minimize these. When shitting onto another person, using a protective cover, like clothing, saran wrap or 'cling film', offers greater protection from pathogens. Also, role-playing using shit-substitutes (e.g. food) reduces or eliminates the risks (see Henkin 1998). Despite vaccines against a few pathogens, health risks become a problem when any amount of shit gets into another person's body, e.g. through the mouth, eyes, vagina, urethra, anus or broken skin. Severe infections such as Hepatitis A, B and C, salmonella, giardia, and dysentery, can be passed from a person with these infections, which may prove life threatening, by leading to blood poisoning (septicaemia), particularly in immuno-compromized (e.g. HIV positive) individuals. Some people might also freeze shit (e.g. in a condom), and use it as a DILDO – inserting ice into bodily orifices can cause its own problems, from damaging soft tissue, to haemorrhoids. As one might expect, state-sponsored sex education programmes – which remain largely EROTOPHOBIC – rarely cover these issues. Although the ABJECT associations of excrement and the ANUS make this a heavily stigmatized SEXUAL PRACTICE, most of us have explored the pleasures of shit-play as children. Thus while psychoanalysts may categorize coprophilia/coprophagia as being a form of infantile fetishism, this formulation assumes – as PSYCHOANALYSIS so often does – that we should renounce childhood pleasures in favour of an adult sexuality which, it is expected, must be reproductive, penetrative heterosexuality. (**David Evans**)

Cosmetic surgery   Cosmetic surgery is a special field of plastic surgery which provides the techniques for surgically altering the appearance of the human body. In contrast to reconstructive surgery as a result of trauma, illness or congenital birth conditions, cosmetic surgery is done purely for aesthetic improvement. As a medical technology cosmetic surgery is used, alongside the beauty, fitness and diet industries, to combat the effects of ageing and includes a range of techniques such as facelifts, breast augmentations, fat removal, body contouring, and the reshaping of genitals. Today, cosmetic surgery makes up 40 per cent of all plastic surgery and is seen by many as a cultural product of a consumer culture which treats the body as a COMMODIFIED vehicle for self-expression. But the beauty system also constrains bodies through the combined pressures of BODY FASCISM and the desire for GENDER CAPITAL. Cosmetic surgery thus has a far reaching impact on questions about subjectivity, identity, agency and morality. Traditionally, social psychology, psychoanalysis, and sociology have looked at women's involvement with cosmetic surgery in terms of conformity, low self-esteem, narcissism or as brainwashed consumers – accounts which have often missed out an analysis of gender and the cultural constraints of the feminine beauty system. Some feminist perspectives have reclaimed cosmetic surgery and have, rather than assigning women to the position of cultural dopes, provided an account which highlights women's agency within the cultural and structural constraints of FEMININITY and the beauty system (Davis 1995). Others maintain that the rhetoric of choice and freedom disguises the cultural colonization of the female body, which represents domination rather than freedom (Morgan 1991). However, the growing importance of cosmetic surgery for the male body, and its use in helping bodies to meet various racial ideals, has ramifications for the concept of cultural colonization beyond gender. (Natalia Gerodetti)

Further reading

Davis (1995).

Cottaging   The practice of engaging in anonymous homosexual sex in public conveniences, or of using public conveniences as CRUISING areas in order to make sexual contacts. In the United Kingdom, public toilets in parks often resembled small houses with sloped roofs, hence the name *cottage*. Most cottaging occurs between men, although there are some cases of women using cottages (the John Waters film *Desperate Living* (1977) features a scene with a lesbian cottage). While the majority of sex that occurs in cottages is gay male sex, some people who cottage may not consider themselves to hold a gay or homosexual IDENTITY and may be termed MSM (MEN-WHO-HAVE-SEX-WITH-MEN). In the United States, cottages are known as tea-rooms or T-rooms. Humphreys carried out an ethnographic study of tea-rooms over several months, coming to the conclusion that his data did not indicate that tea-room activity caused any 'threat to society' (1970: 163).

In many countries cottaging is illegal and can result in prosecution if caught. In the United Kingdom, the 'gross indecency' law that was used to jail Oscar Wilde in 1895 is still being used to arrest gay men for cottaging. Police stings involving mass arrests of men who cottage constitute a form of sexual regulation that guarantees a high rate of convictions and an improved crime clear-up rate. Cottaging may be considered a form of PUBLIC SEX, although the fact that it often occurs surreptitiously in locked cubicles means that it should be better classed as semi-public. One study of men who cottaged (Scott *et al.* 1998) found that 20 per cent started between the ages of 10 and 14, and 32 per cent started between the ages of 15 and 19. The survey also found that 75 per cent of the respondents regularly visited gay social venues and groups, a finding in conflict with the idea that cottagers are CLOSETED, isolated individuals, unable to come to terms with their sexuality. A recent example of prosecution for cottaging occurred with the arrest of British singer George Michael in a Los Angeles restroom in 1998. Despite wide media attention, the incident did not damage his career, suggesting that public attitudes towards cottaging are becoming more tolerant. (**Paul Baker**)

Critical heterosexual studies   Critical heterosexual studies challenge the ways that HETEROSEXUALITY is taken for granted as a form of desire and social organization. The writers in the field may or may not be heterosexual themselves, but all open up heterosexuality to a political analysis conducted on several levels. Some have understood heterosexuality as the basis for women's domination by men, based upon men's appropriation of women's labour power and sexuality. Wittig (1992) goes so far as to suggest that the categories of 'male' and 'female' themselves are products of this heterosexual appropriation and may not exist outside of this context (see SEXUAL DIMOR-PHISM). In partial contrast, Jackson (1999) suggests that while heterosexual practice is often defined in male-dominant terms, more egalitarian forms of heterosexuality are politically possible. Others focus on HETERONORMATIVITY: the ways in which heterosexuality is established as a norm, against which homosexuality is measured and becomes either deviant or only merely tolerable (Rubin 1984). Thus, heterosexuality is socially respectable, legitimate and expected in a way that homosexuality is not. Those influenced by poststructuralism suggest that heterosexuality as a form of sexual identity and social organization cannot exist apart from homosexuality, that both categories rely upon each other for their meaning. Ingraham's (1999) critical heterosexual analysis examines the intersection of gender, sexuality and capitalism. She argues that the embodiment of heterosexuality in the wedding industry interweaves the reinforcement of heterosexuality with increasingly conspicuous consumption, thus supporting both HETEROPATRIARCHY and capitalism (see COMMODIFICATON). Weddings have a part to play in the reproduction of the 'heterosexual imaginary', Ingraham's description for that way of thinking that precludes a critical analysis of heterosexuality as an organizing institution in society. (**Chris Brickell**)

Further reading

Segal (1994).

Cross-dressing   The practice of wearing the clothing associated with members of the other sex. It is a translation of TRANSVESTITE, the term coined by Magnus Hirschfeld in 1910 (see Hirschfeld 1991), which has come to be the less preferred term due to lingering connotations of pathology; transvestic fetishism continues to be listed in the Diagnostic and Statistical Manual (DSM) of the American Psychiatric Association (APA) as a disorder. Cross-dressing is a form of DRAG involving gender and erotic identity issues even as it poses social, psychological, and existential questions. It appears across cultures, in many historical eras, and is prominent in theatrical contexts. It is practised for diverse reasons by a variety of individuals, including transsexuals, female impersonators, DRAG QUEENS, DRAG KINGS, she-males, and all those who bend their gender or are considered transgendered (see GENDERFUCK and GENDERQUEER). The term TRANSGEN-DER better reveals the valued function of ritual cross-dressing as it is part of religious, ritual and cultural modalities in some contemporary (non-Western) societies. There is little in Western society that is analogous to such valuing. Although practised by both women and men, much of the literature on cross-dressing focuses on men (Ekins 1997). Most estimates suggest that many more men than women participate in cross-dressing and that the majority identify as HETEROSEXUAL and do not express a desire to permanently change their sex. It is difficult to verify the accuracy of such statistics due to social stigmas against cross-dressing leading many to keep their practice in the private realm. In terms of clothing and fashion, in numerous Western societies women may wear clothing with clear masculine signifiers in a greater number of contexts than men are allowed to wear women's clothing. In part, this is because in a patriarchal culture, women are appropriating symbols of power, whereas in appearing to relinquish their higher place in the social hierarchy, men face harsher penalties (Garber 1992). (**Karen Lovaas**)

Further reading

Bullough and Bullough (1993).

Cruise   To seek anonymous sexual contacts, usually in public or semi-public places. Cruise originated in the sixteenth century and was first used in connection with the movement of ships in the sea. By the end of the seventeenth century, its meaning had generalized to other types of movement, including people: 'Madam, how would you like to cruise about a little' (Farquhar, 'Love and Bottle', 1698; Cited in *Oxford English Dictionary* 1994). By the twentieth century, the word's meaning had become associated with walking, or driving around, either aimlessly, or to look for casual sex (especially homosexual male) partners. Humphreys (1970) describes how cruising was a popular activity for gay men as a result of the popularity of the automobile and the installation of a comprehensive water system across American towns, which preceded the creation of a number of public conveniences in secluded areas in parks. As well as occurring in or around COTTAGES, cruising can take place in bars, clubs, saunas, parks, on public transport or in urban high streets. Cruising is viewed with different attitudes within the gay community, varying from potentially dangerous to harmless fun. Some gay groups (e.g. Gay Men Fighting AIDS, United Kingdom) have run seminars to advise gay men on their cruising techniques, which are designed to help increase feelings of self-worth, improve a person's ability to get the sex they want or to say no, to negotiate safe sex, and to get over feelings that can be raised when faced with rejection. As well as the 'movement' use of cruise, the word can also be used to describe the intense, interested way that a gay man looks at a potential sexual partner, e.g. 'I've been cruised at least five times since leaving the house this morning'. (**Paul Baker**)

Cuddle buddies   Just as FUCK BUDDIES fulfil a mutual need for sex, cuddle buddies fulfil a mutual need for affection, physical contact, and warmth – but without sex. Either buddy may have other sexual partners, or be single, but wants to take this friendship to a more physically intimate level. 'Cuddling' may include massage, kissing, hugging, stroking, and depending upon preferences these may take place clothed or naked. Sometimes it may thus resemble FOREPLAY very closely, but for the agreement that neither party wants sex to take place. It should be remembered that with sex before marriage being heavily discouraged up until relatively recently, many 'courting' couples practised a type of cuddle buddy relationship long before the term was coined. The need for cuddle buddies can therefore be read in two very different ways: either as a compensation for the fact that sex is now expected and permitted at an earlier stage in relationships, thereby taking more playfully tactile relationships out of our lives; or as part of the new range of sexual explorations that has been generated by the SEX RADICAL movements of the twentieth century, a new type of para-sexual practice that has erotic elements but which does not resemble sex as we have previously understood it. (Jo Eadie)

D

Daddy The historical use of the term by heterosexual women to refer to wealthy male lovers – or even to their husbands within nuclear FAMILIES where the term signified the 'head of the household' – carries connotations of dependence and infantilization: a recognition that under the economic inequalities of HETEROPATRIARCHY a woman's relationship to a male lover becomes childlike by virtue of her relative lack of power, and a sly reference to the fact than an older man's wealth may be his only attraction. While still used to describe relationships based on economic inequality, the term has recently become a more playful signifier within sexual role-play – particularly, but not exclusively, within SM (see Califia 1995). Here the 'daddy' may earn the term because they are older, stronger, bigger, have a higher social status – or merely because they temporarily adopt the role within a SCENE. As a TOP the daddy can hold out sexual rewards and punishments, while in turn their 'boy' or 'girl' has the challenge of pleasing and teasing them, or masochistically choosing to offend in order to be punished. In such encounters the boy/girl is both more knowing and more active than in the baby-role taken in INFANTILISM. A daddy can come in either sex: women may adopt the role as a type of FEMALE MASCULINITY (particularly for lesbians within BUTCH cultures), with a male or female lover positioning themselves either as a 'boy' or 'girl', depending on their own tastes. PSYCHOANALYSIS reads the power of the father figure as fundamental to identity – and always as SEXUALIZED, since part of his power is the privileged sexual access that he has to the mother. While in the traditional OEDIPUS COMPLEX the boy longs to become a daddy, while the girl longs for a daddy of her own, QUEER rewritings of Freud point out that a boy may desire a daddy of his own (Bersani 1995: 110–12), and a girl may want the power of becoming a daddy herself without in any sense wanting to be a man (Duncan 1996: 100–1). (Jo Eadie)

Daisy chain Gay male slang for GROUP SEX in which each partner is linked to the next either by penetrative anal sex, or ORAL SEX, or a combination of both, thereby forming a circle. A daisy chain can range from a THREESOME, to a much more extended chain of men where there are sufficient numbers – for instance in settings such as bath houses, saunas and SEX PARTIES. Like the CIRCLE JERK, it can be read as embodying 'a sort of Whitmanesque democracy, a desire to know and trust other men in a type of brotherhood far removed from the male bonding of rank, hierarchy, and competition that characterizes much of the outside world' (Altman 1982: 79–80). However as Bersani (1988) points out, any sexual encounter may in practice be fraught with judgements and rivalries, and the daisy chain is no guarantee of utopian sex. Although, like many other practices involving multiple penetration, the daisy chain lost some of its glamour at the height of the AIDS CRISIS CONDOM use ensures it can still be practised safely. (**Jo Eadie**)

Date rape   Koss and Cook (1993: 105) describe date rape as 'a specific type of acquaintance rape that involves a victim and a perpetrator who have some level of romantic relationship between them'. It is part of a typology of RAPE that distinguishes date rape from rape by strangers or by acquaintances with other forms of interpersonal relationships. It has been significant in recent debates around 'communicative sexuality', focused on the problems of sexual communications in determining how sexual CONSENT is sought and given. Communicative sexuality focuses on the verbal and non-verbal communication of consent decisions within sexual relationships, emphasizing the 'messiness' of sexual consent discourse. Archard (1998) has argued that a distinct verbal utterance of sexual consent is necessary to mark the moral transformation of a relationship from non-sexual to sexual, whilst Pineau (1996) has claimed the need for verbal consent consigns women to passivity. Cowling (1998), in contrast, has argued a need to adopt a 'realistic' position about the prevalence of non-verbal sexual communication, whilst remaining aware of its problems. An alternative view is that date rape is just another means by which the violence of rape is blurred now that women's campaigning has led to a greater delineation between consenting sex and rape (McColgan 1996). Whilst the focus on interpersonal communicative problems in negotiating sexual consent is important in developing sexual ethics, the term itself dilutes the political rejection of rape that pushes for more stringent legal sanctions and public sex education (Reynolds 2002). The term 'date rape' is a dangerously deceptive category and the potential source of apologia for more subtle forms of male sexual violence. (**Paul Reynolds**)

Further reading

Cowling (1998).

De-gaying   See AIDS CRISIS; HOMONESS; SAFE(R) SEX.

Dental dam   A small square piece of latex (6 inches by 6 inches), originally designed for dental surgery but adopted by SAFE(R) SEX campaigners for use as a barrier between the vagina or anus and the mouth, to prevent the transmission of HIV. There is an ongoing debate whether or not it is an important sexual health tool (Gorna 1996); on the one hand, it has been proven fairly effective in the prevention of infections and the HIV virus from vaginal or anal secretions during ORAL SEX; on the other, there is some doubt as to whether HIV can be transmitted during cunnilingus (Farquhar 2001: 40–41). This very uncertainty reveals the low priority given to researching the safer sex needs of women in general, and lesbians in particular. Acevedo points out that because dental dams were not designed for use in sex, they may be too thick to allow for pleasure, and not necessarily the best shape to cover the vulva. However, Jeffreys (1993: 163–8) has suggested that the promotion of dental dams was primarily a scare tactic for lesbians during the height of the AIDS CRISIS. She suggests that lesbians came under pressure to model their sexual needs on those of gay men, and that only by formulating a discourse in which their health risks appeared identical, and in need of similar protective technology, could they gain political recognition at a time when the AIDS crisis was overshadowing the concerns of lesbians. (**Alison Smith**)

Desexualization   To treat a group, or an individual, as having no interest in sex, or as not being desirable. Just as certain subjects are SEXUALIZED by the particular tastes of a culture, so others are regarded to be inherently ASEXUAL: in the current climate we might list children, pregnant women, disabled people, older people. Indeed, up until relatively recently it was assumed that 'respectable' women did not enjoy sex with men but should endure it as a reproductive duty (Segal 1994: 75). It has therefore been a political struggle for many of those groups to assert their rights to sexual expression in a society that assumes that they do not, or should not, experience desire and enjoy sexual activity. Many of those same groups who are largely desexualized nevertheless find themselves HYPERSEXUALIZED in certain niche markets of PORNOGRAPHY: children, the elderly, people with disabilities. This suggests that much so-called PERVERSION is the expression of an erotic interest in those body-types which are usually treated as asexual. Whether this makes such desires a political rejection of BODY FASCISM or merely an exploitation of the vulnerable can only be determined from the contexts and degrees of CONSENT involved.

Desexualization is also a positive political strategy, used particularly within FEMINISM to challenge the way in which certain situations sexualize people against their will – the sexualization of secretaries by their bosses or children by their parents – by drawing attention to the realties of SEXUAL ABUSE and SEXUAL HARASSMENT behind situations that are often treated as erotic. (**Jo Eadie**)

Desire   In everyday language, this term is used to refer to the frequency and intensity with which a person wishes to engage in sexual behaviour, with or without a partner. Sexual desire can take many forms, and may be defined in relation to AUTOEROTICISM and the PARAPHILIAS. Desire is also bound up with emotional energies associated with other

states of mind such as love, passion and repulsion. Desire, then, should be seen as socially and culturally constructed, mirroring society's conceptual ordering of the world. Desire plays a very important role in the formation of social and cultural notions of SEXUAL IDENTITY. As this would suggest, desire is not purely physiological; it has, at the very least, a subjective element and, according to certain theoretical perspectives, an unconscious element too. PSYCHOANALYSIS argues that desire is central to our experience of identity. It is produced through repression and is therefore one of the constitutive marks of the unconscious. Lacan (1977c), drawing on Hegel, argues that in desire what we seek is the recognition of the Other. Desire is an effect of the Other, an other with whom it cannot engage, because the Other is not a real person but rather a symbolic place, the locus of law, the symbolic and language. Desire can attain fulfilment at an unconscious level through hallucinations and FANTASIES. These include the fantasies implicit in the OEDIPUS COMPLEX, which, according to psychoanalysis, sets the scene for all other relations. This, in turn, infers that desire comes to be satisfied only through a series of substitute objects premised on what Butler (1990) sees as the HETEROSEXUAL MATRIX perpetuated in dominant ideology. Such conceptions of desire have prompted a great deal of FEMINIST work highlighting the PHALLOCENTRISM that haunts the theoretical paradigms thus far described. French feminism, indebted to psychoanalysis in many ways, has seized upon the notion of JOUISSANCE in relation to the feminine. Cixous suggests that *jouissance* belongs to 'an instinctual economy' that 'cannot be identified by a man or referred to by the masculine economy' (1986: 82). She posits a feminine economy of desire, asserting that woman 'has never ceased to hear what-comes-before-language reverberating' (ibid., 86). In other words, Cixous sets out to claim that repressed feminine *jouissance* can be seen as providing an alternative to the binaristic logic of gender that is implicit in PHALLOCENTRIC systems.
(**Caroline Bainbridge**)

Developmental narrative   Any account of human sexuality which assumes that there is a natural progression through various fixed stages, towards a normative goal. The most commonly cited example is that of PSYCHOANALYSIS. In psychoanalytic theory humans are believed to move through stages from POLYMORPHOUS PERVERSITY, via the OEDIPUS COMPLEX, through a period of LATENCY, and to a full adult sexuality in which the OBJECT-CHOICE is a member of the opposite sex. Since this model assumes reproductive heterosexuality as a final goal it is both HETERONORMATIVE and enforces the COITAL IMPERATIVE. But as Dollimore (1991) has noted, Freud's own work also advances the theory that while heterosexuality is a goal, it is also a goal that none of us will fully attain, and he thus assumes that we will all develop many other types of sexual pleasure and desire. To some extent early pyschoanalysis regarded these so-called PERVERSIONS as acceptable aspects of human sexuality, although many of its later adherents held that they could be 'cured'. The apparent restrictiveness of developmental narratives is thus belied by the fact that they must constantly seek ways to explain and recuperate innu merable exceptions – and thus end up cataloguing examples of their failure. In their attempts to assert their inevitability, they therefore makes themselves look increasingly unconvincing as the definitive route to 'normal' sexuality. (**Jo Eadie**)

Deviance   A wide-ranging term referring to behaviour which conflicts with the dominant norms and values of a society. Traditionally, deviancy has been seen as inherent in certain groups of people, for example, homosexuals and the mentally ill. The influence of early deviancy theory remains evident in some criminological and psychological research, which continues to theorize these groups in terms of their essential deviance. Sociologists however, have critiqued this ESSENTIALIST approach and instead view deviancy as socially and historically specific, and thus subject to social and cultural change. Here there is no single definition of deviancy: acts such as murder or INCEST can be seen to take on different meanings in specific cultures and across varying historical periods.

Émile Durkheim is considered to be the dominant sociological theorist of deviancy. For Durkheim (1893), deviant behaviour emerges out of the state of 'anomie', which induces normlessness during periods of rapid social change. Durkheim's work moves the study of deviancy away from the pathology of a certain type of person and towards an analysis of deviancy as a social system. From this perspective VIRTUAL SEX would be analysed as a substitute form of INTIMACY, practised by people who are socially isolated. Durkheim's work however, can be criticised for negating the ways in which deviancy is transmitted. The Chicago School for example, argued that criminality in gang members was viewed as a regular part of their cultural learning process (Shaw and McKay 1969). More recently, research into subcultures and sexuality has shown how certain sexual practices such as SADO-MASOCHISM acquire their own meanings and statuses within their distinct cultures. Deviancy has also been theorized in relation to social conflict theory. From this perspective, rather than being inherent in the makeup of certain groups of dysfunctional people, deviancy is viewed as a rational response of individuals or groups who are disenfranchized. BUTCH styles within lesbian cultures can be seen in these terms as an alternative expression for women who have been marginalized by HETEROPATRIARCHAL norms. This represents a further shift from the traditional pathological approach to deviancy, whereby the assignation of 'deviancy' is an act of power, in which socially powerful groups stigmatize those whose values and practices conflict with their own. (**Sally Hines**)

Further reading

Walton. and Young (eds) (1998: Chapter1).

Dildo   A dildo, a type of SEX TOY, is an artificial phallus typically used for sexual stimulation. The use of dildos is often associated with lesbians, but women and men of all SEXUAL ORIENTATIONS use the devices. Dildos have been used throughout recorded human history (Panati 1998). Some anthropologists believe the earliest dildos were fertility symbols. Dildos were described in Greek literature dating from the third century BCE (in which two women praise the work of a particular dildo craftsman) and often depicted on pottery. Some early Chinese dildos were carved from ivory or jade, while the Indian *Kama Sutra* of Vatsyayana shows phallic devices made of wood. In the late nineteenth century mechanical dildos – better known as VIBRATORS – made their appearance, originally used to treat female HYSTERIA. By the 1960s and 1970s mass-produced dildos made of rubber or plastic were commonly available in sex shops. Today dildos are often fashioned of newer materials such as silicone and cyberskin. Traditionally made to resemble a PENIS (some are modelled after the genitals of famous porn stars), modern dildos come in a dazzling variety of colours and shapes, including dolphins, human figures, and corncobs. Some abstract dildos made of glass or metal resemble *objets d'art* more than functional sexual devices. In Japan it remains illegal to manufacture sex toys that resemble genitalia, while in the US state of Texas it is unlawful to sell (or possess more than six) devices 'designed or marketed as useful primarily for the stimulation of human genital organs' (Scott 2003). Dildos may be held in the hand or secured to the body using a harness (when used this way, they are known as STRAP-ONS). Devices with a flared based designed for anal use are referred to as butt plugs. In addition to their use for sexual stimulation, dildos may be worn under the clothes to create a bulge, a practice known as PACKING. (**Liz Highleyman**)

Disavowal   A synonym for denial. It functions as a defence mechanism in the psychic apparatus when the subject refuses to admit or recognize a facet of her/his personality or unconscious motivation (Freud 1925). Disavowal is frequently mustered as a defence in situations that provoke a traumatic response. It is a primal defence mechanism that helps us to deal with the difficulties of external reality. In disavowal, there is a simultaneous affirmation of that which the subject seeks to deny. In this sense, disavowal enables us to acknowledge the existence of a repressed wish or fear whilst simultaneously maintaining the REPRESSION itself. As a defence mechanism, disavowal is fundamental to the PSYCHOANALYTIC account of the functioning of the mind in relation to sexual identity. In infantile sexuality, children disavow the lack of a penis in little girls. For psychoanalysts, this is a common occurrence and one that should not provoke neurosis. It is only when disavowal is associated with adult sexuality that it becomes dangerous, often pointing towards the potential for psychosis. In FETISHISM for example, disavowal is regarded by Freud as playing a significant role. The disavowal of a woman's 'CASTRATION' underpins the aetiology of this PARAPHILIA, showing the extent to which it may function in terms of formulating SEXUAL IDENTITY. However implicit in the notion of disavowal is a fundamentally conservative assumption which insists that there is a realm of perversion which it is best to avoid acknowledging. Recently, sexual theory has insisted against this, suggesting that what has been disavowed may come back to unsettle a HETERONORMATIVE culture (see Dollimore's PERVERSE DYNAMIC). (**Caroline Bainbridge**)

Divorce   Divorce is the legal termination of a MARRIAGE. A divorce is distinct from an annulment in that while an annulment confirms that a marriage was never valid, divorce terminates a marriage that was valid but has irretrievably broken down. The ease with which a divorce can be achieved, and the grounds upon which a divorce can be obtained, vary enormously across different religious and national contexts. In the United Kingdom, in order to prove the irretrievable breakdown of a marriage, evidence must be given of either: adultery; desertion; unreasonable behaviour; separation of two years with mutual consent; or separation of five years at the sole wish of the petitioner. Approximately 40 per cent of marriages in the West currently end in divorce.

Divorce is frequently, and perhaps not surprisingly, an acrimonious process, and the courts are frequently involved in the dividing up of assets, and in determining custody and access to any children. As same-sex marriages gain legal recognition, they stand to be embroiled in these same hostilities (see Lehmann 2001). Significantly, the legal protections which are available to divorcing married couples do not always apply to separating cohabiting couples. Many couples, and particularly those with substantial assets, choose to establish a pre-nuptial agreement which determines the division of those assets in the case of divorce. In spite of the legal protections which exist, divorce can severely disadvantage women, and particularly those whose marriages relied upon a traditionally gendered division of labour. These women may lack recent work experience and training, as well as possibly having ongoing caring responsibilities which prevent them from seeking employment outside the home. However, many women continue to find themselves financially dependent on contributions from their ex-husbands, creating a problematic power dynamic. This power dynamic is particularly pernicious in cases where women have experienced violence from their husbands during their marriage, and many choose to forgo financial support in favour of a complete cutting of all ties, although this is not always possible if the ex-husband continues to demand access to the children (see Yalom 2001). (**Karen Throsby**)

Further reading

Freeman (1996).

Dominatrix   The Latin 'dominatrix' simply means 'a woman in control of a situation'. In modern language, the term usually refers to a woman who has the dominant role in an SM relationship (see TOP). This relationship can be either private or professional – professional dominatrixes are SEX WORKERS who offer dominating services which may or not include sexual services. Activities and services vary immensely, but usually include discipline, bondage and humiliation. Usually, but not always, dominatrixes have certain clothes and accessories, including leather garments and whips and other discipline equipment, in order to look dominant and in control (see LEATHERSEX). As McClintock notes, the dominatrix thus inverts – and therefore challenges – the socially sanctioned male–female power imbalance, but only in a very confined symbolic space: 'in the private security of fantasy men can indulge secretly and guiltily their knowledge of women's power, while enclosing female power in a fantasy land' (1993: 102). (**Ana Lopes**)

Don't ask, don't tell   This phrase refers to the botched result of an effort by President Bill Clinton to end the ban on gays and lesbians serving in the US military. As a candidate, Clinton stated, 'If elected, I would reverse the ban on gays and lesbians serving in the United States Armed Forces. Every patriotic American should be allowed to serve their country, regardless of sexual orientation' (Thompson 1994: 392). Clinton's election promise to issue such an Executive Order, however, met with fierce opposition from the Joint Chiefs of Staff, as well as Congress, which quickly acted to make the ban into law. Once in office, Clinton found himself looking for a compromise, which resulted in the policy named 'don't ask, don't tell'. Under this plan, the Pentagon would not ask about soldiers' SEXUAL ORIENTATION, and gay and lesbian soldiers were advised not to volunteer any particulars about their sexual orientation (Carlson 1993). Dissatisfied, the Clinton Administration added a new aspect to the policy that provided what one official called a 'zone of privacy' for gay and lesbian service members (Carlson 1993). This new 'don't ask, don't tell, don't pursue' law was intended to create a PUBLIC/PRIVATE split in order to respect individual privacy and limit the extent of investigations. While criminal prosecutions and witch-hunts for homosexuals that characterized earlier years have significantly declined, the policy in all its forms is largely seen as a failure. Total discharges of gays and lesbians have steadily increased since 1994, with 1,250 in 2001 (more discharges than any year since 1987) and a total of more than 7,800 since the implementation of the policy at a total cost to taxpayers of nearly $230 million (Servicemembers Legal Defense Network 2002). The term has now come to be used by lesbian and gay activists to describe the common heterosexual attitude which seeks to relegate same-sex desires to a private realm where their visibility does not disturb the heterosexual status quo. As the example of Clinton shows, this position often presents itself as liberal, but in fact seeks to impose HETERONORMATIVE standards on the public realm. (**Linnea Stenson**)

Double standard   In sexuality studies, the term is particularly used of the different sexual standards applied to males and females; for instance the prevalent view that PORNOGRAPHY is harmless fun for adolescent boys but corrupting for adolescent girls; or that having multiple sexual partners makes a man a 'stud', but makes a woman a WHORE. It can also be applied when different standards are applied to people of different sexualities; for instance, cases of SEXUAL ABUSE of boys by men are often held up as 'evidence' that gay men should not be allowed to be responsible for children (as teachers or adoptive parents), but sexual abuse of girls by men is not taken as evidence that all heterosexual men pose a threat. The abolition of the double standard of morality was one of the central aims of the SOCIAL PURITY movement from the second half of the nineteenth century onwards. The central contention was that men were judged by a different standard of morality than women. The men and women in the social purity movement fought the assumption that PROSTITUTION was necessary because of the 'strong male sexual drive' and stated instead that the male sexual urge was a social and not a biological phenomenon. Instead, they adhered to a bourgeois, patriarchal concept of morality trying to uphold virtues such as respectability, honour and chastity. The central demand was directed at men, who should restrain themselves more and enjoin chastity, rather than claiming more moral and sexual freedom for women (Jeffreys 1985). Although different perceptions of sexual conduct are a persistent issue for contemporary FEMINISMS, the terminology of the 'double standard' has been largely abandoned and replaced by claims to 'sexual LIBERATION' which demands that women be allowed the same sexual freedoms granted for men. (**Natalia Gerodetti**)

Douching   Douche: literally to shower; more specifically to wash out the VAGINA or rectum. Douching may be performed with hose attachments to taps, gravity douches (a bag of water held higher than body level, with tubing and a nozzle), or the portable bulb syringe douches. The history of vaginal douching can be found in many cultures, especially associated with myths such as that using acid (vinegar) or alkaline (sodium bicarbonate) can pre-determine the sex of a child, or that it is an effective post-coital CONTRACEPTION. Women are still encouraged to douche as part of feminine hygiene (Carrera 1992), hence the use of disinfectants or perfumes in the douche water. The vagina, however, is really comfortable about cleansing itself, and whilst the instantaneous rush of water and cleaning agents might appear attractive to some, generally, vaginal douching may predispose to more problems than solutions (Evans 2000). The commercial drive to impose these supposed 'improvements' may therefore derive from the non-acceptability of natural female hygiene, a misogynistic suspicion of the female body, and the constant consumerist emphasis on 'fresher than freshness'. Rectal douching is different in that it is to evacuate the lower bowel, for instance prior to anal sex (such as intercourse and FISTING) (Gayle 1994). It might also be part of a repertoire of scat play (see COPROPHILIA). Rectal douching, enemas and colonic irrigation can also be used as part of cultural belief systems for catharsis, or bodily cleaning of toxins. Important health points to remember: vaginal douching is probably unnecessary; strong force of liquid and incorrect insertion of the nozzle can cause internal damage; sharing unsterilized equipment between orifices or persons is dangerous; tepid water, by itself, is the safest liquid to use; too much douching can change the natural pH balance, *flora*, and protective mucus lining (predisposing to infections); rectal douching prior to anal intercourse can lead to greater susceptibility to sexual pathogens, including HIV. (**David Evans**)

Drag king   A drag king theatrically performs male impersonation. When Esther Newton noted the existence of female counterparts to male DRAG QUEENS in her anthropological study, it was only to note that they were few and far between (1972: 5). Since the arrival of 1990s QUEER culture, however, drag kings, seen as female exponents of the (popularly) assumed gay male practice of CAMP, and of FEMINIST readings of Bakhtin's theories of carnivalesque (Cleto 1999a: 32) have become of great cultural interest. Delimitations between the drag king, the BUTCH dyke, and various TRANSGENDER identities are ambiguous and contentious. Reich (1999) suggests that lesbian GENDERFUCK (in which she includes both drag *per se*, and the specifically sexual 'drag' of DILDO use,) transgressively disrupts the symbolic order. Davy, however, suggests that only the butch DYKE (and not the drag king) has the potential to retain both social power and femaleness, without simply 'reinscri[bing] heterosexual ... paradigms', (1994: 138) maintaining that both male and female impersonation articulate male voices: the woman who 'appropriates [her] "opposite" is simultaneously effaced' in the unequal representational economies of gender (ibid., 1994: 133). By way of synthesis, we might consider that 'Drag King performances are neither essentially rebellious and inherently transgressive, nor are they ... [an] attempt to dress up the feminine in new garb ... Above all, they are contradictory, confusing – and intentionally so' (Volcano and Halberstam 1999: 41). (**Alex Evans**)

Further reading

Volcano and Halberstam (1999).

Drag queen   A drag queen theatrically performs female impersonation. Heavily associated with CAMP, drag is usually seen as distinct from other forms of TRANSVESTISM in that the drag queen does not necessarily attempt to 'PASS' as a woman – 'Drag means, first of all, role-playing ... it is an act or show' (Newton 1999: 105). Male versions of drag have long been recorded in Western culture, from the substitution of boys in the place of women on the Renaissance stage, through the mock marriage and birth ceremonies held by seventeenth-century 'Mollies' (see Baker 1994: 99–107). The twentieth century saw drag performance used as a cultural expression of community in the underground gay life of the 1950s, and its radical political use in the street activism of the 1970s, and the in-your-face sexual politics of 1990s AIDS activism and QUEER demonstrations (see Lucas 1994). Butler (1990) notes drag's 'parodic' nature, and claims that 'in imitating gender, Drag implicitly reveals the imitative structure of gender itself'; in other words, both drag and *gender itself* are 'performances' of gender (ibid., 31). Despite its potential for subversion, drag takes many guises, some of them socially conservative and misogynistic – not least in the implicit suggestion of some drag queen performance that nothing could be more ridiculous than the socially powerful man choosing the role of the subordinate feminine 'other'. Such political fragility might remind us of drag's cultural contingency – that 'parody is not by itself subversive' and that care should be taken to select performance which is 'disruptive, truly troubling' and does not simply become 'recirculated as [an] instrument ... of cultural hegemony' (Butler 1990: 139). (See also DRAG KING; EFFEMINACY.) (**Alex Evans**)

Further reading

Lucas (1994).

Dyke   Sometimes spelt 'dike'. This word refers to a tough, masculine woman, and commonly although not exclusively connotes lesbianism. It is usually considered working-class slang. While used pejoratively by the heterosexual mainstream, the word enjoys self-referential popularity among lesbians, and 'dyking' is a contemporary slang term for TRIBADISM. The origins of this word are, at best, obscure. The Oxford English Dictionary cites the term's use as early as 1851, which refers to a man dressed with extra care and stylishness. It is easy to imagine the word slipping in meaning to refer to a woman CROSS-DRESSED as a man. Poet Judy Grahn suggests two possible sources for the word. A minor Greek goddess, Dike, functioned as the balancer of forces. When matriarchal religions gave way to patriarchal ones, she was an avenging figure against those who were breaking woman-centred traditions (1984: 47). Grahn also suggests that 'dyke' is a shortening of 'bulldyke', and that this word is a homonym of the pronunciation of Celtic queen Boudica's name: "'Boo-uh-*dike*-ay'" (1984: 137), who led her people in revolt against the Romans in AD 61. The name could have been a ceremonial title as well, meaning 'bull-slayer priestess', who performed sacrifices on 'the sacred altar-embankment, or dyke' (1984: 139). Grahn's critics argue that there is no historical or linguistic evidence to support the etymology that she proposes, appealing though it is. The link between masculine-acting women and bulls is found in African-American culture. A black cowboy introduced the rodeo event of 'bulldog-ging' in the 1920s and this word likely transformed into 'bulldagger', which refers to one bull mounting another. As Bogus notes, 'the black woman who assumes the male sexual prerogative is called a bulldagger by the genteel as well as by the ignorant' (1990: 276). The recording of 'B.D. Woman's Blues' by Lucille Bogan (aka Bessie Jackson) in 1935 supports this African-American etymology, as 'B.D.' is alternately recognized as either 'bulldagger' or 'bulldiker' (Garber 1988: 52). (**Linnea Stenson**)

E

Early modern sexuality   The early modern period is classed roughly to extend from 1500 up to 1800, bringing society from the medieval period through the

Renaissance and the Enlightenment into the industrial age (see MEDIEVAL SEXUALITY and MODERN SEXUALITY). During this period several factors combined to create a more conservative view of marital sex and also a tightening of laws regarding non-marital sex. The sacrament of MARRIAGE became the only acceptable institution in which sex could take place. Self-purification as sexual restraint was promoted by both the Catholic and the emerging Protestant churches. Laws regarding PROSTITU-TION, adultery, fornication and especially SODOMY were revised and heavily enforced. However the central influence during this time span was the growing relationship between the church and the state, the pastoral and the patriarchal, which directly affected the development of the family as a social unit and established the domi-nance of the husband in the home. While the writings of St Augustine were still very much influential at the beginning of this period, by the late eighteenth cen-tury, literature regarding sex had become increasingly liberal.

After the Council of Trent, 1545–63, where the Catholic Church redefined its doc-trines and beliefs while distancing itself from the growing Protestant faith, both Catholic and Protestant churches in Europe endeavoured to promote a new and puri-fied sexual morality within society. Marriage was the only institution in which sex was acceptable and then only in the interests of procreation. Luther, heavily influenced by the writings of St Augustine, believed that CELIBACY was impossible for all. The best Christian life was therefore one in which sexual activity was channelled into marriage (Wiesner-Hanks 2000: 63). The requirement of a church marriage took over from the feudal practice that recognized RAPE as the beginning of a relationship to be quickly followed by a proposal of marriage. Women especially were expected to control sexual urges; moralistic literature from the late sixteenth to the early eighteenth centuries promoted the ideas of chaste, humble and faithful wives, however there was some lib-eral reaction against this concept.

The influence of Church–state relations saw a strengthening of the legal and moral authority of fathers and banned forms of sexual conduct which threatened the patri-archal hierarchy in society and in particular in individual homes (see SEXUAL CONTRACT) By the start of the eighteenth century the Church's influence had begun to wane, espe-cially in the larger cities of London, Paris and Philadelphia (Nye 1999: 58–70). The work of John Locke had challenged the traditional view of patriarchy, however Foyster argues that by this time its implications for domestic conduct had become the main-stay of household manuals (1999: 3). While a growing liberalism within literature and popular culture emerged in the late eighteenth century, laws concerning non-vaginal non-marital sex still held force and allowed persecution of those found breaking them.

Prostitution, adultery and fornication were classed as equally abhorred crimes and punishable by fines, however the crime of SODOMY came to be seen as the worst kind of sexual sin during this period. In 1533 Henry VIII issued a so-called 'BUGGERY' law making sodomy punishable by hanging while Holland adopted a similar way of deal ing with sodomites. Between 1730 and 1732, 75 men were executed by the Provincial Court of Holland after a nationwide network of sodomites was uncovered. In previous years the crime had been denounced, however the growing importance of procreative sex bestowed semen with an almost sacred status, not to be wasted on recreational or non-vaginal sex. This move towards a PHALLOCENTRIC society and the establishment of the male–female relationship as the only natural union contrasted with the MEDIEVAL and CLASSICAL attitude that male passivity rather than sodomy was a sin. Works such as the anonymously produced *Onania* and Tissot's *Onanism* instructed against the sins of MASTURBATION, COITUS INTERRUPTUS and sodomy. Fornication also referred to SEDUCTION which was not only a moral matter but one of economic significance to the family of the girl involved.

Despite this strict puritan atmosphere of the sixteenth and seventeenth centuries Hitchcock has proposed a transition in the eighteenth century to a greater prevalence of sexual activity, which he supports with demographical evidence (Hitchcock 2002: 186–9). It is also suggested that the secular authorities, especially in France, withdrew from the task of enforcing standards of morality defined by the clergy (Fout 1991: 172). This was accompanied by a greater cultural awareness of sex, for example the rise of PORNOGRAPHY, publications such as Cleland's *Fanny Hill* (1748–9) and the novels of de Sade and the emergence of the radical pornographers of London and pre-revolutionary Paris. (This contrasted with Madame de Lafayette's 1678 novel *La Princesse de Clèves*, In which the main character's only obstacle to true love is her own conscience). Despite this decline of earlier Tridentine influences Hitchcock has also contends that patriarchy had not only subordinated women 'it had also imposed men with a restrictive form of masculinity, which was policed by a highly effective public and print culture' (Hitchcock 2002: 197). (**Linda Kiernan**)

Further reading

Wiesner-Hanks (2000).

Effeminacy   Effeminacy is often used of men who are perceived to be too soft, gentle or 'feminine'. Historically, there has been a connection between feminine men and passive homosexuality. In the Roman world, which tolerated active male homosexuality (in which the dominant partner penetrated a slave, boy, or male of lower status), men who accepted the passive role were stigmatized as *molles* or 'soft' (Cantarella 1992: 108; see also CLASSICAL SEXUALITY). This term was later used to designate members of the first recorded urban subculture of homosexual males to emerge in the EARLY-MODERN era, the so-called Mollies of eighteenth-century London (Norton 1992) who CROSS-DRESSED at private parties. However, as Dowling (1994: 6) has pointed out, the use of the term effeminacy at this time was highly complex, signifying a man's failure to perform his civic duties through his overindulgence in 'luxury'. She argues that the 'effeminatus' in early-modern discourse was a largely rhetorical figure signifying not so much a propensity for deviant sexual acts but rather a self-absorbed, frivolous individual who (like all women) was considered incapable of assuming the responsibilities of the mature, adult male citizen. Sinfield (1994) suggests that it was not until the late nineteenth century that effeminacy in males became inescapably linked with homosexuality, largely as a consequence of the Oscar Wilde trials in which Wilde's 'decadent' behaviour, CAMP sense of irony and love of luxury became associated in the public mind with the same-sex practices for which he was imprisoned. Before the gay liberation movement of the 1970s impacted on the wider media, practically the only visible 'gay' characters embodied this effeminate stereotype – including figures such as Liberace, Kenneth Williams (of the *Carry On* films) and John Inman (*Are You Being Served?*). In contemporary gay culture, the stereotype of the effeminate homosexual has been challenged by the emergence of the hyper-masculine CLONE – gay men who adopt a BUTCH style in dress and mannerisms. (**Mark McLelland**)

Ejaculation   The rapid emission of semen by the male accompanying ORGASM, is often held up as the end point of a sexual encounter, especially in heterosexual sex, and this partially derives from the ideas adopted by sexologists Albert Moll (1933) and Havelock Ellis (1931) who argued that there were two essential components of the normal sexual impulse: a process of being aroused, and a process which led to orgasm. This point was further reified by Sigmund Freud (1991a), who argued that sexual PERVERSIONS fell into two main categories: perversions of object (i.e. homosexuality, BESTIALITY, etc.), and perversions of aim (where orgasm was not the aim of the sexual impulse). Ejaculation is perceived to be the mark of authentic sex, an idea which is more than illustrated in the current focal point in PORNOGRAPHY: the ejaculation scene or MONEY SHOT in which the male ejaculates into the face or over the body of the recipient. This status has been challenged by FEMINISM, arguing that on the one hand the primacy of ejaculation within heterosexual sex defines sex only from the perspective of male participants, yet on the other that men themselves – both gay and straight – may be limiting their range of sexual pleasures through this obsession (Dyer 1985). (See also FEMALE EJACULATION; SAFE(R) SEX.) (**Ivan Crozier** and **Jo Eadie**)

Epistemology of the closet   This term was coined by Sedgwick in her book of the same name (Sedgwick 1991), to describe common knowledge that relies on the silencing or devaluing (CLOSETING) of homosexual experience. For Sedgwick, what we know is often structured by an implicit heterosexual/homosexual opposition that precedes other binaries. For example, we might talk about a PUBLIC/PRIVATE divide as problematic in terms of gender roles in the workplace and in the home, but we do not so easily ask why we assume what is 'private' is to do with our interpersonal relationships in the first place. Thinking through Sedgwick's epistemology of the closet, HETEROSEXUAL PRIVILEGE can only remain an unmarked presumption *because* homosexuality is hidden or

PASSES as heterosexuality. Her approach might help explain why when we use a term like FAMILY we automatically think of a heterosexual family unit with a mother, father, one or two children and possibly a grandparent or two. The term 'family' here is coded through a heterosexual/homosexual opposition that does not need to be made explicit.

Sedgwick's term has been taken up by theorists of sexuality studies and QUEER studies in a number of important ways. Methodologically, the epistemology of the closet challenges social science methodology that relies on empirical evidence as visible or self-evident. Knowledge is instead governed by silence, secrecy and what is hidden, rather than by what is said, declared or on the surface. In this respect the term echoes Foucault's (1990) re-evaluation of the status of CONFESSION as truth. It is perhaps unsurprising, then, that Sedgwick's term is more popular within literary criticism than the social sciences. Theoretically, the term has also been adapted somewhat playfully by bisexual theorists concerned to identify the erasure or incorporation of bisexuality as a prerequisite for the stability of the heterosexual/homosexual binary (Eadie 1994; Pramaggiore 1996): hence the term EPISTEMOLOGY OF THE FENCE. (**Clare Hemmings**)

Epistemology of the fence A conscious reworking of Sedgwick's (1991) more familiar term EPISTEMOLOGY OF THE CLOSET, which plays on the popular dictum that bisexuals 'sit on the fence' between heterosexuality and homosexuality. Where Sedgwick argues that everyday as well as scientific knowledge is governed by a heterosexual/homosexual BINARY, an epistemology of the fence focuses on the slash ('/') that ensures these two terms remain exclusive. An epistemology of the fence, in its focus on the space or line between categories, aims to highlight what is left out of sexual opposition, what is uncomfortable, challenging or partial. The term is associated with bisexual theory.

Pramaggiore (1996) focuses on the bisexual erasure that sexual opposition produces and relies upon. As well as highlighting bisexual silencing, for Pramaggiore, 'fence-sitting' also describes a uniquely bisexual vantage-point from which to analyse sexual relations (3). Eadie (1994) proposes the epistemology of the fence as a way of beginning to provide a critical rather than simply descriptive history of bisexuality. Following Sedgwick again, the epistemology of the fence allows us to ask what the category of bisexuality does, rather than what it essentially is or has been. Both Eadie and Pramaggiore playfully QUEER the accusation that bisexuals are fence-sitters who cannot make up their mind which side of the fence they are, or want to be, on, taking it up as a critical rather than irresponsible location. (**Clare Hemmings**)

Erection The erect PENIS is pictured as embodying idealized MASCULINE qualities: hedonistic, asocial, independent, heroic, tireless – and often violent (Woods 1987). However as Segal (1994: 117–64) suggests, this PHALLIC fantasy may in fact be a way of staving off the reality of male psychic and social life: a fear of vulnerability and failure, the uncertainty of male roles and power, and a primal separation anxiety which the child feels in striving to become a separate entity from his mother. That the erection has become the defining signifier of male sexuality leads to a number of erroneous assumptions in everyday thinking: both that there can be no desire without an erection – and that an erection *per se* is proof of willing desire, whereas in fact erections may result from non-consensual experiences. The sexual SCRIPTS that men learn thus focus on the erect penis as the only legitimate site of pleasure and ORGASM as the only satisfactory goal – with the result that IMPOTENCE is seen as a loss of the ability to have or enjoy sex, which is far from the case since a host of other sexual body parts remain pleasurable (Kimmell 1990). Women have recently begun to challenge the ways in which men have used the identity-defining connotations of 'their' erections by applying the term to an engorged CLITORIS – a move echoed by FtM transsexuals who speak of the testosterone-enhanced erections they acquire. While these new discourses risk PHALLOCENTRISM, by taking the erection as the standard model for desire (Chisholm 1995), and repeating earlier beliefs in which lesbians were read as women with unnaturally erect clitorises (Trumbach 1994), the erection may come in time to be thought of not simply as evidence of phallic power, but rather as merely one of a number of non-gender-specific physical expressions of desire, on a par with hard nipples or a wet mouth. (**Jo Eadie**)

Erogenous zones   The erogenous zones are those sexually sensitive areas of the body that respond to the sensation of touch. In theory, any part of the body can be seen as an erogenous zone if it contributes to a state of sexual arousal when it is stimulated. In practice, there are several key areas of the body, including the buttocks, genitals, BREASTS, NIPPLES and inner thighs, that respond to touching because they are filled with many sensory nerve endings. Stimulation of the erogenous zones is usual in context of FOREPLAY. Advocates of PANSEXUALITY invite us to expand our sense of our erogenous zones by recovering the full bodily erotics of POLYMORPHOUS PERVERSITY. (**Caroline Bainbridge**)

Erotica   A notoriously unclear term, used to refer to sexual imagery (visual or literary) whose producers or consumers wish to demarcate their material from PORNOGRAPHY. For instance, some writers have insisted that we need the category of 'erotica' to mark the difference between respectful representations of sexuality and exploitative ones (Russell 2000: 48). Offering a definition, Williams (1990: 277) suggests the difference is that pornography emphasizes satisfaction (always showing sex to the point of ORGASM in the MONEY SHOT), whereas erotica arouses our DESIRE often by setting limits to how much it shows (by stopping short of depicting sex, showing individuals aroused but alone, or using lighting and scenery to partly conceal sexual organs and acts). Erotica is often claimed to have an aesthetic or 'tasteful' dimension, appealing to the intellect, while pornography (particularly hard core) supposedly appeals merely to the sexual appetites. In this way, we can see a class division at work in the definition: the consumer of erotica claims to be enjoying with taste and restraint, and conforming to a bourgeois notion of pleasure, while pornography is defined in terms that suggest a stereotypically working-class lack of those qualities. Erotica is thus defined so as to be a part of what Bourdieu (1984) has called 'cultural capital': the supposedly refined sensibilities that allow the middle-classes to claim their pleasures as superior. (Jo Eadie)

Erotophobia   Erotophobia is literally a fear of sex, from the Greek *eros* (sexual love). However, like many other so-called sexual 'phobias' – HOMOPHOBIA, BIPHOBIA – it can rarely be considered a genuine 'phobia' in the psychiatric sense of the word. Whilst personal or internalized erotophobia might be true for some individuals, for example in those who have been sexually traumatized or abused, the term more appropriately describes cultural and institutional ways in which certain sexualities and expressions are morally regulated or proscribed. An example of this, and its converse, is in sex and relationship education for children and young people in countries as different as the Netherlands and the United Kingdom (see Schalet 2000). In the former, sex and relationship education is integrated holistically into the natural development of children and young people. The result is that first intercourse tends to take place at about 19 years of age in a committed relationship, with accurate use of SAFER SEX practices and with few or no regrets. Conversely, the United Kingdom still has evidence of a mentality that prefers not to effectively educate children and young people about sex, sexualities and sexual health, in the vain hope that they will not commence an early or 'unacceptable' sexual career. This is driven by a fantasy of 'childhood innocence', i.e. pre-sexual awareness, or ASEXUALITY (Callery 1998). It also treats sexuality and SEXUAL PRACTICES, especially those outside of marriage and marital procreation, as immoral and, in some cases, illegal. This leads to an invisibilization of certain people and their needs, and hence a denial of their equal rights of citizenship, and concomitant STIGMATIZATION of all non-'normalized' sexual expressions (Evans 2001). Erotophobia, from this perspective, is therefore not to do with an irrational fear of sex for oneself, but the cultural enthronement of particularly restrictive sexual mores, which hinder human sexual well-being and development (Richardson 2000). (**David Evans**)

Essentialism   Essentialism is a key concept in cultural studies, a discipline developed in response to social movements like FEMINISM and labour, and civil rights. In affirming that differences are culturally constructed, theorists emphasized that certain physical characteristics are not per se the cause of the social differentiations that ensue from them. A paler complexion is not the cause of higher social status – the way in which society views and constructs skin colour is. Women may believed to be unfit for intellectual work due to alleged mood swings related to their period. This idea attributed an essential quality to women based on their anatomy. Cultural studies specialists pointed out that this very idea was a cultural construction (Parlee 1994). Not all women have PMS, and the very symptoms of PMS could be due to societal expectations of them, rather than to anatomical necessity. In emphasizing how differentiations are culturally constructed, the discipline's founders did not intend to cast the study of anatomical differences aside, but rather to emphasize that these differences are not essential to the understanding of how society operates around them. However, SOCIAL CONSTRUCTIONISTS wanted to subsume everything under their paradigm, sometimes at the price of discounting common sense and facts. Those who insisted in the old ways were constructed as 'essentialists'. It was a way to discount their sometimes well-taken arguments. Acknowledging that women's reproductive capabilities are part of our psychophysical make-up is more realistic than ignoring the fact, which unfortunately results in constructing women as men *manqué*. In feminist debates of the 1980s essentialism was often used as an insult against French or otherwise non-Anglo feminists to discount their arguments. The Romance feminist concept of SEXUAL DIFFERENCE, a historical parallel of the Anglophone 'gender', was considered essentialist because it dealt with female embodiment in a way that was perhaps distasteful to some feminists raised in an English-speaking environment. At one point, constructionists came to affirm that 'everything' is culturally constructed. The dogmatism of this statement proves that, in its excessive zeal, constructionism defeated its own purpose, that of calling attention to the cultural component in any physical fact, and analysis thereof. (**Serena Anderlini-D'Onofrio**)

Further reading

Fuss (1990).

Ethnic model   The 'ethnic model' of gay identity, sometimes referred to as 'identity politics', describes gays and lesbians (and sometimes bisexuals, transsexuals, and transgendered individuals) as a clearly defined minority similar to oppressed racial or ethnic groups. Following the example of the African-American Civil Rights Movement, gay and lesbian activists have sought to obtain rights equal to those enjoyed by the heterosexual majority, including freedom from employment and housing discrimination, the right to marry, and the right to adopt children. The ethnic model stands in contrast to the liberationist model espoused by activists in the early 1970s, who believed that sexual LIBERATION would be achieved through the return to POLYMORPHOUS PERVERSITY; the lesbian FEMINISM of the 1970s, which proclaimed lesbianism as a political choice potentially including all women; and QUEER THEORY, which pursues a radical critique of identity (Jagose 1996). The historical roots of the ethnic model can be found in the SEXOLOGY of late nineteenth- and early twentieth-century Europe, and in the HOMOPHILE movement, but it has also been linked more generally to the political structures of liberal democracies (Weeks 1985: 195–200), and to the effects of commercialization (Altman 1982) (see MODERN SEXUALITY). Activists and intellectuals of colour have criticized 'gay ethnicity' as a male, white middle-class ethnicity and challenged the notion that sexual orientation is the primary component of an individual's identity to which other elements such as race and gender are added. Bisexuals and advocates of non-gender-specific sexual practices such as SM have criticized the ethnic model for its obsession with gender as the crucial category of SEXUAL ORIENTATION. Viewed from this perspective, the ethnic model serves a homogenizing and normalizing function (Seidman 1993: 120ff.). Some SOCIAL CONSTRUCTIONISTS caution against the ESSENTIALISM of an ethnic model that uncritically claims homosexual minorities to have existed in all times (D'Emilio 1986: 112ff.); however, others affirm the creation of a modern gay and lesbian subculture as the prerequisite to effective political action, suggesting the possibility of non-essentialist models of ethnicity (Epstein 1998). (**Gary Schmidt**)

Exhibitionism   Exhibitionism is the practice of exposing oneself in order to gain sexual pleasure. It encompasses both consensual and non-consensual acts. The latter include 'flashing', or exposing one's genitals to unsuspecting victims, generally those less powerful than the flasher, such as schoolgirls and isolated women. In these contexts it can create a climate of fear in which women feel unable to use relatively isolated public spaces (Burgess 1998: 123–4), and although punishable by law, authorities often fail to take seriously what in fact constitutes a threatening form of SEXUAL HARASSMENT. It can also involve PUBLIC SEX, parading around the house naked with the blinds open so that people can see, or having sex in a place where people might notice – again including in rooms with open windows. Gay activists in particular have argued that sexual activity should be recognized as a legitimate use of public space, and that watching others having sex has been an important consensual pleasure in CRUISING grounds (Bell 1997); exhibitionism may therefore challenge a prevalent DESEXUALIZATION of the public. At the same time, sex clubs designated to allow the pleasures of exhibitionism have flourished – particularly within SM culture – creating contexts where visible sex does not impinge on others against their will, blurring the PUBLIC/PRIVATE demarcation so prevalent around sexuality and the naked body. Exhibitionism is different from NUDITY, in that the nudist believes in the purity of the body in its naked form, whereas the exhibitionist achieves a sexual thrill from being seen performing sexual acts or from exposing their genitals. (**Ivan Crozier** and **Jo Eadie**)

Fag hag   An American slang term widely used within English-speaking gay cultures to describe a HETERSOSEXUAL woman who spends most of her leisure time in the company of gay men. The term may be derogatory or inclusive depending on the context of its usage. Moon (1995) outlines two principal ways in which the term is used: (i) a heterosexual woman who is sexually attracted to gay rather than heterosexual men; (ii) a heterosexual woman who prefers the social company of gay men to that of women or heterosexual men. The phenomenon shows STRAIGHT women's dissatisfaction with the currently available modes of heterosexual MASCULINITY, while the term reveals much about gay men's ambivalent relationship to straight women and their capacity for misogyny alongside admiration. (**Iain Williamson**)

Fag/Faggot　Generally used as a pejorative term for a gay man, someone suspected to be gay, or a man who appears effeminate or weak. The word can also be used as an all-purpose insult towards any man. However, as with many pejorative terms, 'faggot' has been reclaimed as an affectionate term within the gay community. Rutledge (1996) suggests five possible etymologies of the word: a bundle of sticks used as fuel and linked to the practice of burning heretics or 'sodomites' alive at the stake (although no evidence has been produced to support this etymology); a term for disagreeable women from the 1500s; in nineteenth-century British public schoolboy slang, to 'fag' was to perform duties for older boys such as polishing boots, running errands, warming a cold toilet seat for them, etc. – this system contained some sexual overtones; in the First World War cigarettes were referred to in British slang as 'fags' and were regarded by some as unmanly in comparison to pipes or cigars; Grahn (1984) writes that the faggot was a wand for divination and sacred fire-making and has belonged to the province of gay male wizards, sorcerers and priests for thousands of years (again, no evidence exists for this claim). More recently, the term fag has been used as an acronym of Factory Accessorized Gay meaning an FTM transsexual who is also gay. (**Paul Baker**)

Family　The family is a social institution which presumes a group identity based on privileged forms of relatedness. Within the dominant discourse, biological and marital ties delineate family membership, at the heart of which sits the nuclear family – *the* family – comprised of a heterosexual, MONOGAMOUS, married couple with children. The nuclear family is necessarily reproductive, and the familiar question 'Do you have a family?' highlights this by rendering children and family as synonymous. The use of the term 'family planning' to refer to CONTRACEPTION also points to the ways in which the family functions as a regulatory mechanism, confining sexuality within a reproductive, heterosexual framework.

The nuclear family is both produced by, and productive of, a profoundly gendered set of power relations, and some feminists have identified the family as a central locus of oppression, violence and SEXUAL ABUSE for women (Daly 1978). However, black feminists have argued that for many black women, the family can offer a highly valued refuge from a racist society (hooks 1986). Although the nuclear family retains its normative dominance, it is by no means the dominant familial arrangement, and alternative family structures continue to proliferate (Gittins 1993; Weston 1991). These include, for example, step-families whose constitution is often dynamic, with children moving between families; same-sex and opposite-sex partnerships outside of MARRIAGE; those who choose not to, or cannot, have children; those living communally; those living singly, or raising children alone; or those raising children in co-operative parenting arrangements involving more than two SOCIAL or BIOLOGICAL PARENTS. Reproductive technologies such as IVF or ARTIFICIAL INSEMINATION have also contributed to the formulation of novel family structures. This proliferation illustrates the extent to which the institution of the family, though wielding considerable normative potency, is constantly being resisted and reformulated (Wright and Jagger 1999; Weeks *et al.* 2001). (**Karen Throsby**)

Further reading

Gittins (1993).

Family values   A phrase that names a particular set of values ascribed to the traditional nuclear FAMILY (defined as a middle-class married heterosexual man and woman with children). The phrase came into popular use in the early 1980s when it functioned as a sentimental and conservative rallying cry to 'go back' to a mythic-yet-normative time in which women did not work outside of the home, divorce was uncommon and/or impossible, and heterosexuality was all but mandatory. To insist on and to legislate family values would ostensibly remedy the social and cultural ills of late-capitalist democracy and, in the process, would further the conservative agenda. Margaret Thatcher, Ronald Reagan, and Jerry Falwell were among those who referred to family values on a regular basis throughout the 1980s and 1990s. Its reputation within Western contemporary culture reached a peak during then-US Vice President Dan Quayle's infamous attack on television single-mother Murphy Brown (Walkowitz 1993). Hunter (1995) suggests that the family functions as a cultural screen onto which various discourses are projected, and this explains why the discourse of 'values' is attached to 'family' at all. In reaction to the conservative and most common definition of family values, some feminists and leftists projected their own 'pro-family' discourses, including same-sex marriage (Schulman 1994), and the acceptance of gays in the military, thereby calling for a wider definition of what counts as a family. (See also ASSIMILATION.) (**Rachael Groner**)

Fantasy   Fantasy is a form of self-stimulation or AUTOEROTICISM. Fantasies may occur by themselves or may be prompted and/or fuelled through MASTURBATION or sexual engagement with another. The function of fantasy is to heighten the enjoyment of sexual activity. Fantasies have a considerable amount in common with (day) dreams. They refer to a private, internal world forged through the imagination and are often associated with pleasure and DESIRE. In most fantasies, the subject plays a starring role, leading to the PSYCHOANALYTIC contention that fantasy is central to our sense of identity to the extent that fantasy has been called 'the fundamental object of psychoanalysis' (Laplanche and Pontalis 1986: 14). According to Freud, fantasy originates in infantile hunger. As the human child is incapable of seeking its own nourishment, it is entirely dependent on another to provide food. Once hunger has been sated for the first time, Freud contends that a model is formulated for the infantile response to subsequent bouts of hunger. The infant takes solace in the memory of its satisfied need for food and thus begins the human propensity for fantasy. Fantasy, then, is associated with the fulfilment of wishes. However, Freud insists that it is not merely the imagined objects of desire that provide the foundation for fantasy and the pleasure it entails, but rather the setting in which such objects are seen. In fantasy, it is the pursuit of objects and the setting in which this is played out that matters. Fantasy can be both conscious and unconscious: for example, Freud suggested that unconscious fantasy lies at the root of HYSTERIA and also plays a crucial role in dreams. Fantasy can also reveal REPRESSION and it thus relates to defensive processes such as DISAVOWAL. This insight has been important in the cultural analysis of repressed HOMOEROTIC desire within self-consciously hetero-sexual narratives. (**Caroline Bainbridge**)

Further reading

Cowie (1997).

Feltching   A slang term used to refer to the activity of eating SEMEN from the VAGINA or ANUS of a partner after EJACULATION (Pranzarone 2001). It is similar in some ways to a RAINBOW KISS. Like many non-reproductive sexual practices, it is STIGMATIZED, perhaps more so because it breaks the traditional narrative whereby ejaculation is seen as the end-point of sex, thereby violating the cultural taboos that insist that the point of sex is for semen to find its proper resting place once in the body of a recipient (see Roberts *et al.* 1996). Feltching supplements this narrative, violating the assumption that semen is a gift from one partner to the other, extending sexual pleasure after ORGASM, and crossing and recrossing the highly charged boundaries of the body. There may also be an AUTOEROTIC element to feltching, since it involves taking one's own semen back into the mouth – and therefore in a sense has a HOMOEROTIC element even when practised by a STRAIGHT man. The impact of AIDS has raised new concerns since feltching can only occur after unprotected sex. Current evidence from epidemiological statistics on sex-ually acquired infections point to a recent increase in rectal infections, such as gonor-rhoea. This is symptomatic of a failure in SAFE(R) SEX messages to increase and maintain condom use for anal intercourse (see BAREBACKING). Feltching is a high-risk activity and the possibilities of infections with this practice are open to all participants, from the penis and semen of the penetrator, from the insertee's vagina/anus, and into the mouth of the 'feltcher'. However, MONOGAMOUS couples and TRIADS may manage these risks by systematic STD and HIV testing, in order to ensure that they can pursue these pleasures safely. In NON-MONOGAMOUS relationships, it is not uncommon for couples to elect to practise risky activities only with each other, ensuring their safety by practising extremely safe sex with other sexual partners. These strategies depend – perhaps naively – upon high levels of trust. (**David Evans**)

Female ejaculation   An arching spurt, gush, or trickle of clear fluid at peak sexual response that has been equated to male EJACULATION. In women, this fluid is produced in the labyrinthine network of glands embedded in erectile tissue surrounding the urethra and is ejected from the twin paraurethral (Skene's) ducts on either side of the urethra (Zaviacic 1999). Female ejaculate is alkaline and contains prostate specific antigen (PSA), which does not appear in urine. The presence of PSA indicates that the ejaculatory fluid is *not* urine. About 75 per cent of women produce some ejaculate during sexual response and the amount of fluid varies enormously from a few drops to multiple gushes (Cabello-Santamaria 1997). It is not known why some women do not ejaculate, but various researchers suggest that they may have small or few glands or arteriosclerosis; have had prior infections or genital surgery; or they fail to become fully aroused. Historical references to female ejaculation abound (Chalker 2000: 117–24). 'Copious emissions' that 'exude outward' are described as early as 500 BCE in Chinese sex advice literature. Greek medical documents mention female 'seed' or 'ejaculate'. The Dutch anatomist de Graaf asserted that the female prostate generates 'a pituito-serous juice'. Medical commentators in the nineteenth and twentieth centuries exhibited little interest in the subject, although references frequently appear in PORNOGRAPHY/EROTICA, and literary sources. Modern anatomy texts rarely illustrate the erectile tissue surrounding the female urethra.

Males produce a single, explosive ejaculation at ORGASM, but female ejaculation may be released once or multiple times at peak sexual arousal, with or without orgasm. There is controversy over whether pressure on the G spot, a hypersensitive area on the anterior wall of the vagina, is required to elicit ejaculation, and many critics still question whether female ejaculation occurs at all (Feminists Against Censorship 2001). Unaware of the possibility of ejaculation, many women mistakenly assume that the fluid comes from the vagina or bladder. Fearing that it is urine, some women suppress arousal or avoid orgasm to prevent fluid expulsion. Ejaculation is emblematic of male sexual primacy and the idea that women ejaculate directly challenges this paradigm. Ejaculation is also intimately linked to male potency, whereas it is not an essential component of female reproduction, thus, female ejaculation may often be discounted, because reproduction is still widely considered to be the essence of female sexuality. (**Rebecca Chalker**)

Female masculinity   A term that refers to a spectrum of masculine-inflected IDENTITIES and IDENTIFICATIONS. Elaborating extensively on earlier analyses (Burana and Due

1994: Newton 1984), Halberstam (1998) argues that the analytical labour at stake in theorizing female masculinity is geared towards unhinging the relation between MAS-CULINITY and men. From a QUEER perspective, Halberstam proposes a female masculin-ity continuum that may encompass lesbian and trangendered masculine-inflected subjectivities, including ANDROGYNY, soft butch, BUTCH, STONE BUTCH, TRANSGENDER butch, and FTM. Female masculinity includes contemporary performers of masculinity such as DRAG KINGS, as well as the youthful masculine identification of tomboys. 'Female masculinity' sets out to challenge HETERONORMATIVE cultural judgements that patholo-gize gender variance in general, and women's masculine gender anti-conformism in particular. Moreover, 'female masculinity' takes issue with feminist analyses that con-demn masculine identifications as complicity with patriarchal systems of domination, control and denigration of women, to expose complex cultural histories of female virility and masculine experience. (**Silvia Posocco**)

Femininity   Unlike Freud (see OEDIPUS COMPLEX), most contemporary scholars view femininity as a culturally constructed ensemble of gendered subject positions gener-ally associated with women. Taking Beauvoir's (1953) statement 'one is not born, but becomes a woman' as her starting point, Butler (1990) argues that femininity is never simply given – it does not issue forth naturally from a woman's biology. Femininity is, instead, an acutely social phenomenon that must be worked at, achieved and contin-ually renewed by the subject. Like Butler, Brownmiller argues that femininity is not merely the social elaboration of innate femaleness, but rather an ideological impera-tive that compels women to ritualistically enact their status as man's 'other': feminin-ity serves to give masculinity 'its romantic validity and its admiring applause' (1986: 4). While femininity may be culturally constructed, its performance is not straightfor-wardly optional – particularly in the arena of human sexual relations. As Brownmiller writes: 'to fail at feminine difference is to appear not to care about men, and to risk the loss of their attention and approval. To be insufficiently feminine is viewed as a failure in core sexual IDENTITY' (2–3). It is important to note, however, that while most recent scholarship on the question of femininity focuses on the restrictions it introduces into women's lives, there remains a critical mass of research (e.g. Davis 1995) devoted to how femininity can enable the women who 'do' it to resist the very domination their presentation of self is said to evidence. While femininity is generally considered the province of heterosexual women, it is also an important facet of the lesbian commu-nity as embodied by the FEMME. The femme, however, is often at pains to assert her presence as both a feminine and a lesbian woman as her femininity is often misread as a form of PASSING (that is, as a heterosexual female) rather than as a viable form of les-bian expression (see Martin 1996). (See also FEMALE MASCULINITY.) (**Marc Lafrance**)

Further reading

Brownmiller (1986).

Feminism   Feminism is premised on the fact that women face inequality, which feminists seek to correct (although have yet to fully achieve). The term itself emerged in mid-nineteenth-century Europe (Andermahr, Lovell and Wolkowitz 2000: 93), though there have arguably always been examples of women challenging gender conventions. The emergence of an organized feminism developed directly after the French Revolution in 1789 – including the formation of a number of women's groups – and was based on the revolutionary 'ideals of freedom and equality' (Giddens 1992b: 178). In Great Britain feminism was facilitated by its position amid the European Enlightenment (Andermahr, Lovell and Wolkowitz 2000: 93), and also by the Industrial Revolution. The latter represented the first mass shift of lower-class women into paid employment and, while there were few immediate changes in women's status, it was the beginning of further changes (see MODERN SEXUALITY).

Feminism, particularly in Western industrialized countries, is usually loosely divided into three periods or 'waves'. The first-wave – largely enabled by the earlier abolition movement – was centred in the late nineteenth and early twentieth centuries, and focused on issues relating to women's suffrage, particularly in the United States where feminism initially developed more quickly (see Giddens 1992b). In many ways, the abolition movement prompted first-wave feminist interest in trying to bring an end to sexual slavery, which is when 'women and children are sexually used by men in conditions of slavery' from 'child SEXUAL ABUSE in the family home, through forced marriage, to trafficking of women into PROSTITUTION' (Jeffreys in Kramarae and Spender 2000: 1827). First-wave feminism 'was deeply marked by its Western and bourgeois roots' (Andermahr, Lovell and Wolkowitz 2000: 93), as subsequent waves have been. This is evident in first-wave feminist notions about the inherent purity and domesticity of female sexuality that could (and should) tame the baser sexual instincts of men through marriage (see SOCIAL PURITY). This co-existed with a more radical critique of the institution of compulsory MARRIAGE and was part of a broader shift, including some of the earliest arguments for the need for reliable CONTRACEPTION, which aimed not only to validate women as sexual beings, but also to increase women's social and sexual agency. By the late 1930s more androgynous conceptions of FEMININITY were becoming evident in popular fashion and Hollywood cinema, such as in the 'Euro-ANDROGYNY' of Greta Garbo and Marlene Dietrich, and represented women's negotiation of modern identities after their mass movement into the workforce and resulting increased social and economic agency (Berry 2000).

The second wave marks the next boom period of feminism in the late 1960s and 1970s. Other contemporaneous movements – such as the civil rights movement, student activism, and gay and lesbian liberation movements – heavily influenced the secondwave of feminism that, as a result, covered an enormous range of issues including abortion, education, sexual freedoms, and workplace equality. Indeed, second-wave feminism was positioned within a larger social context of sexual exploration and experimentation (Stewart 1995: 232). These included heterosexual FREE LOVE and an emerging experimentation with bisexuality as a bohemian ideal, which were both associated with exceeding the boundaries of conventional heterosexual MONOGAMY. A major precursor was the arrival of the PILL, the first oral contraceptive. Feminists were initially excited about the potential of the pill to allow women the same social, economic, and sexual freedoms as men, though there were later (justified) concerns about its safety (Seaman and Eldridge in Kramarae and Spender 2000: 1549). ABORTION and SEXUAL HARASSMENT were also major issues and, like the pill, were part of second-wave feminism's attempt to allow women greater control over their own bodies. Part of feminism's approach to the serious problem of male sexual violence involved undermining conceptions of women as victims, such as through Take Back the Night marches. Feminists, especially radical feminists, have linked sexual violence to cultural products such as PORNOGRAPHY, which OBJECTIFY women. Consequently, there have been a series of anti-pornography feminist campaigns that have been controversial not only in wider society, but also within feminism where there are groups campaigning both for and against pornography (Stewart 1995: 86; see SEX WARS).

Second-wave feminism witnessed the development of many feminist organizations, but was also the site for much controversy. One of the largest organizations was the US-based NOW (the 'National Organization of Women'), which started in 1966, and became controversial in the early 1970s for its rejection of lesbian members (derogatorily labelling them the 'lavender menace') (Stewart 1995: 176). Alongside the development of gay and lesbian liberation movements, this was one of the catalysts for the emergence of lesbian SEPARATIST groups. Many lesbian separatists and other radical feminists countered the 'lavender menace' controversy by arguing for women-only communities through slogans such as 'feminism is the theory, lesbianism is the practice' (Stewart 1995: 85–6). While black feminists such as Sojourner Truth had played important roles in the early stages of feminism, particularly in the United States, they continued to face racism not only from mainstream society, but also from feminists who were (and, in many groups, continue to be) predominantly white and middle to upper class (see hooks 1986). This was (and is) an important area of feminist inquiry, but also represents the reason many groups have rejected the label of 'feminism'. For instance, African-American writer Alice Walker describes herself as a 'womanist' rather than a feminist (Andermahr, Lovell and Wolkowitz 2000: 93). During the second wave, feminism sparked changes internationally, including a broader shift towards internationally aware feminisms, reflected by the United Nations' 1975 declaration of an 'International Decade for Women'. Other global initiatives included the SEX WORKERS' rights movement and a growing concern over SEX TOURISM.

The third wave of feminism is generally considered to have peaked in the early 1990s, and has been influenced most heavily by the academy, with POSTMODERNISM, poststructuralism, and postcolonial studies among the most significant stimuli. Judith Butler's *Gender Trouble* (1990) has been particularly significant in destabilizing conventional gender categories and rendering all identity categories 'permanently problematic' (Butler 1990: 128). Part of this shift in scholarship for destabilizing identity, gender, and sex conventions, has been a broader shift towards a more diverse approach to sexual pleasure (see SEX POSITIVE). Much of the work of third-wave feminist activists has been consumed with trying to convince young people that feminism still has much to achieve. Susan Faludi's *Backlash* (1992) was influential in the early stages of the third wave by arguing that not only has feminism *not* yet achieved its early goals, it is also facing some extremely pervasive anti-feminist campaigns (notably from religious fundamentalisms). (**Kelly McWilliam**)

Further reading

Kramarae and Spender (eds) (2000).

Femme   The term FEMME describes a feminine woman whose gendering is a central way of embodying her DESIRE for other women. Femmes have not been understood as emblematic of lesbian desire in the same way as BUTCHES, because their desire for women is not seen as visibly subverting heterosexual norms. In order for a femme to signify as lesbian she is understood to need the presence of another woman, usually a butch. Following Butler's understanding of gender melancholy (see LESBIAN GENDER) a femme's FEMININITY is not the sign of her simultaneous desire and loss in the same way as a butch's MASCULINITY (Butler 1997). In this reading, since a femme does not adopt the gendered traits of the lost male object as a butch does, her femininity casts suspicion over whether she has in fact repudiated HETEROSEXUALITY at all. Her desire for other women has been explained as temporary and therefore untrustworthy in similar ways to bisexual women's desire (Martin and Lyon 1972: 67).

Femme writers and activists have challenged this problem of femme representation in a number of ways. Nestle has written movingly of the importance of femme courage and persistence throughout lesbian history (Nestle 1987), reclaiming key femme figures such as Una Troubridge (1887–1963) from relative obscurity. And recent collections have highlighted the PERFORMATIVE aspect of femme femininity, emphasizing its strategic voicing of lesbian strength (e.g. Munt 1998b). Because of the 'bisexual slur' attached to femmes, most writing insists on the lesbian specificity of femme desire and history, although Hemmings has argued that an account of cultural instead of OBJECT-CHOICE repudiation in the form of NON-HETEROSEXUAL subjectivities would allow for a more expansive vision of both feminine and masculine queerness (Hemmings 1998). (**Clare Hemmings**)

Further reading

Nestle (1992).

Fetishism   Generally, a fetish is an object associated with primitive religions that is believed to be invested with magical power. In terms of sexuality, fetishism is understood as a PARAPHILIA in which an individual experiences sexual arousal in response to an inanimate object or body part (e.g. foot) instead of in relation to a partner. Inanimate objects taken as fetishes are most frequently items of clothing, such as underwear or footwear, although, for some fetishists, the material from which the object is made is of more importance. In such cases, leather, rubber, silk and fur are amongst the most popular choices. The fetish object is used to stimulate sexual arousal during masturbation, or as a component of sexual activity with a partner. The fetish is not a substitute for its owner. Instead, the object is significant in its own right. As Stoller suggests, this is because it is 'safe, silent, co-operative, tranquil and can be harmed or destroyed without consequence' (1977: 196). Self-organized fetish communities dispute this interpretation, arguing instead that sexual play with costume and equipment constitutes a mode of human sexuality which, while it may have its origins in childhood experiences, can also be part of an intense emotional interaction between participants (see SM and LEATHERSEX).

In the PSYCHOANALYTIC account (Freud 1991a), fetishism originates during infantile sexuality. It centres on the belief in the early stages of sexuality that the mother has a penis. For Freud, fetishism is an exclusively masculine PERVERSION that comes about when the little boy witnesses SEXUAL DIFFERENCE for the first time. The little boy is horrified by what he sees and seeks to DISAVOW it. He wants to continue believing that the mother has a phallus, and so he takes a fetish object as a replacement or substitute for it. The fetish object enables the little boy to deny the evidence of castration with which he is faced. He is thus able to preserve the FANTASY of the maternal PHALLUS and maternal omnipotence while refusing the threat of castration. Freud suggests that the fetishist experiences a horror of real female genitalia and is able to achieve sexual satisfaction only in relation to the object that stands in for them. Freud's understanding of fetishism relies on his theories of the OEDIPUS COMPLEX, female castration, male castration anxiety, PHALLOCENTRISM and oculocentrism (the primacy of the visual). Fetishism in this sense contributes to the ideological tendency to privilege the phallus. But it also highlights the fragility of these ideas, because it is a constant reminder of the boy's uncertainty about maternal lack. (**Caroline Bainbridge**)

Further reading

Gamman and Makinen (1994).

FGM   An acronym for 'female genital mutilation', also commonly referred to as 'female CIRCUMCISION'. It refers to the removal of varying amounts of the female genitalia, and is generally performed between the ages of four and twelve. The most common form, 'excision', comprises the removal of the CLITORIS and part of the labia minora. The most severe, 'infibulation', involves the complete removal of the external genitalia and stitching together of the remainder of the vulva, leaving only a small hole. The removal of the clitoris (considered an overly masculine organ and hence a source of undesirable ANDROGYNY) is considered to 'enhance' a woman's genitals, to repress excessive DESIRE and thus to make girls marriageable. In some contexts it is linked to the observance of Islam, however most Muslims do not practise FGM. FGM is found most commonly in Africa and the Middle East, where an estimated 100–130 million women have had some form performed. The removal of the clitoris was also practised on a smaller scale in Western countries from the mid-nineteenth to the mid-twentieth centuries as a cure for 'excessive MASTURBATION' and 'nymphomania', and in more contemporary contexts 'labia reduction' and 'hymen repair' are sometimes performed as forms of COSMETIC SURGERY (Dorkenoo 1994).

In recent decades FGM as practised in developing countries has received attention in the context of international FEMINISM. The Hosken Report (1982) brought the issue to the attention of a wide audience, and called for immediate eradication of the practice. Hosken and other Western feminists characterized FGM as a significant support to patriarchy. While African activists were also working to end FGM, these broad statements by Westerners were considered by many to reinforce stereotypes about non-Westerners as 'primitive' and 'barbaric' (Walker and Parmar 1993). Debate still lingers over whether FGM is a matter of universal rights for women or a matter for individual cultures to decide for themselves, but a broader range of voices are evident in ongoing discussions. (**Julie Wuthnow**)

Further reading

Dorkenoo (1994).

Fidelity   See MARRIAGE; MEDIEVAL SEXUALITY; MISTRESS; MONOGAMY; NON-MONOGAMY; POLYFIDELITY.

Fisting   The SEXUAL PRACTICE of inserting the whole hand, plus part of the wrist and sometimes forearm, into the rectum or VAGINA. In order to be fully accommodated, the hand must be wrapped into a fist as it fills the cavity – hence the term 'fisting'. Damage to skin, nerves and muscles is possible, therefore amongst its practitioners fisting is seen as an art, more safely acquired if taught by an expert, than if discovered for one-self. Since there is usually no exchange of body fluids, the risk of HIV transmission is small; however, if hands have cracked skin or wounds, latex gloves may be used as a SAFE(R) SEX precaution. Although often assumed to be part of an SM repertoire, Califia (1997a: 193) suggests that there can be a divergence of needs and interests between fisters and SM practitioners, since the aggressive element of an SM SCENE may be incompatible with the care and concentration needed for fisting. Sedgwick (1994: 99–103) suggests that fisting within a male–female couple is a democratic practice in that the partners can always reverse roles (although in some cases only one partner might want to be fisted), and argues that the act has powerful meanings attached to it: reaching into the soul of another, filling up a lover's body, exploring or discovering a secret space. Because it has these symbolic connotations, and because of the element of physical risk, fisting often generates particularly intense bonds of trust between part-ners. These elements of skill, meaning, and intimacy mean that – like many other STIG-MATIZED practices – fisting can become both a key node in a sexual identity, and a point of COMMUNITY with other fisters, that may cut across lines of gender and sexual orienta-tion. (**Jo Eadie**)

Flaneur/Flaneuse   Deriving from the nineteenth-century use of the word defined as a person who walks in a leisurely manner around the city, enjoying its pleasures and will-ing to risk dangerous areas, its sexual usage denotes a person who wanders about and/or through sexual encounters without necessarily being a participant, or while CRUISING (see Pile 1996: 226–37). As with VOYEURS, there is a strong visual component to the sex of the male flaneur or female flaneuse, although there may also be a physical component to such sex (e.g. cruising). Some might use flaneur/flaneuse to describe a person who is a sexual tourist, that is, a person who wanders through and participates in multiple varieties of sexual experiences and activities. Finally, the mainstream use of 'flaneur' has a consumerist connotation, describing a person who wanders about look-ing at (and not necessarily purchasing) consumer items, a potential customer; there may be a similar connotation attached to the flaneur or flaneuse to describe someone who is visually consuming, but not necessarily purchasing, sex. Munt (1998a: 30–53) suggests that the flaneuse is a useful concept for thinking about modern lesbian sexu-ality since she is urban, takes back control of the streets, and is independent of men, while being on show *to* women and on the look out *for* women. (**Rachael Groner**)

Fluidity   When taken in its most literal sense, fluidity refers to the nature and signifi-cance of bodily emissions (e.g. tears, sweat, mucus, menstrual blood, breast milk, faeces, SEMEN). Grosz (1994), drawing on the work of Irigaray (1985a) and Kristeva (1982), has shown how the 'metaphorics of fluidity' have been traditionally associated with FEMININITY. Indeed, insofar as the female body has been and continues to be con-structed primarily as the site of reproductive processes (and thus MENSTRUATION and lac-tation), 'womanhood' has remained tied to notions of leakiness, uncontrollability and borderlessness. In contrast, however, men's relationships to bodily fluidity are largely disavowed in Western accounts of MASCULINITY. While the dawn of the AIDS CRISIS fuelled medical interest in the question of male flow – and particularly that of gay male flow – generally masculinity remains bound up with the thematics of solidity, imperme-ability and self-containment rather than (and in opposition to) those of indetermi-nacy and flux. The concept of fluidity can also be used in a more metaphorical sense, referring to the relative malleability of one's SEXUAL ORIENTATION – see for instance HET-EROFLEXIBLE. The idea that human sexual experience is fluid and changeable rather than stable and fixed was first introduced to the sphere of Western social science by Kinsey (1948; see KINSEY SCALE) and is now a basic tenet of most feminist and QUEER theory (see, in particular, Rich 1986). (**Marc Lafrance**)

Foreplay   It is often claimed that men regard foreplay as the 'difficult bit' that comes before 'proper sex', and women regard it as the 'pleasurable bit' too briefly engaged in before male ORGASM, demonstrating male ignorance of women's pleasure. Such a view seems to confirm the popular cultural claim that 'men are from Mars, women are from Venus' (see Potts 2002). Foreplay is a general term for those sexual activities that precede heterosexual penetrative sex with the intention of arousing the sexual actors. Whilst foreplay can be used to imply initial play before other forms of sexual behaviour, such as gay sex, its meaning derives from its heterosexual construction. It focuses on the activity that generates the 'warming' up of desire prior to penetration and orgasmic sex, and came to prominence with the idea of the female orgasm as decoupled from male penetrative vaginal sex. It often consists of ORAL SEX, mutual masturbation and the stimulation of EROGENOUS ZONES. Foreplay can involve a range of activities including anal sex, light spanking, BONDAGE, use of sex toys – its definition as foreplay rather than a particular sexual pleasure simply denotes its subordinate ordering in a hierarchy for the forms of heterosexual pleasure. Foreplay is therefore a signifier of the way in which sex is culturally constructed around the centrality of heterosexual penetration and male orgasm/EJACULATION from a HETEROPATRIARCHAL and HETERONORMATIVE conception of sex rooted in the medico-moral discourses of sex for procreation within heterosexual couples, where pleasure was alternately subjugated or denied. It has been, at the same time, the means by which different and diverse sexual activities and pleasures have been introduced into heterosexual sex-play and led to its diversification, and indirectly to a greater understanding of the range of sexual pleasures and desires. (**Paul Reynolds**)

Free love   While the phrase free love may be interpreted as having numerous meanings, it has generally meant that individuals should be at liberty to love the persons they choose to love without the requirement of entering into marriage or limiting oneself to one lover. It represents a rejection of conventional beliefs about love, sexuality and MONOGAMY and the accompanying relationship models and legal arrangements as well as the conception of love as a limited resource. Most often, free love has been used in reference to social experiments in utopian communities in Europe and the United States in the nineteenth and early twentieth centuries. Some of these movements have had a religious foundation, others have been political in nature, but all have involved some critique of the socially sanctioned structure of the family and have advocated that sexual relations should not be limited to monogamous relationships in the context of heterosexual marriage. While some communities were strictly heterosexual, others involved same-sex relationships. Many proponents of free love were involved in other movements such as FEMINISM, abolitionism, socialism, anarchism, and spiritualism (Cott 1987; Nordhoff 1875). One of the best known and longest lasting examples is the Oneida Community, a utopian religious community founded by John Humphrey Noyes. From 1848 to 1879, Oneida's members practised a system of 'complex marriage', in which the approximately 200 adult members were in committed heterosexual relationships with one another (Noyes and Foster 2001). Many of the communities and individuals involved in free love faced strenuous opposition and personal castigation for their beliefs, which were often misinterpreted and represented as arrangements lacking in morality and meaningful connections (Spurlock 1988). Diverse forms of intimate relationships and alternative sexual communities continue to emerge with POLYAMOROUS communities growing in visibility since the 1990s (Jansen, Kesler and Poldervaart 2002). (**Karen Lovaas**)

Frigidity   See ASEXUALITY; IMPOTENCE.

Frottage   A form of non-penetrative sex involving rubbing parts of the body (usually the genitals) against someone or something (see also TRIBADISM). The word comes from the French *frotter*, meaning to rub. Forms of mutually consensual frottage that have traditionally involved one male thrusting his penis between the thighs of another male have been referred to as the 'Princeton rub', 'Harvard style', 'English method', 'college fuck', 'dry fuck', 'leg fuck', 'irrumatio' or 'hump'. Frottage can therefore be a SAFE(R) SEX alternative to penetrative sex. However, other forms of frottage can be non-consensual, typically occurring on crowded public transport, when bodies are tightly packed together and physical contact can be excused as coincidental. In this sense, non-consensual frottage is considered to be one of the PARAPHILIAE and is illegal in many parts of the world as a form of SEXUAL HARASSMENT. (**Paul Baker**)

FtM   A term meaning female-to-male. The term is commonly used to describe a person who was born with female physical characteristics but who identifies as male. The term FtM includes transsexuals who take male hormones and/or have surgery to physically change their bodies, as well as those who express their male gender in ways which are not connected to body modification practices, for example by changing dress or behaviour. An FtM may also identify as a TRANSMAN, or simply as male. Recently the term has also come to be used by women whose gender *expression* is male, although their *identity* is female: some BUTCH DYKES or DRAG KINGS for example, may describe themselves as FtM, but not as transsexual. Although female-to-male transition has a long history in the West, until recently TRANSGENDER men have not been as visible as MtFs largely because historical writers and anthropologists have incorrectly identified transgender men as lesbians. (Cromwell 1999). Some lesbian critics have criticized transmen by positioning them as 'unhappy' lesbians. Thereby many writers have mistakenly collapsed gender identification with sexuality. Although historically and contemporarily there are some connections between butch lesbians and transmen, many transmen do not identify with this group. Likewise, although some FtM individuals have a past lesbian identity, others have always identified as heterosexual. As with transgender and transsexual people, there is no immediate relationship between gender identity and sexuality. FtMs have also been the subject of feminist criticism, with some feminist writers arguing that transmen have negated their political responsibilities as women by opting for male privilege (Greer 1999). Other critics however, dismiss such arguments as instances of TRANSPHOBIA.

There are debates surrounding the aetiology of female-to-male gender identification or expression: while, some FtMs articulate a corporal male identification from childhood, for example as tomboys, for others FEMALE MASCULINITY is seen as a PERFORMATIVE hybrid gender choice. The murder in 1993 of FtM Brandon Teena and the subsequent film of his life story *Boys Don't Cry*, was a significant development in terms of the visibility of transmen. (**Sally Hines**)

Further reading

Halberstam (1998)

Fuck buddies   A term originating in the gay male community, but now used by people of all sexualities and genders, to describe a friend with whom one has sex on a casual basis, free from the expectation that any more established relationship will develop. This might be a long-term – even lifelong – form of NON-MONOGAMY, co-existing with, and even outlasting, other more formal sexual relationships, or a temporary arrangement that might terminate when one or other buddy becomes part of a MONOGAMOUS couple. Fuck buddies can thus be important parts of one's sexual and emotional life, or casual playmates. This might be seen as a type of PURE RELATIONSHIP, in which each partner is entirely honest about their needs and wants, there is an agreed goal of mutual pleasure, and the relationship can be dissolved at any time by either partner without recrimination. The temporary nature of the bonds also allows for experimentation that is not seen as having any implications for the SEXUAL ORIENTATION of participants: for instance, some lesbians and gay men might become fuck buddies without it being taken to render them either heterosexual or bisexual (see also BICURIOUS). (**Jo Eadie**)

G

Gay   While there are multiple readings of the sense components and extensions of 'gay', it most commonly refers to the male subset of the whole class of homosexuals. Less often, it refers inclusively to the entire homosexual system, in which case it includes women. When applied to women, 'gay' is used euphemistically in place of the inherently feminine – hence more charged – term 'LESBIAN'. As such, 'gay' functions in a double capacity, as both male-specific and (pseudo-) generic. English borrowed 'gay' from Old French 'gai'. Its ancestral meaning is 'happy, carefree, hedonistic', qualities historically associated with male homosexuals. In time the term came to denote the 'effeminate, pretentious male character roles' of Middle French burlesque theatre (Kramarae and Treichler 1992: 173). In nineteenth-century England, 'gay' was applied to PROSTITUTES of either sex, such that, for example, 'gay women' led 'gay lives', worked in 'gay houses' and were all-around 'gay in the arse' (Rawson 1995: 190). It was also used interchangeably with 'copulate' (to 'gay it', which either sex could do). The twentieth-century sense of 'gay' may be traced back to John Saul, a prostitute and key player in the 1889 Cleveland Street Scandal, which involved young male postal workers in a brothel in London's West End. In a police deposition, Saul referred to his male homosexual friends as 'gay' (Rawson 1995: 191). Others attribute the currently primary (male-specific) sense of 'gay' to a semantic extension of the American slang term 'gaycat', 'a boy, often one involved in PEDERASTY, who acts as a lookout for criminals and tramps' (Ayto 1990: 251). In the late 1930s and early 1940s, it emerged as the preferred self-referent among homosexual men, but remained coded language until the 1950s at which time it came into general usage. It was not, ironically, until the advent of 1960s ACTIVISM, in the form of the Lesbian and Gay Liberation Movement, that it acquired its dual function.

Contemporary FEMINIST discourse posits that (pseudo-) generic masculine word-forms and their underlying thoughts promote male visibility at the expense of both female identity and stature (Stanley 1977: 50–66). Many feminist language activists argue that 'gay' when used pseudo-generically is no exception in that, being at root masculine, it conjures up predominantly male images and, thus, can and often does result in lesbian erasure (Cohen 2002). As such, it contributes to the framing of human experience in terms of males' experience and the concomitant neglect of women's.

'Gay' (in its contemporary capacity) and 'homosexual' are semantically related in such a way that the applicability of the latter is a condition for the applicability of the former (i.e. all gays are by definition homosexual). In the same way, the applicability of 'homosexual' is a condition for the applicability of 'lesbian' (i.e. all lesbians are by definition homosexual). The same, however, cannot be said of 'gay' with respect to 'lesbian' for the simple reason that the applicability of 'gay' is not a condition for the applicability of 'lesbian', and vice versa. Whereas the meaning 'homosexual' is included in the meaning of both 'lesbian' and 'gay', the meaning of 'gay' is not included in the meaning of 'lesbian', nor is the meaning of 'lesbian' systematically included in the meaning of 'gay'. As such, while 'gay' remains the preferred term of SELF-DEFINITION for some women, this choice may be related to misogynistic associations with 'lesbian' (On gay male history and culture, see also: ANTI-GAY; CAMP; CLONE; COTTAGING; INVERSION; SODOMY; STRAIGHT ACTING; THIRD SEX; POLARI; POST-GAY). (**Tamarah Cohen**)

Gay brain   This became a frequently used term after in 1991 Simon LeVay, a neuro-scientist, published a study showing a physical difference between heterosexual and homosexual brains. He cited a difference between the nucleus of the hypothalamus which appeared larger in heterosexual men than in gay men (Rixecker 2000). LeVay's ideas were further promoted in his book *Queer Science* (LeVay 1996), which also encouraged research about the GAY GENE. LeVay's work has been particularly amenable to popularization and the reinterpretation of the scientific findings, leading to the belief that there are fundamental and potentially innate features that distinguish homosexuality. This is relevant to LeVay's view that identifying a biological cause for homosexuality would disable discrimination towards gay men and lesbians. The idea that there are structural differences in brains between heterosexual and homosexual reflects a long history of research into structural differences between male and female brains (SEXUAL DIMORPHISM); a similar historical project carried out on racial differences has been curtailed owing to moral and ethical considerations. A key response by feminist scientists (see Fausto-Sterling 2000) is that the notion of a 'gay brain' presumes a relationship between brain structure and behaviour or IDENTITY which is overly simplistic and underplays important work on the complex interaction between biological systems, or interactions with other social and cultural forces. Those who take a genealogical approach to sexuality view the involvement of science in identifying a physical basis for (male) homosexuality as an issue of power – and the status of science in the debates is a reflection of the production of that power (Turner 2000). The question asked by QUEER THEORISTS then is: for what gains is this research being carried out? (**Sara MacBride-Stewart** and **Stefanie Rixecker**)

Gay father(s)   Gay men can become biological or social fathers in number of ways. Some men may be the BIOLOGICAL PARENTS of children conceived in previous relationships with women; others may have contracted the services of a surrogate. Gay men can also become biological fathers by establishing individually negotiated co-parenting relationships with LESBIAN MOTHERS, based either on existing friendships and acquaintances, or through advertising in the classified ads in gay magazines (Hogben and Coupland 2000). Paternal involvement in the upbringing of the child may be limited to conception, or extend to varying degrees of SOCIAL PARENTING. The partners of gay men who become biological fathers may also identify as the social parents of those children.

In the United Kingdom, the 2002 Adoption and Children Bill aims to place cohabiting heterosexual, lesbian and gay couples on an equal footing with married heterosexual couples in relation to adoption and fostering, although prior to the legal changes, only married couples or single people were eligible. Oppositional voices in the parliamentary debates around the bill drew heavily on a range of persistent prejudicial assumptions about the suitability of gay men to be fathers, relying on negative stereotypes of gay men as incapable of sustaining stable relationships, as posing a threat to children, and as providing an environment which may endanger "normal" development. By taking reproduction out of its normatively heterosexual context, gay fatherhood fragments the familiar and unitary categories through which reproduction is conventionally understood. As such, it offers valuable insight into power relations within which the heterosexual nuclear FAMILY is constituted as a regulatory norm against which other family structures are measured (Wright and Jagger 1999; Lehmann 2001). (**Karen Throsby**)

Gay gene   A term popularized in the mid-1990s when Dean Hamer published research proposing genetic linkages on the X chromosome of 40 gay brothers. The research undertaken by Hamer and his team is regarded as scientifically thorough and careful, and led to their conclusion that at a particular location on the X chromosome there could be identified a statistically significant particular 'marker' (Xq28) for homosexuality. This finding however must be carefully interpreted to acknowledge that this does not mean that it is solely responsible for homosexual expression; other influences (e.g. hormonal) also affect the expression of homosexuality, and Hamer's finding is specific to male homosexuality (see Rixecker 2002). As with the GAY BRAIN, scientific research on the 'gay gene' must contend with the social and popular reinterpretation that knowing where the genetic markers are is evidence of an innate biological cause of homosexuality. For supporters of the 'gay gene', scientific determination of the causes of lesbian and gay identity is regarded to be able to resolve the BINARY between nature (ESSENTIALISM) and nurture (SOCIAL CONSTRUCTIONISM) – although Butler (1993) has argued that this is a false binary that cannot be resolved. However, the contentious nature of this debate is not so much that proof of the genetic innateness of homosexuality is assumed to resolve prejudice over homosexuality, but is more complexly related to its very political effects. Those who believe that homosexuality is a choice (including some of the religious right) reject the idea of a gay brain because of the political value of arguing that homosexuality is a sin and can be refused (Fausto-Sterling 2000). Turner (2000) further characterizes the debate over the 'gay gene' as representing a potential conflict of liberal values between the right to ABORTION and the concerns over designer foetuses. (**Sara MacBride-Stewart** and **Stefanie Rixecker**)

Gender blending   A tem referring to the mixing of culturally assumed gender characteristics. The term incorporates the practices of TRANSGENDER, TRANSSEXUALITY, TRANSVESTITISM and ANDROGYNY, and relates to both FTM and MTF identities. The concept relates to individuals who cross gender through the use of surgery and/or hormones and those for whom cross-gender identification is less permanent or visible.

Gender Blending theory rejects the medicalization of gender-mixing practices and the medical category of GENDER DYSPHORIA. Critics argue that medical discourses pathologize gender blending practices and 'limit our gaze to a narrow view of cross-dressing/sex-changing phenomena and hide from view the behaviour of all except those who are seen as problematic' (Ekins and King 1997: 1). Connected to the recently developed field of TRANS THEORY, gender blending theory aims to move beyond the pathologizing tendencies of medical and psychoanalytical studies of cross-gender practices and rejects their assumptions of DEVIANCE. Rather, gender blending theory explores cross-gender practices in relation to the social construction of gender itself. Gender blending theory aims to articulate the experiences of individuals who mix gender in a diversity of ways and looks at the ways in which transgender practices are variably socially patterned. Thus the term enables the articulation of a range of cross-gender states and provides a critique of the ways in which cross-gender practices have been traditionally theorized by 'those who blend the gender of others' (ibid., 2). (**Sally Hines**)

Further reading

Devor (1998).

Gender capital   Just as capitalism rewards economic achievements, so HETEROPATRI-ARCHY rewards men and women for successfully 'achieving' the appropriate character-istics of their gender – and STIGMATIZES those without them. The successful PERFORMANCE of FEMININITY and MASCULINITY – via dieting and make-up in women or muscles and deepened voices in men – brings social and, more particularly, sexual status. Like SEXUAL CAPITAL, gender capital is a mixture of the innate (certain facial features, such as a 'strong jaw' being seen as masculine), the learned (such as posture), and the artifi-cially acquired (COSMETIC SURGERY). Within TRANS STUDIES gender capital is understood as those attributes which trans people are often said by mainstream culture to lack, since TRANSPHOBIC accusations often centre on the notion that the 'real' (i.e. birth) gender is visible in the size of hands (in MTFS) or fineness of facial bones (in FTMS). These are therefore attributes that transsexuals might seek to access in order to PASS successfully as their chosen gender (see Shapiro 1991). But gender capital is not simply rewarded – very feminine women may face additional discrimination or stereotyping, and while to pass successfully as a woman may win gender capital for a MtF transsexual, it will also render her the target of SEXUAL HARASSMENT by STRAIGHT men. While it is possible to seek to appropriate gender capital, it is also possible to reject as HETERONORMATIVE the very system that allocates value on the basis of conformity to gendered characteristics. GENDERFUCK flouts the values of gender capital, combining attributes that are validated in men (muscles, beard) with those validated in women (shaved legs, make-up), draw-ing attention to arbitrary and oppressive classification. Similarly, ANDROGYNY is a polit-ical refusal to take up a place in the hierarchies of gender. (**Jo Eadie**)

Gender dysphoria   A term used by the medical profession to describe the disquiet TRANSSEXUAL individuals feel with the gender they are assigned at birth. TRANS THEORY has suggested an opposite term to describe the state of feeling wholly comfortable with one's assigned (or chosen) gender: gender euphoria (Bornstein 1994). The incongruity between assigned gender and 'gender of choice' relates both to an individual' body and the expected social roles of their assigned gender. The medical diagnosis o gender dysphoria states that it is 'characterized by a strong and persistent cross-gende identification which does not arise from a desire to obtain the cultural advantages o being the other sex' (Whittle 2000: 62). Further, the diagnosis clearly distinguishe between the 'condition' of gender dysphoria and CROSS-DRESSING practices such as TRANS VESTISIM, TRANSGENDERISM and male or female DRAG, by stating that it should not be confused with 'simple nonconformity to stereotypical sex role behaviour' (ibid., 63). The diagnosis of gender dysphoria by a psychiatrist is needed before an individual is considered for hormone therapy and/or surgery within the NHS. Psychiatric diagnosi. remains crucial for both state and private surgical procedures in both the United Kingdom and the United States. The diagnosis of gender dysphoria is strongly criticized by transgender organizations. Individuals, for whom transgender practices are a choice rather than an essential function, argue that the diagnosis stigmatizes them with a mental illness. Critics also argue against the practice of diagnosis being used to erase cross-gender practices amongst children. Transgender organizations argue tha the prerequisite diagnosis, which is needed before 'treatment', assigns psychiatrists the power of 'gatekeeper' and instead press for diagnosis to be reclassified as physica rather than psychological. (**Sally Hines**)

Gender euphoria   See GENDER DYSPHORIA.

Genderfuck   Zita (1998) describes four strategies for undoing sex and gender cate gories as 'active readers of the body': postoperative transsexuality; transgendering; gen ital de-essentializing; and 'genderfuck'. She describes engaging in genderfuck as 'takin seriously the centrality of meaning-in-sex-acts as a sufficient criterion for sex categor membership', where you 'construct sex scenes in which your sex acts take on the mean ings of acts performed by the "opposite sex"; ask that others agree to these readings and to this criterion for sex category membership' (99). This might include practices such as DRAG, ANDROGYNY, and PACKING (see Reich 1999), and identities such as LESBIAN BOY Genderfuck represents an articulation of QUEER THEORY strategies for deconstruction PERFORMATIVITY and transgression in thinking about the physical ways in which peopl engage in sex free of gendered categories – a sexual strategy for POSTMODERN times. Th term has gained currency in the cultural performance of sexual difference by people o diverse sexual identities, and the political articulation of sexual freedom from bot HETERONORMATIVITY and from categories such as lesbian, gay and transsexual and the cul tural and sexual expectations they place on the individual subject. It has the sam strengths as queer theory in refusing and disrupting sexual categories and the sam weaknesses in its representation of the body in cultural and discursive form rather tha material, physical and social form. Where genderfuck has value is in its moment of dis ruption and liberation, to think differently and act differently from regulatory norms – Zita's MALE LESBIANS, drawing from Stoltenberg's (1989) refusal to be a man. Where Zita's analysis is worthwhile is in understanding that such a strategy has limitations and that the dissolving of sexual categories within genderfucking works within philosophical and social contexts that require further critical examination before it is celebrated as a means of sexual emancipation. (**Paul Reynolds**)

Further reading

Wilchins (2002).

Genderqueer   An identity descriptor mostly adopted by young people coming of age in the early twenty-first century. It refers to a combination of gender identities and sexual orientations. One example could be a person whose gendered presentation is sometimes perceived as male and sometimes as female but whose gender identity is female, gendered expression is BUTCH and sexual orientation is lesbian. It suggests non-conformity or mixing of gendered stereotypes, conjoining both gender and gayness and 'pluralistic challenges to the male/female, woman/man, lesbian, butch/femme constructions and identities' (Nestle 2002: 9). Genderqueerness is both unintelligible and ABJECTED in the BINARY sex/gender system:

> Our embodiments and our subjectivities are abjected from social ontology: we cannot fit ourselves into extant categories without denying, eliding, erasing, or otherwise abjecting personally significant aspects of ourselves . . . When we choose to live with and in our dislocatedness, fractured from social ontology, we choose to forgo intelligibility: lost in language and in social life, we become virtually unintelligible, even to ourselves. (Hale 1998: 336) (**Jill Weiss**)

Ghetto   See COMMUNITY; ETHNIC MODEL; HETEROFLEXIBLE.

Golden showers   See WATERSPORTS.

Group sex   See CIRCLE JERK; DAISY CHAIN; *MÉNAGE À TROIS*; SEX PARTIES; TRIAD.

Hard core   See PORNOGRAPHY.

Hermaphrodite   This historical term was coined by Victorian medical practitioners after the Greek mythical figure of Hermaphroditus, who had both 'female' and 'male' genitals. At this time, European doctors – who did not have knowledge of genetics endocrinology or embryology – defined 'SEX' in terms of gonads (ovaries and testes) 'True hermaphrodites' were defined as individuals who had both ovaries and testes whereas 'pseudo-hermaphrodites' were defined as individuals only having the genita 'appearance' of two sexes (Hird and Germon 2001). Sometimes the qualifiers 'female or 'male' were placed before the term hermaphrodite, with problematic consequence: because these assignments often contradicted the sex assignment of the child. Likewise the terms 'true' and 'pseudo' may be very harmful because they imply an authenticity or illegitimacy to intersex conditions (ISNA 2003a). Some people with intersex conditions have recently reclaimed the term 'hermaphrodite' in a positive way (in a simila way that the LGBT community has reclaimed the term QUEER). However, the term remain. stigmatizing, and has been replaced by the more accurate term INTERSEX by intersex sup port groups, and increasingly, the medical community. (**Myra Hird**)

Further reading

Dreger (1998).

Heteroflexible   A recently coined IDENTITY, used by those whose primary preference i: for opposite-sex partners, but who are open to contact with members of their own se: (see also BICURIOUS). In part, the term can be seen as a response to the perceived restric tions of belonging to a COMMUNITY or 'gay ghetto', as people seek ways of exploring homosexual desire without making it the centre of their identity or lifestyle (Scheid 2002; see POST-GAY). Given that HOMOPHOBIA still encourages individuals not to identif: as lesbian, gay or bisexual, the term may also act as a safe way to explore sexual feel ings for one's own sex without taking up a stigmatized identity. While this may vali date same-sex desire for a wider number of individuals, it also encourages them to se their sexuality as a private choice, rather than as part of a political movement, an hence may impede social change in some areas even while it hastens it in others (**Jo Eadie**)

Heteronormativity   Describes a BINARY gender system in which only two sexes are accepted and sex is equated with gender identity, gender role, and heterosexuality: 'th assumption that everyone is heterosexual and the recognition that all social institu tions . . . are built around a heterosexual model of male/female social relations' (Nage 2003: 49–50). A heteronormative scheme excludes gay men, lesbians, bisexuals, inter sexed and transgendered people, insofar as it implies the consistent pairing of wome and men. On a heteronormative paradigm, the term 'man' is rendered meaningles unless it includes 'desiring women' and vice versa. Thus, heteronormativity represent the idea that heterosexuality is the preferred and acceptable SEXUAL ORIENTATION. A other orientations are viewed as DEVIANT. Warner suggests that heteronormativity organizes *all* patterns of thought, awareness, and belief around the presumption of a universal heterosexual desire, behaviour, and identity (1993: xxi–xxv). Heteronormativity thus acknowledges no variations or exceptions to heterosexuality and simply becomes the lens through which we perceive the world. It is thus a further reaching concept than HETEROSEXISM, since it implies that everyday institutions and metaphors (such as 'a marriage of ideas') impose heterosexual standards. In this way, heteronormativity permeates social institutions, marking the unquestioned and invisible presumption of a universal heterosexual desire. Sanctions follow for those who deviate from the societal standard. Heteronormativity should not be conflated with patriarchy, since even some patriarchal systems do not have binary gender systems (for example, some contain a THIRD GENDER). Moreover, as Seidman points out, 'from a poststructuralist perspective, gay identity constructions maintain the dominant hetero/homosexual code, including its normative heterosexuality' (1997: 132). That is, some scholars argue that gay politics must move away from a concern with the ETHNIC MODEL of gay identity, since to focus on 'gay identity' is to problematically replicate the hetero/homo binary and sustain heteronormativity (see MONOSEXUALITY). (**Mary Bloodsworth-Lugo**)

Heteropatriarchy   Defined as a framework which combines male supremacy and heterosexual supremacy to establish patriarchy and heterosexuality as the 'natural' order. In a heteropatriarchy, maleness, MASCULINITY, and heterosexuality are joined together; thus, sexism, misogyny, and HOMOPHOBIA become conceptually and practically linked. Heteropatriarchies thereby maintain HETERONORMATIVITY and sustain the HETERO-SEXIST binary of masculinity and femininity – with related expectations according to biological sex – and portray heterosexuality as the only approved form of sexual expression. At this moment in time, heteropatriarchy remains the dominant social structure across the globe, except for pockets of SEPARATIST exception. Via heteropatriarchal systems, anti-gay and anti-lesbian prejudice may be explained by the perceived threat that gay men and lesbians pose to the established gender order.

Irigaray (1985a; 1985b) and others have referred to this order as HOM(M)OSEXUAL, since it represents a male-ordered economy in which women are objectified and exchanged. Similarly, Frye states that heteropatriarchy 'consists of cultural and economic forces and pressures in a culture and economy controlled by men ... which work to keep at least local culture and economy in male control' (1983: 13). While lesbians have clearly been rendered powerless within heteropatriarchies – being neither heterosexual nor male – the place of gay men has been the source of some debate. For instance, some scholars have argued that gay men, like lesbians, threaten heteropatriarchal systems in that they fail to maintain 'the FAMILY' and male power in the usual, sanctioned way. Others have suggested that while gay men do not enjoy HETEROSEXUAL PRIVILEGE within heteropatriarchies, they nonetheless do benefit from male privilege, and that male privilege positions gay men as complicit with these structures in a way that lesbians are not. (**Mary Bloodsworth-Lugo**)

Heterophobia   Heterophobia is variously understood as the fear of being emotionally or sexually intimate with the opposite sex, fear of heterosexual people, or fear of being perceived as heterosexual. As with HOMOPHOBIA, heterophobia also refers to the violence, rage or hatred that is a response to that fear, particularly where the fear itself is seen to be an indication of repressed desire. Heterophobia, then, indicates fear or hatred of heterosexuality and heterosexuals, but may also indicate repressed heterosexual desire. Again, like the term 'homophobia' it may be used to refer to institutions, groups and communities as well as individuals, so that an organization rather than its individual members might be accused of heterophobia. Where heterophobia is the property of an individual it is understood to be irrational or unconscious; where heterophobia describes an institution or group it is usually understood to be systematic.

Klein understands homophobia and heterophobia as linked expressions of a larger societal fear of intimacy (Klein, 1978). For Klein COMPULSORY MONOSEXUALITY prevents us from reaching the desired state of 'One Hundred Per cent Intimacy', where our relationships with other people are completely free. Similarly, Hutchins and Ka'ahumanu (1990) define the term as 'the fear of closeness and/or intimacy with those of the other sex' (369). These authors all see heterophobia as one of the main causes of BIPHOBIA in gay and lesbian communities, identifying an often-unacknowledged homosexism as one of the reasons why gay and lesbian people fear being perceived as STRAIGHT. For bisexual writers, homosexism and its concomitant heterophobia are always negative, while for many lesbian and gay writers and activists, a dislike and hatred of heterosexual culture and privilege is an understandable and necessary response to historical and contemporary endorsement of violence against homosexuals (see QUEERBASHING). In this context homosexism might be re-named lesbian and gay PRIDE, and heterophobia a strategic necessity (see SEPARATISM). (**Clare Hemmings**)

Heterosexism and homophobia   Two closely linked terms, describing attitudes and policies in evidence when heterosexual norms are used as a yardstick to judge other ways of thinking and being. Heterosexism is a neologism, coined by comparison with 'sexism', and used to describe those varieties of prejudice which are characterized by the (often tacit) assumption of heterosexual norms – an example might be the assumption that one's status as a father or mother was a clear sign of one's heterosexuality. 'Heterosexism' is sometimes deployed as if it is synonymous with the term 'homophobia'; but a distinction between the two is, equally, often observed. One difference is that 'homophobia' tends to denote a greater aversion to, active hatred of, and even violence towards the fact of same-sex desire and those who experience it than is conveyed by 'heterosexism'; it describes a more powerful animus against homosexual ity than that term, one that may be deliberately acted on, but also, importantly, one that may be viscerally experienced. Thus a significant difference between heterosexism and homphobia lies in the former's avoidance of the suffix 'phobia', which connotes an *irrational* antipathy, perhaps deriving from and/or evidencing a psychological condition (in certain psychoanalytic models homophobia is taken as a sign of, and is therefore seen as being caused by, repressed homosexuality). The concept of heterosexism therefore allows for the articulation, exploration and analysis of bias or prejudice which is rooted in an implicit or explicit adherence to heterosexual norms and standards, while avoiding diagnosing that bias or prejudice as being rooted in irrationality or sickness. Another difference between the two terms is that while homophobia might be glossed as 'anti-gayness' or 'anti-lesbianness', heterosexism does not necessarily manifest itself in relation to homosexual people. To return to the example given at the start of this entry: one might be a bisexual parent. In this case, the assumption that one is STRAIGHT might more accurately be labelled heterosexist than homophobic.

It could be said, then, that heterosexism implicitly references a kind of alliance: gay men, lesbians, bisexual people and others may all suffer discriminatory treatment that ultimately derives from the elevation of one way of being sexual to *the* way of being sexual. Bristow has noted this; however he criticizes 'heterosexism' for implicitly overstating the degree to which anti-gay and anti-lesbian sentiments are the same: '"heterosexism" wrongly lumps together lesbians and gay men as the *same* object of sexual discrimination' (1989: 57, my emphasis) he says (and obviously we might add other identity categories, like bisexual, in thinking about this point – hence the coinage of 'BIPHOBIA' and 'lesbophobia'). It is worth noting that Bristow makes a similar charge against 'homophobia', which marks one similarity between the terms; it is also worth noting that a virulent homophobia might in fact underlie a more overt heterosexism: in many cases it might be difficult to decide which is the more appropriate term to use. (Chris West)

Heterosexual matrix   Coined by Butler (1990), a set of norms and structures through which we must all pass and which seeks to construct us as heterosexual. She argues that sex, gender and sexuality are forced to cohere in order to uphold the fiction of stable identity: the myth being that biological males/females are naturally masculine/feminine and desire each other exclusively. Rejecting gender as a core identity or role, Butler turns the normative sex/gender/sexuality trajectory on its head: the law of heterosexuality is covertly set in stone through the gender citation that disguises the ideological construction of 'sex' (Butler 1993). This matrix is the crux of Lacan's (1977a) structuralist account of the psyche: sexed positions are assumed through fixed positioning around the PHALLUS. This psychic account of gender construction Lacan (1977b) sees as a comedy – these positions are fantasy ideals, impossible to inhabit coherently. On this Butler follows Rose's reading of

Lacan which underlines the *failing* of sexual identity (Rose 1986). Butler agrees that 'sex' is a fantasy ideal, but asks further political questions: how does it consti- tute legitimate/illegitimate identities and by whom is this 'law' enshrined? Following Rubin's (1975) early influential feminist reading of Lévi-Strauss and Lacan (the sex/gender system works by transforming biological POLYMORPHOUS PER- VERSITY into culturally mandated heterosexuality, policed by the heterosexual family and a rigid notion of SEXUAL DIFFERENCE), Butler argues that Lacan's law is presup- posed by a prohibition on homosexuality. Heterosexual identity is established through a DISAVOWAL of homosexuality and of cross-gender identification, what Butler sees as a form of gendered melancholy, or the psychic incorporation of unresolved same-sex attachments. Butler's main gripe with Lacan is that the matrix forecloses the possibility of lesbian and gay subversions: the examples of the femi- nized FAG and the phallicized DYKE. Lacanian critics claim Butler misconstrues Lacan: Dean argues that Butler ignores the Lacanian 'real'; sexual difference is not a pre-symbolic, non-negotiable framework, but an open question (Dean 2000). Butler's reply is that this recourse to the real is apolitical: the emptiness of sexual difference gives it a transcendental status, above its socio-cultural applications. (**Nicholas Rees-Roberts**)

Heterosexual privilege   Described by Hutchins and Ka'ahumanu as 'the benefit of basic civil rights and familial recognition that heterosexuals accord themselves as the norm' (1990: 369), this describes the legal, moral and social structures that treat het- erosexuality as more valid than homosexuality, and that reward heterosexuals accord- ingly with tax privileges, cultural VISIBILITY, adoption rights, and public acceptance. Within SEXUAL POLITICS the term has particularly been used as a challenge to bisexuals, whose critics have argued that they possess heterosexual privilege that renders their oppression less than that of lesbians and gay men. Hemmings (2002: 78–9) describes the charges as including: the option to PASS as STRAIGHT when with an opposite-sex lover; the possibility of marriage; and greater authority given to public speech.

Critics of the application of the concept to bisexuals have pointed out that by 'pass- ing' as straight bisexuals in fact do violence to their identities by silencing themselves and refute the notion of a hierarchy of oppressions, pointing out that all sexual sub- jects have different privileges over one another – a MONOGAMOUS gay couple may receive validations that that a POLYAMOROUS bisexual TRIAD does not (see BIPHOBIA). It is also a heavy expectation to demand that individuals tackle large social structures in isola- tion, thus some bisexuals may be in situations where it is not safe for them to chal- lenge heterosexual privilege – just as some lesbians and gay men may opt not to COME OUT. As Udis-Kessler (1992) argues, while privilege may accrue to some bisexual choices, bisexuals have historically been aware of this risk and elected to fight it – as have many heterosexuals – both as an act of solidarity with lesbians and gay men and as part of the making VISIBLE of their own sexual identities. Debates about strategies to dismantle it thus figure prominently in Tucker's (1995) and Weise's (1992) key anthologies. (**Jo Eadie**)

Heterosexuality   Historically, heterosexuality has not been subject to the same academic scrutiny as homosexuality, although it has been argued by SOCIAL CONSTRUCTIONISTS that sexuality, including heterosexuality, cannot be understood as an essential human attribute, rather it is culturally, historically and spatially contingent and rooted. Biological determinists, on the other hand, view sexuality as prefixed, definable and explicable in terms of a reproductive norm and the reproduction of the species. Although heterosexuality has a history of being problematized by individual feminists, a consistent problematization of heterosexuality has only emerged since the 1960s when radical FEMINISM put heterosexuality at the centre stage by proclaiming that 'the personal is political'. In addition, the economically and socially constructed basis of heterosexuality has been exposed through concepts such as COMPULSORY HETEROSEXUALITY or the SEXUAL CONTRACT. Heterosexuality, and its role in the control and exploitation of women, has been a subject of heated feminist debate with some women maintaining that women cannot have autonomy while they are in heterosexual relations, thus proclaiming the need for SEPARATISM. Other strands of feminism reassert the possibility of egalitarian and pleasurable heterosexual relations (Segal 1994).

Heterosexuality has often been naturalized by linking it with reproduction, but CONTRACEPTION and reproductive technologies have disrupted the reproductive model of sexuality. Whereas FAMILY has often been equated with heterosexuality, the history of family and intimate relations has pointed to the economic, social and political basis of the family. It has recently been claimed that the transformation of INTIMACY (trends in marriage and cohabitation) has disrupted and destabilized heterosexuality, and efforts to allow marriage for lesbians and gay men, or alternatively the legislation brought in to prevent this, are indicators that the naturalized status of heterosexuality is being challenged and that heterosexuality is only one of many SEXUAL ORIENTATIONS. The way in which heterosexuality has encoded and structured everyday life and has been normalized and institutionalized by the law, the state and social conventions has been conceptualized by feminist and queer theory as HETERONORMATIVITY: this is embodied in a range of practices which privilege heterosexuality, including greater public recognition of heterosexual relationships (e.g. through wedding ceremonies), legal rights (e.g. AGE OF CONSENT laws, adoption and immigration), and greater cultural visibility in the media.

However, heterosexuality does not infer a given set of SEXUAL PRACTICES, rather heterosexuals can be sexually unorthodox in some or all of their sexual practices such as POLYAMORY, SM or CROSS-DRESSING. Some heterosexuals thus face ostracism, or legal sanctions, over their sexual preferences, producing SEXUAL STRATIFICATION between the less and more socially acceptable forms of heterosexual sex. Bisexual and QUEER activists have also pointed out that male–female sexual interactions need not necessarily be STRAIGHT, so that some male–female relationships need to be included amongst what have recently been termed NON-HETEROSEXUALS. (**Natalia Gerodetti**)

Further reading

Jackson (1999).

HIV   Discovered in 1983 and named the Human Immunodeficiency Virus in 1985, HIV is almost universally regarded as the causative agent for a deterioration of the immune system which may culminate in various opportunistic conditions and AIDS-defining illnesses. SEMEN and blood appeared 'prime suspects' of infectivity, even though public and media hysteria preferred blaming 'high risk groups' and all bodily fluids (Bloor 1995) (see AIDS CRISIS). HIV infection occurs when sufficient quantity and quality of virus – present in semen, blood and to lesser degrees vaginal secretions and breast milk – effectively enters the bloodstream of another person. The virus infects human cells identifiable to it by specific characteristics ('CD^4 markers'), including macrophage and T^4 lymphocytes (white blood cells). Macrophages and T^4 (or *T-helper*) cells normally orchestrate an immune response to deal with non-self-pathogens. In this particular condition these essential cells are infected, and frequently destroyed, predisposing to immune-system deterioration. Despite meeting the internationally agreed 'Koch's Postulates on Disease Causation'(NAIAD 1999) certain 'AIDS dissidents' disagree with the above aetiology on grounds that the patterns of spread around the world, coupled with the heterogeneity of illnesses attributed to AIDS, cannot causatively correlate with each other (Duesburg 2001) and vital efforts in disease prevention and treatments have been diminished due to scientific and political disagreements over whether or not HIV leads to AIDS – notably in the case of the South African President Thabo Mbeki who adopted the position that HIV did not cause AIDS as the basis for state AIDS policy.

Unlike health conditions that are treated compassionately, HIV infection and disease attract high levels of hostility, frequently due to their link with primordial notions of life, sex and death (Sontag 1990). People with multiple forms of STIGMA and oppression are particularly vulnerable, e.g. due to gender, sexuality, poverty, poor health, lack of SAFE(R) SEX awareness, skills and resources, and the inability to adequately protect oneself from means of transmission (Carlisle 2001). Great advances have been made in treatments for HIV infection and disease since the advent of 'combination therapies' (1996 onwards), and many more will be made. To date, however, these therapies are not always suitable for every individual, and are far too costly for the majority of people in the world who need them (AIDSmap 2001). Essential points to be recalled in the third decade of this pandemic are: HIV infection is largely preventable; prevention is more humane and cheaper than treatment; and as yet, there is still no effective vaccine or cure for HIV infection and disease (SFAF 2001). (**David Evans**)

Further reading

Bloor (1995).

Hom(m)osexual 'Hom(m)osexual' is a term coined by French philosopher and psychoanalyst Luce Irigaray (1985a; 1985b), whose attack on the exclusion of female sexual subjectivity from philosophy and psychoanalysis has largely influenced debates on SEXUAL DIFFERENCE within Anglo-American feminist theory. According to Irigaray, man has reduced otherness to a relationship with himself; sexual difference is in fact a screen for the operations of 'sexual indifference' whereby woman is defined solely by, for and in relation to man. Sexual indifference is a phallic order, a sexual contract between men; 'hom(m)osexuality' is her term for this all-male domination cemented by a supposed repressed HOMOEROTICISM. Accordingly, because they eroticize the 'same', gay men reveal the true stakes in the heterosexual economy. Many critics view this as HOMOPHOBIC: Dollimore (1991) sees the metaphor as a scapegoat in her analysis of heterosexual difference. De Lauretis, who previously found Irigaray's concept useful to formulate patriarchy's indifference to the other sex and its denial of lesbian representation (De Lauretis 1993), later abandons the term for its inability to think of gay sexuality as anything but assimilable to the normal (De Lauretis 1994). For heterosexuality to be an alibi for the displaced structure of male erotic bonding, sexual difference must be a totalizing social division. Such a move ultimately hinders Irigaray given the empirical evidence against any social alliance between gay and straight men; whilst there are many gay men who defend what foothold they have in heterosexist society at the expense of women, there is no reason to assume the inevitability of such a connection (Earl Jackson 1995). Indeed, 'hom(m)osexuality' and 'sexual indifference' form part of Irigaray's later heterosexist fundamentalism; her conservative engagement with what amounts to an ideal of heterosexual difference means that she ignores any relations or identifications (cross-gender for instance) outside her rigid paradigm. (**Nicholas Rees-Roberts**)

Homoeroticism Also known as homosocial desire (Sedgwick 1985), homoeroticism refers to the sexual tensions that exist in HOMOSOCIAL (same-sex) environments such as public schools, the armed forces and sports teams. Analysts such as Dundes (1985) use Freudian arguments about human beings' basic BISEXUALITY to suggest that homosexual desire in same-sex environments is expressed through sublimation and displacement. For instance, the very vocabulary of sport overlaps with sexual slang, terms such as 'make a pass', 'score', 'dribble' and 'rim shot' having clear sexual reference. The hazing of new recruits and the physical intimacy (hugging, kissing, groping) that takes place on the sports field or between 'buddies' in war movies are symptomatic of what Bech (1997) refers to as 'absent homosexuality', that is, the consciousness that these actions might really be homosexual has to be repressed and denied at all costs. Hence, homosocial environments can become sites of HOMOSEXUAL PANIC (Sedgwick 1991) where the disavowal of homosexual desire must be constantly rehearsed.

However, Sedgwick (1985) and Dollimore (1991) have suggested that homosocial desire is not *repressed* in same-sex environments but actually *created* by the social forces at work there. They look at literary scenarios of man–woman–man love triangles where they argue that the men are as erotically invested in each other as they are in the woman. Also, the idea that men value male company over that of female has been argued in relation to the male bonding in 'buddy movies' and TV serials where intense emotional involvement is always in danger of spilling over into homoerotic attraction. In women's SLASH FICTION this implicit homoeroticism is made explicit (Penley 1992).

Female homoeroticism has received less analysis than that between men, perhaps because women are allowed greater freedom to express themselves physically and emotionally with other women. Rich (1986) for example, speaks of a LESBIAN CONTINUUM that links the experience of all women who are brought together by the disadvantages they face within patriarchy. Also there have been comparatively fewer 'buddy' movies featuring female couples, although *Fried Green Tomatoes (1991)*, *Thelma and Louise (1991)* and, of course, *Xena Warrior Princess* provide clear examples of female homoerotic tension. (**Mark McLelland**)

Homoness   Coined by Bersani (1995) to counter the tendency in SOCIAL CONSTRUCTION-IST theories of sexuality to 'de-gay gayness' by which he meant the denial of erotic specificity to same-sex desire. Homoness means rejecting the heterosexual obsession with difference for a form of relationality based on sameness: 'Homosexual desire is desire for the same from the perspective of a self already identified as different from itself' (Bersani 1995: 59). Bersani takes as his starting point Wittig's STRAIGHT MIND, the social contract based on naturalized heterosexual relations, which Bersani psychoanalytically transposes as the sublimation of the traumatic privileging of SEXUAL DIFFER-ENCE in heterosexuality: accordingly, the childhood origins of our hierarchy of difference lie in the boy's flight to the father following a retreat from women. Sameness for Bersani is not an ESSENTIALIZING definition of sexuality, but a means of exploring how desire gets attached to persons or identities through fantasy, implying a potential discontinuity between sexual fantasy and political identity: gay men's erotic investment in the PENIS might or might not suppose investment in structures of male domination. Ironically the forms of the homosexual's possible desire are inevitably imprisoned within the PSYCHOANALYTIC paradigm in which the only similarity between gays and lesbians is failed psychic identifications, and in which the erotics of sameness for gay men are reduced to phallic identification in sex. Bersani's earlier example was passive anal sex: the gay man's 'suicidal ecstasy of being a woman'.

(Bersani 1988: 212) in which a shattering of the ego reveals the inherent masochism in all sexuality. This cross-identification takes Woman as the ground for gay male fantasy and positions her as heterosexual, thus eliding lesbian sex (Hart 1998). Bersani wants homos to have the subversiveness of 'femininity' in sex without being female or EFFEMINATE (Garlinger 1999). (**Nicholas Rees-Roberts**)

Homophile   The term homophile was popularized in the 1950s and 1960s, particularly in the United States of America (Stewart 1995: 121). It was used generally as an alternative to homosexual, though homophiles used it to emphasize the emotional aspect of same-sex relationships – given that the root of 'homophile' is 'the Greek *philos* for love' – over the sexual focus of homosexual (Stewart 1995: 121). The term is also used to describe various organizations that emerged during this period, as well as the collective 'homophile movement' of which these groups were a part. Organized homophile groups emerged in the 1950s and were largely sex-segregated. Among the largest were the (female-dominated) Daughters of Bilitis, the (male-dominated) Mattachine Society, and the (male-dominated) ONE, though females were welcome at the latter two and often played pivotal roles within the groups (Blasius and Phelan 1997: 240). D.O.B. – with their female-dominated membership, combined with the rise of FEMINISM in the late 1960s – would also come to be remembered as one of the birthplaces of 1970s lesbian-feminism (ibid.). Each of these groups had influential publications – *The Ladder*, *The Mattachine Review*, and *ONE Magazine* respectively – which proved to be important sites for gay and lesbian writing and writers (Blasius and Phelan 1997: 239). In the 1960s national groups also emerged, such as NACHO (the North American Conference of Homophile Organizations), which would organize conferences around shared objectives (ibid.). These groups were an important precursor to the gay and lesbian groups of the 1970s. Though homophile groups, and the movement as a whole, were considerably more conservative than later gay and lesbian groups, this was largely out of necessity given the considerable bias gays and lesbians faced during this period. This necessary conservatism is highlighted by many of the political goals and strategies of the movement – such as inviting 'experts' (like doctors or clergy) to meetings, and demanding that group members dress conservatively to these meetings (women were asked to wear dresses and men business suits) – which were usually collectively focused around ASSIMILATION with the white, heterosexual mainstream (Blasius and Phelan 1997: 239–40; Phelan 1998: 193). This is perhaps unsurprising given that most of the larger homophile groups were comprised predominantly of middle-class whites (ibid.). (**Kelly McWilliam**)

Homophobia   See HETEROSEXISM.

Homosexual panic   A popular label for a strategy employed by HETEROSEXUAL criminal defendants (mostly male) trying to justify their violent action against lesbians or gay men. The theoretical framework for this strategy suggests that individuals who are LATENT homosexuals may, due to the fear of their own homosexuality, have a violent response to people they perceive to be homosexual. In practice, the 'homosexual panic' defence is most frequently used to argue that the defendant acted in self-defence upon perceiving themselves to be subjected to a homosexual advance rather than as an argument that the defendant is a latent homosexual (Dressler 1995). Although in the United States no appellate court accepts the homosexual panic theory as a complete defence in the case of a serious, violent crime against a victim who is or is perceived to be gay, the strategy has been successfully used to convict them of less serious offences than charged by the prosecution or to acquit defendants in less serious circumstances. In Britain, the defence of 'homosexual panic' has been used at least 15 times between 1896 and 1996 to reduce charges from murder to manslaughter. As lesbian and gay groups have organized to combat HOMOPHOBIA and have educated courts and law enforcement officials the homosexual panic theory has become more controversial. Yet despite the trend towards disallowing evidence concerning the homosexuality of the victim or the psychiatric or psychological evidence in support of homosexual panic theory, unless there is corroborating evidence about the circumstances of the attack, in many cases such evidence is still introduced. (**Natalia Gerodetti**)

Homosexuality   Homosexuality is a compound noun combining Greek *homos* ('same as') with Latin *sexualis*. It appears to have first been used with its current understanding in 1869 by Karl Westfal, a German SEXOLOGIST seeking a more liberal attitude to same-sex desire. However, in the psychiatric environs in which the term was taken up, and psycho-pathologizing institutions of societies in which it is continually perpetuated, homosexuality was regarded as an INVERSION, a non-realization of the 'epitome' of sexuality as perceived by normative, procreative, patriarchal, heterosexuality (Lewes 1989). Homosexuality has been pathologized and criminalized, with all forms of punishments and discriminations condoned by Church and state, in a misguided attempt at deterrence. The connotations of the term draw on centuries of traditional (mis-) understanding and repression, especially in cultures whose developments are founded on Judaism, Christianity and Islam (Weeks 1991b). Female homosexuals – LESBIANS – so frequently denied their identity, are sometimes assumed not to be included in this term. This is because of (a) a misunderstanding of the prefix homo- as being the Latin noun *Homo*, meaning 'man'; (b) misapprehension of female sexuality per se and (c) cultural invisibilization of Sapphic identities and lifestyles (Kitzinger 1989).

Homosexuality, as it is generally understood today, barely existed in this form prior to its naming (Foucault 1990), instead, a range of same-sex activities were classified in very different manners. Included in the term were notions of PEDERASTY and SODOMY, earlier forms of male–male sex that had formerly been regarded as activities which *any* man might perform (see CLASSICAL SEXUALITY); with the concept of 'homosexuality', it became assumed that these activities stem from a fixed SEXUAL ORIENTATION (see also MONOSEXUALITY). Its naming has been retrospectively applied to various sexual practices and lifestyles 'obscuring the difference between ancient pederasty and modern mutual androphilia' in a way which is called 'naive essentialism' (Donaldson and Dynes 1990). As a pseudoscientific STIGMATIZING marker, the term is now being transformed by many through self-adopted labels such as GAY and the reclaimed QUEER. In essence, *the* 'homosexual' is a psycho-pathological descriptor imposed by others. Contrariwise, 'lesbian' and 'gay' are terms of self-affirmation embracing notions of SEXUAL CITIZENSHIP, cultural and political sexual identities. The concept of 'homosexuality' thus remains inadequate for conceptualizing the many forms of same-sex desire that exist – as shown by the need for supplementary terms such as 'MSM' (MEN-WHO-HAVE-SEX-WITH-MEN), a neologism that refers to men who would not label themselves as gay, but whose SEXUAL PRACTICE is sometimes with other men (see also SITUATIONAL HOMOSEXUALITY). (**David Evans**)

Further reading

Dynes, Johansson and Percy (eds) (1990).

Homosocial   A term made famous in LESBIAN AND GAY STUDIES by Sedgwick in her pioneering work, *Between Men: English Literature and Male Homosocial Desire* (1985). Sedgwick draws on Adrienne Rich's (1986) notion of the LESBIAN CONTINUUM and hypothesizes its male equivalent: the homosocial continuum. This is an imaginary construct which charts an area containing all male–male relations, both social and sexual. However, Sedgwick's conceptualization of this continuum is uneasy. In the first place: the strict taboos on certain kinds of male–male relations evidenced in certain societies at particular historical conjunctures mean that at the moment of writing, unlike the lesbian continuum, it suffers from what she calls 'a prohibitive structural obstacle' (3) – on one side of this lie condoned male–male behaviours, while on the other lie condemned male–male behaviours. The continuum, on this view, is in fact 'radically discontinuous' (5). In the second place: at a different point in her argument Sedgwick apprehends this radical discontinuity differently, calling it 'an invisible, carefully blurred, always-already-crossed line' (89). The problem, loosely, is that certain behaviours are acceptable in certain situations, while in others the same behaviours are not – Sedgwick cites the tactility displayed by men during football games and 'what goes on' in fraternities at American universities as examples. The problem can be approached from a different angle by remarking the effects of the long-lasting tension between conceiving of homosexuality as a specific identity (one example of a MINORITIZING model of homosexuality) and conceiving of it as a specific practice (one example of a UNIVERSALIZING model) on Sedgwick's continuum: depending on the understanding of 'homosexuality' deployed, the homosocial continuum assumes a different shape. When understandings of homosexuality are deployed in which 'homosexuality' refers to a minoritized identity, the homosocial continuum tends to accommodate a radical discontinuity. When understandings of homosexuality are deployed in which a UNIVERSALIZING model is in operation, the continuum's rupture may fade into invisibility. (**Chris West**)

Honeymoon The honeymoon is the early period immediately after a wedding, and historically, was the time when the MARRIAGE would be consummated and the couple would have their first opportunity to spend time alone without a chaperone. Contrary to the construction of the honeymoon as a pleasurable time (i.e. *honey*moon), for women with little or no knowledge or understanding about their own bodies, or of sex, this could be a terrifying experience. In contemporary society, the term 'honeymoon' has come to refer specifically to the post-wedding holiday, celebrated in popular discourse as a time of heightened romance, and bawdily, as period of prolific sexual activity (Bulcroft 1999). However, the term 'honeymoon' also implies the inevitable waning (i.e. honey*moon*) of that heightened romance, to reveal problems, incompatibilities and the mundane realities of everyday life. Therefore, honeymoon is also often used outside of the context of marriage to refer to the optimistic early stages of a new job or a new relationship, for example. The 'honeymoon period' in this context, then, refers to the period of optimistic newness which is to be enjoyed, but which is ultimately unsustainable. (**Karen Throsby**)

HRT HRT or hormone replacement therapy regulates levels of oestrogen and is offered to women in mid-life, often upon MENOPAUSE or following gynaecological surgery. Like the contraceptive PILL it emerged during the 1960s. It is seen as a wonder drug capable of protecting against osteoporosis (demineralization of bone), heart disease, and breast and uterine cancer, whilst also slowing down ageing. Many doctors connect menopause with disease or potential danger in the form of osteoporosis and prescribe HRT as a preventative treatment, despite criticisms of its benefits to health. The preservation of sexual attractiveness and beauty as well as the general prevention of the 'decay of femininity' can also be a reason for women to take HRT.

HRT provokes significant debates as the biomedical discourse, with its reliance on the hormonal body, portrays the female ageing body predominantly in terms of deterioration and in need of intervention, while the classic feminist discourse attempts to underline more positive aspects of the menopause and refutes a medicalization of women's bodies (Lupton 1995). Other approaches stress that HRT presents women with possibilities for agency in a world which associates FEMININITY with youth and body maintenance, or conceptualize menopause as the remarkable adaptability of women's bodies to encounter changing bodily circumstances (Harding 1997). The so-called threat of ageing and deterioration to femininity and beauty conceives strategies such as HRT exclusively within a HETERONORMATIVE framework which eradicates differences between women, such as sexuality, race, class or disability. On the other hand, the hormonal body seems to have made an emergence for men in recent years with the discovery of the male menopause and VIAGRA. (**Natalia Gerodetti**)

Hybridity   Hybridity refers to the combining of separate elements to form a new entity. The term has been in force since the nineteenth century and has been used within a number of disciplines including biology, cultural studies, sociology and sexuality studies. Hybridity implies a number of key features. Firstly, the process of hybridization links the past with the future, by using established entities to create new ones. Secondly, hybridization challenges the apparent stability of each constituent element. These two features may be illustrated by examples drawn from sexuality, gender, SEX and biology. For instance, Eadie (1993) applies the concept of hybridity to BISEXUALITY. Eadie argues that recent bisexual politics represents a hybridization of lesbian, gay and heterosexual culture and identity. As Eadie states 'the hybrid acknowledges the part that the past has played in constituting new cultures and identities, and then displaces the dominant (and dominating) culture's attempt to enshrine itself in "an eternity produced by self-generation", by supplementing it and thereby rewriting the future' (1993: 159). Eadie points to the ways in which hybridization represents IDENTITY and politics as a process in constant motion, and thus opens up a range of possible futures that the 'original entities' do not express on their own. Hybridization might also be usefully applied to TRANSGENDER insofar as transgender identity signifies a desire to both acknowledge FEMININITY and MASCULINITY, but at the same time move beyond the fixity of these ideologies and practices. In yet another example, hybridization is particularly useful in theorizing INTERSEX identities. People with intersex conditions may have a range of physical characteristics traditionally associated with female and male bodies. Through an examination of the *cultural* basis upon which children with intersex conditions are assigned to the female or male sex, Hird (2000) argues intersex necessitates reflection upon the current definitional boundaries between 'sex' and 'gender'. In other words, 'the *authenticity* of "sex" resides not on, nor in the body, but rather results from a particular nexus of power, knowledge and truth' (2000: 353). Further, the history of intersex prompts us to consider that the current two-sex (female and male) template of SEXUAL DIMORPHISM on which contemporary gender and sexual identities are based is a recent shift from an early modern understanding of SEXUAL DIFFERENCE as a matter of degree rather than kind. That is, for much of our history, all human beings were thought to share a single sex, with some members (women) containing their genitals internally and others (men) displaying their genitals externally (Laqueur 1990). (**Myra Hird**)

Further reading

Eadie (1993).

Hydraulic model   A term coined by Foucault (1990) to describe the dominant Western understanding of sexuality. SOCIOBIOLOGY, SEXOLOGY, PSYCHOANALYSIS and humanistic psychotherapy all regard sexuality as comprised of a set of primal urges which are to some extent thwarted by existing social arrangements. Foucault thus points out that LIBERATIONIST narratives share with their opponents the notion that sexual desire is the deepest and most authentic part of human existence, and that it is inherently opposed to the existing social order. While conservative positions hold that these hydraulic ordering forces are needed to keep sexuality in check (see SOCIAL PURITY), so-called SEX RADICAL positions argue that sexuality is a positive force that must overturn these restrictions in order to find expression. Foucault suggests that both positions are mistaken: in fact, our desires are produced by, and largely suit the aims of, modern social structures (see REPRESSIVE HYPOTHESIS). For instance, the more we feel that we need help discovering our true sexual selves, the more we will pay the professions of sex therapists and psychoanalysts to accomplish this so-called 'discovery' (see CONFESSIONAL SOCIETY). In the face of this sexual obsessiveness, some feminists have argued that CELIBACY is a positive step to free ourselves from the expectation that we organize our lives around sexual pleasure, in favour of more creative and diverse life choices (Densmore 1968). Foucault himself argued that the alternative was to experience our bodies in a more directly physical manner – regarding our sexual pleasures as intense, but without meaning (Foucault 1997), citing gay casual sex as an example (see COT-TAGING and CRUISING). (**Jo Eadie**)

Hyperfemininity   See HYPERSEXUAL; FEMININITY.

Hypermasculinity   See HYPERSEXUAL; LEATHERSEX; MASCULINITY; PARODY.

Hypersexual   A stereotype of excessive, predatory sexuality applied to ABJECTED groups, such as gay men, lesbians, transsexuals, transvestites, blacks and Jews. It has also been used to refer to a self-presentation of one's self mainly or exclusively as an object of sexual attraction based on masculine or feminine stereotypes; also seen as hyperfeminine or hypermasculine. Its pejorative connotation stresses the ESSENTIALIST, reductionist nature of stereotypical gender presentation, stripping the person of other human qualities. For instance, describing this process in relation to the dominant rep-resentations of Filipinas in the United States, Arguelles (1991) notes:

> their sexuality is increased to the point that they become creatures of their contrived sexuality and nothing more. . . . The Filipino, whom we have already seen stripped of his sexuality, could not possibly constitute a suitable partner for the hypersexual Filipina; this is what American society would have us believe.

Similarly, Hoad says of the roots of contemporary white representations of black people:

> Post Abolition imperial cultural representations hypersexualize blackness, particularly along the lines of simultaneously feminizing and hypervirilizing

black men – the general lasciviousness of savages is a trope that cuts across genres and disciplines throughout the nineteenth century (1998:8–9). (**Jill Weiss**)

Hysteria   For over 2,000 years, hysteria has been in use as a medical term. Its frame of reference, however, has shifted many times with the result that contemporary perspectives on the illness emphasize the difficulty of defining its meaning with any clarity. It usually refers to a disorder in which the patient (most frequently a woman) experiences physical symptoms that seemingly have no physical or bodily origin. The symptoms are regarded as emanating from psychological difficulties and are often associated with heightened states of emotional disturbance. The name itself derives from the Greek *hystera*, meaning 'womb'. This indicates the extent to which hysteria has been associated with FEMININITY. Indeed, throughout the nineteenth and early twentieth centuries, it was assumed that hysteria was a female malady, and therapy often involved barbaric treatments of the female genitals. Symptoms associated with hysteria include feelings of suffocation; nervous coughing; fantasised paralysis of a limb; linguistic difficulties and excessive fainting spells. Such symptoms are regarded as irrational and difficult to control. The connection with femininity is often articulated along similar lines with the effect that patriarchy has frequently sought to dismiss hysteria as a female complaint that merits little attention. Hysteria largely ceased to be diagnosed in the latter half of the twentieth century. Hysterical symptoms, however, persist, and there is much discussion of diseases such as anorexia nervosa, bulimia and chronic fatigue syndrome in the context of hysteria today.

Hysteria played an important role in Freud's discovery of PSYCHOANALYSIS, and many of Freud's early patients were hysterics. Together with Breuer, Freud made the pioneering suggestion that hysteria was not a physical disease of the uterus, but rather, a psychic disease of the mind. Freud (1905a) traced the symptoms to sexual disturbances in the psychosexual development of the sufferer. The symptoms were seen as displacements of sexual FANTASY and DESIRE onto the patient's body. The psychoanalytic definition of the symptom as a signifier of repressed material has its origin here, and it is possible to argue that psychoanalysis has its roots in hysteria. More recently, feminist thinkers have sought to reclaim the discourse of hysteria. Showalter (1997) articulates a useful critique of the apparent alignment of femininity with the disease when she highlights the fact that hysteria suddenly became prevalent amongst male soldiers during the First World War. For Cixous (1986), hysteria offers a form of resistance to patriarchy for woman, enabling her to speak through its alternative and highly ambiguous discourse in order to express her experience of and response to the oppression she has suffered under patriarchy. (**Caroline Bainbridge**)

Further reading

Showalter (1997).

Identification   The most basic PSYCHOANALYTIC definition of identification, via Laplanche and Pontalis (1974), is that it is a 'psychological process whereby the subject assimilates an aspect, property or attribute of the other and is transformed, wholly or partially, after the model the other provides. It is by means of a series of identifications that the personality is constituted and specified' (206). Identifications are mobile, shifting, and often partial processes in which we work out who and what we want to be within the larger social order. To put it yet another way, identification is a process that 'inhabits, organizes, [and] instantiates identity' (Fuss 1995: 2). Identification is as much a process of refusal as it is of acceptance, for as one identifies with 'man', for example, part of the identification is as 'not-woman' ; as one identifies with 'homosexual', part of the identification is as 'not-heterosexual'. There is no consensus about how identification works, however, and contemporary psychoanalytic, film, literary, feminist, and QUEER theories draw on the proliferation of forms of identification to demonstrate that identification is never seamless or complete, but is always already failed and complicated, since we never fully attain a perfect 'fit' with those ideals with which we seek to identify. In doing so, these theories suggest that 'woman', 'man', 'heterosexual', 'homosexual', and other key concepts in sexuality studies, are highly problematic since those who feel they are these things, may also feel they have not fully become them (see Dean 2000; Fuss 1995; Sedgwick 1991). A self-identified heterosexual may still have same-sex fantasies, and a self-identified man may worry that he is not MASCULINE enough.

A recent addition to the study of identification is the formulation of disidenti-fication, a process by which a subject identifies with or as something other than his or her prescribed identity category. Muñoz argues that disidentification is a process that 'scrambles and reconstructs the encoded message of a cultural text in a fashion that both exposes the encoded message's universalizing and exclusionary machinations and recircuits its workings to account for, include, and empower minority identities and identifications' (1999: 31). Disidentification not only challenges identity and identification as normative, but also alters them in the process. For example, a transsexual might be considered disidentificatory because he/she challenges and redefines existing gender roles by creating a new identity. Tomboys or MALE LESBIANS might similarly be considered disidentificatory. In some cases disidentification is a voluntary operation, a conscious choice that one makes to separate from identifications that are politically problematic (e.g. the POLITICAL LESBIAN who disidentifies from her former heterosexuality). But in many cases, disidentification is like identification in that it is not necessarily conscious or voluntary. (**Rachael Groner**)

Further reading

Fuss (1995).

Identity   The term 'sexual identity' is sometimes used to avoid the ESSENTIALISM/SOCIAL CONSTRUCTIONISM debate, since 'identity' implies neither essentialism (in the way that SEXUAL ORIENTATION does) nor constructionism (as SEXUAL PREFERENCE does). The term 'identity' reflects the important element of SELF-DEFINITION, suggesting that one's sexual identity is a matter of self-naming. Some scholars and activists have used the term 'identity' to convey that 'gayness' cannot be reduced to matters of sexual desire or behaviour, but includes culture, ritual and history. While both attraction and action are significant in determining one's sexuality, it is argued that how one identifies oneself is perhaps of greater consequence. Thus, one can have same-sex desires or one can participate in homosexual practices, but this in itself does not imply a gay *identity* (see MSM; SITUATIONAL HOMOSEXUALITY). Rather, to identify as gay is to organize one's desires and behaviours in relation to a COMMUNITY; it is positively to claim an identity. In turn, that identity must be signalled publicly by PERFORMANCE of appropriate codes of speech and dress – which may sometimes be experienced as stifling if they are too rigid – and inflected according to one's particular tastes (e.g. electing to be BUTCH rather than FEMME if a lesbian, or a CLONE rather than STRAIGHT ACTING if a gay man). According to Epstein (1998), being gay can be interpreted as a quasi-ethnic identity. That is, being gay can be seen as analogous to being Black or Latino/a (see ETHNIC MODEL).

    Within the history of the gay and lesbian rights movement, however, 'identity' has come to be considered a problematic concept. So-called 'identity politics' have been criticized for constructing gay men and lesbians as members of an oppressed minority – an essentialized minority that is both more contained and easier to oppress, some have argued, in virtue of this very construction. This way of seeing 'lesbians' and 'gay men' has sometimes been referred to as MINORITIZING (Sedgwick, 1991). Within POST-MODERN and QUEER THEORY, gay and lesbian identities have been rendered FLUID, in recognition of the diversity that such identities take over time, and the contradictions that they contain. Rather than focusing on identities, some scholars have claimed that attention should be centred on the interrogation of HOMOPHOBIC and HETEROSEXIST systems and structures (Gamson 1998). (**Mary Bloodsworth-Lugo**)

Further reading

Blasius (2001).

Imitation   A process by which one adopts, whether consciously or not, the characteristics of some specific person or model. Within the study of sexuality, DRAG is the form of imitation that receives the most critical attention. Newton (1972), for example, argues that drag demonstrates the falsity of gender, for when a drag performer wears the accessories and behaviours of a different gender, he or she is utilizing the very structure of gender in order to create the drag performance. That is, in imitating gender, drag is exposing gender itself as just another kind of PERFORMANCE, neither more real nor ontologically true than drag. Butler builds upon Newton's theory of gender impersonation by arguing that gender has no ontological basis and is a PERFORMATIVE process rather than a stable entity (1990, 1993). The products of gender imitation, 'man' and 'woman', are social fantasies. If we accept this argument we must also recognize that heterosexuality and homosexuality are not ontologically real; rather, heterosexuality and homosexuality posture as the normative measure of the real in Western culture (see also COMPULSORY HETEROSEXUALITY; NORMATIVITY).

The history of imitation in relation to theories of sexuality and gender spans the twentieth century, most notably within psychoanalysis, feminist theory, and queer theory. Within PSYCHOANALYSIS, imitation is one way in which children learn to become gendered persons. In brief, for a young girl to become a woman, she must shift PRE-OEDIPAL IDENTIFICATION from wanting to *have* the mother to a post-oedipal identification with the mother/woman/object in wanting to *be* the mother. The young girl physically and psychically imitates the womanly characteristics she sees in her mother, and she rejects the manly characteristics she sees in her father. Within feminist theory, Riviere articulated how imitation shapes gender and sex as early as 1929. Riviere defines 'womanliness' as a characteristic that can be worn much like a mask; it can be put on and taken off at will. Further, she argues that there is no difference between 'genuine' womanliness and womanliness as masquerade: 'whether radical or superficial, they are the same thing' (Riviere 1986). The theories of Riviere and Butler led to the development of QUEER THEORY, within which imitation has become a valuable theoretical term. Butler argues that to imitate normative sex or gender in a slightly altered manner is to slowly change the normative over time. Critics argue that queer theorists attribute too much power to performativity, as though changing sex norms is as easy as changing one's pair of pants. This critical conversation in feminist and queer theory has raged since the 1990s. (**Rachael Groner**)

Impotence   Impotence is literally the inability to be potent, although in current usage it is a condition that prevents male sexual arousal. This prevention can be either physical or psychological, and can be either permanent or temporary. The definition of the term thus blurs the distinction between the inability to have an ERECTION, or more generally the inability to feel sexual desire. The social and psychological significance of impotence therefore depends on a PHALLOCENTRIC assumption: that there can be no heterosexual sex without erection, therefore ruling out, say, cunnilingus and VOYEURISM as not being 'adequate' forms of sexual interaction. Impotence pertains to the male only; the equivalent in women is referred to as 'frigidity' – a term which implies coldness of reception of sexual overtures, although the physical condition of vaginismus (a contracting of the VAGINA caused by either physical or psychological means which makes penetration impossible) is the true analogous condition in the female. In the nineteenth century, definitions of impotence included desire for homosexual encounters, as the man who desired sex with other men was not aroused by women, and was thus considered a type of psychological impotent. In this way, a man's ability to have sex with a woman was very much considered the basis for his masculinity – and the distress that men feel regarding impotence is at least partly because the inability to achieve erection is seen as fundamental to 'real' MASCULINITY (Kimmell 1990: 104–6). Impotence was also a matter of considerable medico-legal interest, not least because it could be used as a defence against a rape charge. (See also VIAGRA.) (**Ivan Crozier** and **Jo Eadie**)

Incest   Incest is sex between members of the same family. This can be parents and their children, brothers and sisters, or avuncular relations. Legislation varies widely between states, such that definitions of legally prohibited incest can include relations by marriage (e.g. between step-parents and stepchildren or between siblings-in-law), and may exclude some biological relations, most commonly cousins. Anthropologist Edward Westermarck (1921) suggested that it was the early period of growing up together that prevented brothers and sisters forming erotic relationships in later life. Such a speculation carries weight in current ethnology, yet the counter-argument can also be made: that the sharing of childhood space creates opportunities for sexual encounters between siblings.

Although incest has been mythologized, most famously in the story of Oedipus Rex, who kills his father and unknowingly marries his mother, incest is a taboo in many cultures. The notion that incest is against nature is enforced in SOCIOBIOLOGIST thinking by appeals to the genetic risks of resultant pregnancy. However, as Weeks points out, prohibitions on incest are more about social factors (such as the importance of creating economic alliances between families) than about any natural aversion – hence the very different relationships tabooed in different societies (1985: 97–116), and the instances of incest as the preferred means of retaining power within a clan or family (in ancient Egyptian dynasties for instance). Indeed, the stress on pregnancy in debates about incest only demonstrates how fully heterosexualized the notion of incest has become. Describing her lesbian relationship with her sister, Lydia (1995) argues that sex between siblings may constitute a little discussed pool of consensual relationship, while anecdotally many gay men describe sex with brothers as an important starting point in defining their own identities, and differentiate such encounters from cases of SEXUAL ABUSE. (**Ivan Crozier** and **Jo Eadie**)

Incest taboo   Incest is the term used to refer to sexual relations that take place within certain structures of close kinship. The structures of kinship involved vary from one society to another, although most societies maintain prohibition against incest. Typically, incest is defined as taking place across heterosexual kinship structures such as parent/child; brother/sister; or between cousins. The taboo on incest underpins social and legal perspectives on systems such as marriage and entailment. There is a widespread view that the incest taboo impedes genetic inbreeding. However, there is little scientific evidence to support this. The incest taboo also lies behind Freud's account of the necessary REPRESSION of the OEDIPUS COMPLEX, and has been used by anthropologists as the basis for understanding the complexity of kinship relations in a diverse range of societies (Lévi-Strauss 1969). The incest taboo is implicitly HETERO-SEXIST in its conceptualization, as many theorists suggest. For example, Butler (1990) argues that the incest taboo is a crucial part of the HETEROSEXUAL MATRIX since it focuses our subjectivity on a question of opposite-sex desire. (**Caroline Bainbridge**)

Infantilism   A term first coined by SEXOLOGIST Wilhelm Stekel in 1922 (see Stekel 1952), to describe the practice of taking on the role of a baby for sexual pleasure. Most often practised by men, activities typically include having a nappy/diaper changed, being breast-fed or bottle-fed, and being put to bed in a cot; for some participants there may be an SM element involving being spanked or punished; and SCENES may include masturbation: but infantilism exists on the borderline between sexual and non-sexual roleplay, and need not include explicitly erotic activities. Henkin (1989) notes that as with other FETISHES, we can distinguish between those for whom infantilism is a sexual pleasure to be enjoyed occasionally as the mood suits; and those for whom it is a major component of identity, and who might seek to spend as much of their life in role as possible. Stekel (1952) saw this as a continuation of the childhood desire for attention and approval – or, as McClintock (1993) suggests, a way of taking control over childhood trauma and exploring the pleasures of regressing away from the highly regulated bodily control of (male) adulthood. As with almost every PARAPHILIA in the West, the shift away from the sexological model of PERVERSION-as-pathology, and the criminal model of perversion-as-deviance, has enabled infantilism to take its place as one specialized pleasure amongst many. Self-identified 'adult babies' have linked together for support, and a commercial industry has sprung up around manufacturing 'adult-sized' items. (**Jo Eadie**)

Infertility   See ARTIFICIAL INSEMINATION; IUD; SPERM DONOR.

Infidelity   See DIVORCE; MARRIAGE; MISTRESS; MONOGAMY; NON-MONOGAMY.

Innocence   See EROTOPHOBIA; PAEDOPHILIA.

Intercourse   See COITAL IMPERATIVE; CONTRACEPTION; HETEROSEXUALITY; FOREPLAY; MEDIEVAL SEXUALITY; PERVERSION; RAPE; SEX WARS; SEXUAL PRACTICE; VIRGINITY.

Intergenerational sex   A descriptive term for sex between people with different ages. Given the wide international variance in AGES OF CONSENT, both heterosexual and homosexual, it is impossible to fix the ages to which this refers, but it includes sex between adults and ADOLESCENTS; adults and pre-pubescent children; and between young people with a substantial age difference. It is also, but less frequently, used to refer to relations between adults where there is a substantial age difference. The term's critics have argued that it is simply an attempt to lend a respectable veneer to preda-tory adult sexual attention against minors, while its proponents hold that it is a posi-tive validation of the otherwise heavily regulated sexuality of young people. Although the term overlaps with the more charged PAEDOPHILIA, while paedophilia focuses on adult sexuality, and represents young people as powerless victims of adult attention, the concept of intergenerational sex recognizes that young people may seek and initi-ate sexual contact with people older than themselves, and that for some young people this may constitute a form of SEXUAL PREFERENCE. The deliberate – and controversial – neutrality of the term is a tactic to assert that encounters between people of different ages need each to be assessed on their own merits, rather than all being assumed to be coercive (see Altman 1982: 199–202). Nevertheless, given the high rates of SEXUAL ABUSE of children, most cultures choose to define points at which sex between adults and children must be regarded as always emotionally damaging. Some countries, such as the Netherlands, have sought to address this by defining age limits within which young people may legally have sex with each other, but where it would be illegal for older people to have sex with them. (**Jo Eadie**)

Further reading

Edwards (1994: Chapter 3).

Internalized oppression   The process and outcome of making a damaging accep-tance of the prejudices, STIGMAS and discriminations levelled by others (the oppressors) at people like oneself. Internalization can lead to SHAME, a fear of being so identified or labelled (see STRAIGHT ACTING), and the perpetuation of the same oppressions on to others like oneself – e.g. by opposing progressive legislation out of a fear that others should not be encouraged to adopt one's own sexuality. Oppression on the grounds of sexuality can include oppressions based on gender-specific sexual behaviours, SEXUAL ORIENTATION, particular SEXUAL PRACTICES, TRANSGENDER and INTERSEX status and health status. Other demographics that can compound sexual oppressions include age, eth-nicity, socio-economic, religio-cultural and educational indices; other forms of stigma such as physical or mental health problems, can also exacerbate the oppres-sions (Mason *et al.* 2001). Thus, for example, to be poor, black, female and lesbian, may bring not just the individual oppressions of each of these characteristics, but the consequences of each separately and accumulatively. Accordingly, internalized oppression can be overwhelmingly synthesized by the recipient (McFarlane 1998).

External acts of oppression may take several overt and/or covert forms, including violence and abuse, invisibility, and lack of civil rights. These may be directed from other individuals, and so be interpersonal, or from cultural and societal institutions (Herek 1998). Internalized oppression is therefore an agreement with these external forces of negativity. Consequences of this might include poor psychological perceptions of self, such as low self-esteem, depression and even suicidal ideation. Perpetuation of these negativities is not essential. Many people who suffer from internalized oppressions try to improve the situation by challenging the beliefs they have inherited – for instance, in consciousness-raising groups; witness the various egalitarian movements for racial, gender and sexual emancipation. (**David Evans**)

Interracial sex Interracial sex refers to sexual interaction between members of two different races. Anxieties about racial mixing run deep in Western civilization, going back to Jewish prohibitions on marriage with gentiles and later Christian prohibitions on marriage with Jews. In the colonial period, sexual interaction between white colonizers and their colonial subjects was officially discouraged because 'mixed-race' children were difficult to classify in the colonial hierarchy that placed the 'white' races at the top, although this was less of a concern within the Spanish and Portuguese empires where intermediate racial categories such as 'creoles' and 'mulattoes' were acknowledged (Young 1995). In the United States where eugenicist arguments for 'white superiority' were strong, miscegenation or 'race mixing' was illegal in some southern states, marriages between 'whites' and 'blacks' being forbidden.

The tragic legacy of colonialism lives on in various stereotypes about the different races and their sexual capacities, such as the myths of the enormous black penis, the sexual voraciousness of black women and the compliance of 'oriental' women. These unfortunate stereotypes continue to be fed by a pornography industry that fetishizes race resulting in interracial sex being overdetermined for many people. A DOUBLE STANDARD also frequently applies in the manner in which interracial sex is evaluated, it being considered more deviant for white women to seek out non-white (especially black) partners (note the controversy over Spike Lee's movie *Jungle Fever* (1991)). This derives from colonial constructions of white women as chaste and virtuous as opposed to the sensually unrestrained women of other races. White men, however, have had more freedom to transgress racial boundaries – their sexual 'conquest' of other races seen to mirror their political domination.

Among some gay men, too, interracial sex is much fetishized and there are a number of faintly derogatory terms describing gay males who organize their sexuality around racial types. These include dinge queens (white men who prefer black partners), snow queens (black men who like white males), rice queens (white men who like East Asians), potato queens (East Asians who seek out white partners) (Hagland 1998). Most of this terminology assumes the centrality of the white subject whose privileged position in the colonial and sexual hierarchy enables them to objectify (and consume) racial otherness (Mercer 1993). However in recent years terms such as 'sticky rice' for East Asians who prefer other East Asians, suggests that the gay scene is becoming less focused on the centrality of white desire. (**Mark McLelland**)

Further reading

Hodes (1997); Young (1995).

Intersex   According to the Intersex Society of North America (ISNA), the term intersex refers to 'a set of medical conditions that features [a] congenital anomaly of the reproductive and sexual system' (ISNA 2003b). The most important feature of intersex conditions is that they do not conform to socially sanctioned definitions of 'sex' and 'gender'. That is, Western society, through the medical profession, has established norms about 'appropriate' sex chromosomes, external genitalia and internal reproductive systems for females and males. For instance, the medical profession has standardized the 'medically acceptable' length of a clitoris and penis at birth, and babies' genitals are measured against these standards (Hird 2000; Hird and Germon 2001). It is important to note that intersex conditions are common in nature, and in the vast majority of cases, are not life threatening. Chase (1998) estimates that one in every 100 births shows some morphological 'anomaly', observable enough in one in every 2,000 births to initiate questions about a child's sex. Intersex conditions are therefore about as prevalent as Down's Syndrome or albinism. The sexologist John Money founded surgical sex 'reassignment' of infants with intersex conditions in the United States in the 1960s, and his protocols remain standard practice today. In contemporary Western societies, infants born with intersex conditions are routinely subjected to multiple surgeries in an attempt to make their bodies conform to the norms of femaleness and maleness defined by society (Hird 2000; Hird and Germon 2001). However, because Western society is not used to questioning SEXUAL DIMORPHISM, the similarities between surgery on intersex infants and children, and FEMALE GENITAL MUTILATION, have only recently been recognised.

People with intersex conditions radically confront assumptions about the 'immutability' of sex. A growing political intersex community identifies many problems with the current 'management' of children with intersex conditions including: the variability of sexual IDENTIFICATION, the a priori assumption of 'FEMININE' and 'MASCULINE' behaviour, the PHALLOCENTRIC bias in sex re-assignment, and the problem people with intersex conditions often experience in 'belonging' to sexually identified communities (Hird 2000; Hird and Germon 2001). ISNA presently lobbies to abolish all unnecessary surgery and ensure that what surgery is still performed is with the full understanding and consent of the person with the intersex condition. (**Myra Hird**)

Further reading

Preves (2003).

Intimacy   As Jamieson remarks at the opening of her book, *Intimacy* (1998: 1), this 'has become a fashionable word both in the social sciences and in popular self-help books advising on the art of good relationships'. The self-help and therapy industries have had a profound effect on how we think about love, sex and relationships, and the discourse of intimacy is a prime manifestation of this. Intimacy does not (just) mean physical, sexual intimacy – it means interpersonal intimacy, literally the sharing of secrets about the self. In line with the broader therapeutic agenda, this 'new' intimacy is as much about talking and listening, as it is about physical, bodily closeness – although this too is often stressed as a necessary component of intimate relations. Moreover, as Jamieson points out, intimacy can embrace not only the couple form but also other significant relationships, with family and with friends. It therefore invokes different kinds of love, but levels them out to show their equivalence in terms of their role in self-making. In one of the central texts on this way of thinking, Giddens's *The Transformation of Intimacy* (1992a), intimacy becomes a shorthand for the 'democratization' of relationships and of the private sphere. Here interpersonal relations are built afresh using democratic principles – trust, sharing, equality, rights and respect – bundled together by Plummer (1995) under the banner 'intimate citizenship'. Giddens himself develops a new vocabulary to describe these transformations: PURE RELATIONSHIP, confluent love and PLASTIC SEXUALITY. In combination, these concepts reflect a rewriting of the previous SEXUAL CONTRACT, giving it a therapeutic spin. Outside of Giddens's self-help worldview, however, we might question the extent to which intimacy has in fact been transformed; Jamieson (1999) explores this in the context of opposite-sex couples, noting that the pure relationship might be more of an ideal-type than an empirical reality. (**David Bell**)

Intrauterine device (IUD)   A plastic device inserted into the uterus to prevent PREGNANCY. This modern contraceptive device is based on the ancient practice of inserting stones into a camel's uterus to prevent conception. The IUD interferes with fertilization by altering the normal physiology in the uterus and egg transport tubes (Stewart 1998: 512). In the 1960s, IUDs were marketed without sufficient research on safety. In the case of the Dalkon Shield, the deaths of 17 otherwise healthy women and a high incidence of infection and infertility prompted removal from the US market, although the it continued to be distributed globally (Boston Women's Health Book Collective, 1998: 325–6). Early problems with the IUD continue to cloud its reputation and today, only about 100 million women of child-bearing age use it, and of these, 55 million live in China. In theory, the IUD is an ideal contraceptive, with less than a two per cent pregnancy rate (Stewart 1998: 512). Use is completely separated from sexual activity, so no decision, except for the one at the time of insertion is necessary. Some IUDs are infused with progesterone, which does not greatly enhance effectiveness, but can reduce painful menstruation or heavy menstrual bleeding. In practice, the IUD can cause serious potential health problems, most notably uterine perforation and pelvic inflammatory disease (PID) which often result in infertility. With appropriate screening and rigorous counselling, the incidence of serious complications has been greatly reduced. However, feminists and some family planning specialists continue to raise concerns about the use of the IUD in countries where screening, counselling, and routine health care are lacking. (**Rebecca Chalker**)

Inversion   Inversion, or more precisely sexual inversion, was a nineteenth-century term used by SEXOLOGISTS to denote the phenomenon of homosexual desire. *Sexual Inversion* by Havelock Ellis (1859–1939) and John Addington Symonds (1840–93) appeared in English in 1897. Ellis was intent on making a case *for* homosexuality and, as a committed sexual reformer with a liberal approach, one of his arguments was that homosexual love had always and everywhere existed (Weeks 1990). Like other sexologists, Ellis' perspective accepted that some homosexual predilections were acquired whilst also stressing an element of congenitality. In his final version of *Sexual Inversion* Ellis made a distinction between 'homosexual love', which he defined as a sexual attraction and physical relation between people of the same sex, and 'sexual inversion', which he defined as a congenital but relatively rare condition (Ellis 1897). This double definition was not uncommon as it allowed for both the environment and heredity to be a 'cause' of homosexuality. It was a widespread view at the time that people could be 'corrupted' into sexual aberrations and Ellis later wrote that it was the task of social hygiene to prevent the acquisition of 'homosexual perversity'. Nevertheless, the theory of congenital sexual inversion was used to argue against legal sanctions on the basis of the naturalness and therefore innocence of homosexual behaviour (Weeks 1990). Inversion could best be seen as a technical 'abnormality', a congenital turning away from the opposite sex. Ellis strove to emphasize that 'inverts' were essentially 'ordinary' people in all but their sexual behaviour. Like other early sexological research *Sexual Inversion* said little about LESBIANS. See also THIRD SEX. (**Natalia Gerodetti**)

IUD   See INTRAUTERINE DEVICE

IVF   *In vitro* fertilization (IVF) – literally, fertilization in glass – is named after the procedure of fertilizing eggs outside of the body. The term also represents a wider process, which, prior to the fertilization procedure, involves hormone injections to stimulate a woman's ovaries; the collection of eggs by passing a needle through the vagina into the ovaries; and the male production of sperm by MASTURBATION. After the eggs have fertilized, a limited number of embryos are transferred to the woman's uterus (or to that of another woman, in the case of either embryo donation or surrogacy). Since the world's first IVF baby, Louise Brown, was born in 1978, over 50,000 IVF babies have been born in the United Kingdom, although the live birth rate per cycle of IVF is still less than 20 per cent.

IVF is a highly controversial subject with a high media profile. Non-feminist debates have focused on the status of the embryo, with discussions centring on the point at which an embryo constitutes 'life'. Feminists have brought attention to the ways in which IVF impacts upon women: IVF has been variously interpreted within feminism as a potential escape route out of biological reproduction (Firestone 1971); as violence against women by male dominated medical science (Klein 1989); or as an extension of reproductive choice. Recent popular debates have focused on the ethics of sex selection, designer babies, pregnancies in post-menopausal women, and the development of cloning technologies.

In spite of its legislative construction as a heterosexual couple's technology, IVF constitutes reproduction without sex. It consequently poses a challenge to normative heterosexual standards of reproduction and the ideal of the nuclear FAMILY by facilitating the creation of non-traditional family structures and fragmenting unitary understandings of categories of parenthood through the use of donors and surrogates (Hartouni 1997). (**Karen Throsby**)

Further reading

Franklin (1997).

J

Jack off parties   See CIRCLE JERK.

Jouissance   From the French *jouir* (to have an ORGASM), *jouissance* is the French term for sexual pleasure of the orgasmic type. As a theoretical concept, it was developed by Lacan in the context of his analysis of female sexuality. In his system the term indicates a pleasure incommensurable with more ordinary pleasures like tasting good food, enjoying a good book, or having good sex; an intense erotic pleasure that comes from the person's inner state rather than from an object or partner. *Jouissance* can come from the imagination of a pleasure and one's desire thereof, as well as from its fruition. It can also be described as the communion with one's body and one's desire, a sense of total fulfilment and elation, an ecstasy that comes from one's imagined mystical union with the object of one's desire, enhancing one's sense of embodiedness and sensuality. For his doctoral dissertation, Lacan (1933) worked on the Papin sisters, a case in which two female servants in a bourgeois household had killed the lady of the house and her daughter. His theory was that the sisters had a mystical union, an incestuous jouissance the repression of which led them to the crime. This might have inspired his later work. In his view, women are more inclined towards *jouissance* because the sites of their erotic pleasures are closer to the sites of their inner life. A representation of female *jouissance* is Bernini's statue of St Teresa of Avila, which might have inspired Lacan and has been used by Italian female director Lina Wertmuller in her film *Sotto Sotto* (1984), about a Platonic love relationship between two women. (**Serena Anderlini-D'Onofrio**)

Further reading

Evans (1998).

Kinsey scale   In the late 1940s Kinsey, Pomeroy and Martin conducted extensive research on the sexual behaviour of American adults. Their finding that 'only 50 per cent of the population is exclusively heterosexual throughout its adult life, and ... only 4 per cent of the population is exclusively homosexual throughout its life' (Kinsey Pomeroy and Martin 1948: 656), resulted in the development of the Kinsey scale. The scale sought to plot the range of human sexual experiences from 0 to 6, with 0 being exclusively heterosexual and 6 being exclusively homosexual. A Kinsey 3 would be someone who is equally heterosexual and homosexual, but could also be an indication of equal levels of *lack of* sexual behaviour or interest. Storms therefore adapts the scale to differentiate between ASEXUALITY and bisexuality (Storms 1980).

While the Kinsey scale sought to measure both actual sexual encounters and psychological responses, it has been extended by bisexual therapists and theorists in order to account for a fuller range of human sexual engagements. Most notable of these developments is the KLEIN SEXUAL ORIENTATION GRID that seeks to measure FANTASIES, social and emotional attachments and SELF-DEFINITION as well as SEXUAL PRACTICE, in the past, in the present and as an ideal (Klein, Sepekoff and Wolf 1985). Many bisexual theorists have been enthusiastic about the fact that social scientific research measuring sexual behaviour usually finds that the majority of people have sexual feelings for both men and women over their lifetime. Indeed it is common for bisexual psychological and social theorists to include versions of Kinsey's or Klein's scale in their own work (e.g. George 1993). Despite this evidence, however, these statistics have not resulted in acceptance of bisexuality as a legitimate IDENTITY as well as behaviour. (**Clare Hemmings**)

Further reading

Udis-Kessler (1992).

Kissing   Kissing is usually considered to be the meeting of the lips for erotic pleasure. Other parts of the body can be kissed, although kissing specific EROGENOUS ZONES carries specialized terminology (cunnilingus for kissing or licking the vagina/labia/clitoris; fellatio for kissing or sucking the penis; RIMMING for kissing the anus). When sexualized, kissing is often seen as the first part of FOREPLAY, the first transgression of interpersonal space, more than a touch. Yet the meaning of kisses between individuals is subject to an intense interpersonal negotiation. Holloway and Jefferson (1998) have shown how in heterosexual dating situations, men may regard kisses as a sign of CONSENT to sex, whereas women may regard them as more provisional expressions of interest and affection – a disagreement of interpretation which often lies at the root of DATE RAPE. This highly gendered understanding of kissing plays a prominent role in Western culture, as demonstrated by the artistic tradition in which the kiss is imaged as an act by which men overpower women, and women swoon ecstatically – notably, August Rodin's sculpture *The Kiss* (1886) and the much-imitated paintings of Gustav Klimt (1908) (Harper 1994). Kissing also has a significant social role. It is used as a greeting or farewell in continental Europe more than in other Western cultures; it is also deemed a socially acceptable form of the expression of parental or familial relations, and so can be removed from its sexual context, unlike other sexual acts, such as intercourse. Same-sex kisses – particularly kisses between men – have seen a noted shift in status in the period of MODERN SEXUALITY, moving rapidly in the eighteenth century from a mark of affection to an unwarranted intrusion or sign of EFFEMINACY, as a more self-contained and private model of MASCULINITY came to prominence (Davenport-Hines 1990: 71–2). As Morris (1997) notes, mainstream cinema will go to extraordinary lengths to avoid representing same-sex kisses even in films otherwise about homosexuality, since the kiss between men is seen within the cinema industry as commercial death, indicating an intensity of reaction from a straight audience which parallels the heterosexual violence that often greets same-sex public kissing (see QUEERBASHING). (**Ivan Crozier** and **Jo Eadie**)

Klein sexual orientation grid   The Klein Sexual Orientation Grid is a development of the KINSEY SCALE for measuring human sexuality from 0 to 6, with 0 representing exclusive HETEROSEXUALITY and 6 representing exclusive HOMOSEXUALITY. The scale suggests that most people find themselves somewhere in between 0 and 6, and that therefore most people behave bisexually. The Kinsey scale has been critiqued from a number of perspectives. Firstly, it is understood as rather limited in terms of the behaviours that it measures, not leaving any room for affectional ties, or changes over time and context. Secondly, it conceives of bisexuality purely in terms of a percentage combination of heterosexual and homosexual drives and desires rather than as an IDENTITY in its own right.

The Klein sexual orientation grid was developed by Fritz Klein (Klein, Sepekoff and Wolf 1985) in order to flesh out Kinsey's original scale to attend to the nuances it was not designed to take account of. The grid is filled out using Kinsey's numbered continuum, but also takes account of differences that might exist between past and present desires, as well as actual and ideal desires. So a bisexual woman might have had more sexual encounters with men in the past (Kinsey 2), be sexually involved with a man and a woman in the present (Kinsey 3), but wish that she only had sexual encounters with women (Kinsey 6). Thus she might more accurately be said to be a Kinsey 4 on the Klein grid. The grid is still limited by the original categories of the Kinsey scale, which assumes that desire is in fact either heterosexual or homosexual in the first place. A further problem arises when one considers that FANTASY and OBJECT-CHOICE may in fact not overlap at all, or may contradict one another in interesting ways. Consider the following example: a bisexual woman may have sex with women, but only desire women with pronounced masculine traits, and always fantasize herself to be a boy when having sex. The Kinsey scale, however carefully adapted, cannot take account of this kind of complex gendered and sexual specificity. (**Clare Hemmings**)

Further reading

Udis-Kessler (1992).

L

Latency   The period of time between the dissolution of the OEDIPUS COMPLEX and the onset of puberty is described as latency in psychoanalytic theories of sexuality. During the latency period, there is supposedly a marked decrease in the sexual activity of children and relationships with others are not overtly sexualized. It is also during this phase that societal notions of SHAME begin to take root in the attitudes and behaviour of young people. The period of latency ends once the child enters puberty. At this point there is a return to the sexual organization of the infantile period and the emergent adult sexuality is said to be shaped by the unconscious experiences of that period. It is only at puberty that the libidinal urges cease to be AUTOEROTIC (directed towards the self and masturbatory) and begin to be directed towards other objects and people. Freudian psychoanalysis suggests that the aim of these instincts also shifts at this point becoming predominantly genital, with the result that adult sexuality is channelled into reproductive heterosexuality (Freud 1924). Of course, while this DEVELOPMENTAL NARRATIVE accounts for alternative forms of adult sexuality by seeing them as arrested stages of development, it does not validate them and this is a key failing of the psychoanalytic account. (**Caroline Bainbridge**)

Leathersex   A term to describe a sexual subculture organized around leather clothing – caps, jackets, trousers or chaps, boots, wristcuffs, belts – and the SEXUAL PRACTICES
that they can be used for. For some leather is part of a sadomasochistic identity, and
accompanies a repertoire of aggressive sex and roleplay; for others it is an intensely
CATHECTED erotic material, whose pleasures are physical and aesthetic without an element of roleplay or erotic violence. Within gay male culture the look was popularized
from the 1960s onwards by the drawings of Tom of Finland (the pseudonym of
Touko Laaksonen), depicting muscular uniformed men having sex, often in parks
and woodlands, and this hypermasculinity served as an alternative to dominant connections between gayness and EFFEMINACY (see also CLONE). As animal skin, leather has
connotations of animality and instinct; historically, it has resonances of the cowboy
and the biker, of the wild and the outdoors (Lieshout 1997), which repeat and inten-
sify those associations; in practical terms its texture allows it to survive being grabbed
or bitten, while it has the flexibility to bind or beat another. Although heavily associated with gay and lesbian culture, its appeal cuts across genders and sexualities, even
to the extent that a shared leather erotics can form the basis for sex between men who
identify primarily as gay and women who identify primarily as lesbian (Highleyman
1996). Its critics argue that leather culture may contain the aggression, bonding,
competitiveness, and hierarchy often taken to embody HETEROPATRIARCHAL masculinity
(Bersani 1995: 77–112) – and note its inevitable connections to the animal cruelty of
the meat industry. Polchin (1997) suggests that since leather has been so thoroughly
COMMODIFIED in the catalogues and window displays of gay culture, it no longer
appears to express an authentic masculinity, but rather to be one of a number of fluid
and transitory style choices. Similarly Meyer (1993) argues that leather users are
highly self-conscious in their manipulation of their props and persona. While both
may be right, the contributors to the important anthology *Leatherfolk* (Thompson
1991) frequently describe their desires in terms of a return to nature, an instinctual
animal passion, a discovery of their true self or a tribal/pagan reawakening. In this
split we see the difference between a subculture which prizes sex in the 'raw', and
postmodern theory which is suspicious of any language of authenticity or instinct.
(Jo Eadie)

Further reading

Thompson (1991).

Lesbian   Term derived from Lesbos, the Greek island birthplace of the poet Sappho
(*c*.625 BC), who composed the first known HOMOEROTIC poetry to women; 'lesbian' has
been shown to be in use in writings from as many as four centuries ago, notably in
English and French. The term has been used not only as a self-referential label by
women in the last half century, but also as a pathologizing term by the medical profession. It came into politicized use in the early 1970s in the United States in an iden-

tity movement premised on radically non-patriarchal, woman-centred existence. In contemporary lesbian studies, the term has been used to refer to a range of historically and geographically distributed practices, loosely labelled as affective alliances between women; some inclusions have been criticized for overlooking cultural or historical specificity in the effort to reclaim lesbian history (Faderman 1981). Most historical records remain opaque as to which relations between women were sexual; even more, it remains in question to what degree sexuality is a (pre-eminent) constituent in defining lesbianism.

Lesbian FEMINISM, perhaps the most politically marked movement associated with the term, emerged in the 1970s as a radical response to second-wave feminism's significant hostility to lesbians (Friedan 1963). Lesbian feminists saw patriarchy as founded upon heterosexuality, namely women's primary commitment towards affective ties with men (see HETEROPATRIARCHY). They aimed to redirect women's energies towards relationships with other women, thereby turning the patriarchal foundation on its head. While this radical movement was responsible for many lasting political changes, among them the rape crisis lines and women's shelters which exist today, it has also been criticized for its dismissal of BUTCH/FEMME relationships and working-class bar cultures, traditions that made crucial contributions to political resistance and lesbian community in the 1950s (Nestle 1987). By the late 1970s, many began to shift their energies towards what would later be called 'cultural feminism': a cultivation of women's spaces, including music labels, women's publishers, coffee houses and bars; these were the materialization of women's desires to provide alternatives to patriarchal institutions, but to some critics, they were passively disengaged from the national political sphere. Though sharply contested and itself evolving, lesbian feminist work has continued until today.

While some lesbian feminists often only superficially addressed the struggle to end all systems of oppression, it was women of colour, many of whom were active but uncomfortable participants in the lesbian feminist movement, who most eloquently and powerfully articulated their sense that racial oppressions within the movement were largely being ignored, in some cases perpetuated (Moraga and Anzaldua 1983). The Combahee River Collective (1983) pointed to the dangers of monolithic gender separatism: to privilege sexism over all other oppressions, such as racism, is to ignore the complex interweaving of oppressions, and effectively negates the authors' solidarity with black men in the struggle against racism. Later critiques of lesbian feminism came from BISEXUAL women (George 1993) and TRANSGENDER people (Stone 1991) whose lived experiences challenged the universalist or essentialist delineation of 'womanhood' and 'manhood'; poststructuralist scholarship further problematized the social construction of 'women' and 'men' as categories and emphasized the difficulty of separating these genders on epistemological grounds.

Today, lesbian activism and lesbian identity remain vital in the wake of some reorganizing in relation to QUEER politics and identities (Stein 1992), amid larger tensions about whether lesbians are best served by self-generated political strategies or by coalition organizing (Phelan 1989) (see SEPARATISM). Internationally, lesbian activism, scholarship, and support organizations are widespread and growing in visibility and interconnection: a few examples are the Asian Lesbian Network based in Bangkok; the Sangini Support Project in India; the Serbian group Labrys; and El Closet del Sor Juana in Mexico. (**Melinda Chen**)

Further reading

Faderman (1981 and 1991).

Lesbian and gay studies   An interdisciplinary scholarly field that employs sexuality as a useful category for analysis. Its scope, however, is not limited to the study of gays and lesbians nor to studies engaged in by gays and lesbians. Rather, it works to high-light the ways that an understanding of the intersections of sex, gender, and sexuality is central and enriching to all academic disciplines. As institutionalized today, most lesbian and gay studies programmes and departments include bisexual and TRANSGEN-DER studies under its broad umbrella of work. D'Emilio (1992) locates the birth of les-bian and gay studies in the United States in the wake of women's and racial/ethnic studies programmes that were institutionalized at universities in the late 1960s and early 1970s. Central to the emergence of lesbian and gay studies in the academy was an LGBT political movement that built COMMUNITY infrastructure first, and then turned its attention to gaining power in established institutions, including the academy. While researchers within institutions worked to create courses and conferences centring on lesbian and gay issues, by and large universities were not 'an especially hospitable place for either gay research or gay people' (D'Emilio 1992: 166). Consequently, grassroots scholars and institutions, including community-based archives, provided much-needed resources and research for the growth of lesbian and gay studies, and dissem-ination of this knowledge. Because of the strong connection to its founding political movement, lesbian and gay studies intends to 'express and advance the interests of les-bians, bisexuals, and gay men, and to contribute culturally and intellectually to the contemporary lesbian/gay movement' (Abelove, Barale and Halperin 1993: xvi) Scholars of QUEER THEORY have charged that lesbian and gay studies relies too much on ESSENTIALISM and promoting an ETHNIC MODEL of sexuality, rather than contesting politi-cal and historical identity categories. Scholars of lesbian and gay studies have coun-tered that queer theorists' obsession with POSTMODERN theory ignores the real-life experiences of gay, lesbian, bisexual and transgender people, particularly at a point where 'the voices of previously marginalized groups are beginning to have some impact on the academy' (Beemyn and Eliason 1996: 165). This disagreement is largely (though not exclusively) characterized by a split between social sciences and human-ities disciplines. Nevertheless, since the mid-1970s lesbian and gay studies has con-tributed valuable scholarship across a wide variety of fields including history literature, art, sociology, and, economics. (See also CRITICAL HETEROSEXUAL STUDIES.) (**Linnea Stenson**)

Further reading

D'Emilio (1992).

Lesbian boy   A term that may be associated with the LESBIAN identity of a young or young-looking BUTCH, though with more contemporary connotations that lean towards notions of gender PERFORMATIVITY. Butch lesbian identities have traditionally been viewed by other lesbians as anti-feminist impersonations of MASCULINITY (Jeffreys 1989). From this perspective, role-playing within lesbian culture is seen to signify a masquerading of traditional gender roles, with butchness representing the imitation of male power and privilege. During the last decade however, lesbian culture has diversified and witnessed the development of a range of subcultural identities, which present a deconstruction of the essential categories of gender and sexuality. Alongside 'DYKES with dicks', 'dyke daddies' and 'DRAG KINGS', the identity of lesbian boy can be linked to expressions of FEMALE MASCULINITY, through which sexual symbols and practices are dislocated from BINARY gender categories. Rather than aping a conventional male aesthetic, contemporary forms of female masculinity can be located as a means of PARODYING normative masculinity. From a QUEER perspective, identities such as lesbian boy destabilize the notion that masculinity is the preserve of 'men' and work to fracture ESSENTIALIZING tendencies within gay and lesbian theory which articulate a 'correct' or uniform gay or lesbian identity. (**Sally Hines**)

Lesbian chic   A term used to describe periods where lesbianism has suddenly become fashionable within the mainstream heterosexual media – for instance, the 1990s, where key figures include Sharon Stone's character in the film *Basic Instinct* (1992), and the celebrated 1993 *Vanity Fair* cover where K.D. Lang shaves model Cindy Crawford. It also refers to periods where experimentation with lesbian sexuality has become more accepted – or possibly, merely more visible (such as the very public coupling of Madonna and Sandra Bernhardt). Faderman (1991) points out that there have been a number of periods of lesbian chic: the popularization of Freud's work on sexuality and the rise of an upper-middle-class bohemianism, led to the experimentation of the 1920s, embodied in figures like Virginia Woolf; while a later period of sexual permissiveness led to the 'bisexual chic' of the 1970s. Its critics argue that lesbian chic only promotes selective images – of women who are FEMININE, and happy for their sex-lives to be made public in a way that can be consumed by heterosexual male audiences (Madonna, again). It thus distorts lesbian imagery by marginalizing other types of lesbian identity – BUTCH, POLITICAL LESBIANISM – and by playing into male fantasies that such women may be available for them. While some have seen the rise of lesbian chic as an opportunity to break taboos on lesbian visibility, Smyth

(1994) argues that the phenomenon could only be welcomed in an environment which had otherwise been purged of lesbian representation. Futhermore, she points out that while such a culture may flirt with images of lesbianism aimed at a select straight audience, it remains censorious over, say, lesbians in prime-time television – and particularly hostile to images of lesbianism created by lesbians. Yet even within these limits, it is also the case that greater visibility and experimentation nevertheless enable new generations of women to discover lesbian possibilities (Groocock 1994: 118). (**Jo Eadie**)

Lesbian continuum   This term was coined by poet and essayist Adrienne Rich in her widely influential essay 'Compulsory heterosexuality and lesbian existence', first published in 1980. In the essay, Rich calls the 'fact of the historical presence of lesbians and our continuing creation of the meaning' of those lives 'lesbian existence' (1986: 51). Rich distinguishes this existence from a broader conception of what she calls the 'lesbian continuum' which she connects with a range of 'WOMAN-IDENTIFIED experience' throughout individual women's lives and history (1986: 51). These experiences move beyond sexual desire of one woman for another, and encompass all forms of female interactions, 'from the infant suckling at her mother's breast, to the grown woman experiencing orgasmic sensations while suckling her own child . . . to two women, like Virginia Woolf's Chloe and Olivia, who share a laboratory, to the woman dying at 90, touched and handled by women' (1986: 54). Rich's intent, in broadening out the word 'lesbian' to include more than the sexual, was to unite all women around a female-centred ideal and to break down growing ideological impediments between lesbians and heterosexual feminist women in the women's movement. Rich was criticized for devaluing the real differences between women found along the lines of, for example, race, class, and ethnicity, as well as for making the word 'lesbian' so expansive as to completely desexualize it and make it meaningless. Rich herself noted the use of the phrase 'by women who have not yet begun to examine the privileges and solipsisms of heterosexuality, as a safe way to describe their felt connections with women' (1986: 73). Nevertheless, Rich believed it a useful term that would open heterosexual feminists to an analysis of the institution of COMPULSORY HETEROSEXUALITY of which they are a part. (**Linnea Stenson**)

Lesbian gender   The term lesbian gender references, but is theorized as distinct from, heterosexual gender. Heterosexual gender at its most blunt reinforces the link between FEMININITY and woman, MASCULINITY and man, and posits these locked pairings as oppositional and complementary. Lesbian gender takes the *lesbian couple* as its beginning and endpoint instead, drawing on historical and contemporary evidence of gendering used within lesbian contexts to signal DESIRE.

Theorists of lesbian gender have consistently drawn on Case's 'Towards a Butch-Femme Aesthetic' (1989), in which she argues that BUTCH/FEMME (seen as an indivisible unit) necessarily provides a critique and PARODY of heterosexual gender roles. Lesbian gender thus indicates either interplay between FEMME and BUTCH embodiments and desires, or refers to the specifically butch (masculine) lesbian. Butler highlights a similarly parodic aspect of butch/femme, but also develops an understanding of lesbian gender as melancholia. Unlike heterosexuals, who for societal reasons cannot grieve the loss of a homosexual love object, a lesbian grieves the loss of her heterosexual male object by taking it on as her (masculine) gender (Butler 1997). Her masculinity is therefore experienced as a marker of both lesbian desire *and* the lost heterosexual desire. Munt (1998a) focuses on the spatial aspects of lesbian gender, its constitution in site-specific exchanges of the gaze between women. She emphasizes that both masculine and feminine lesbian subjects are active in this exchange such that the gaze is reciprocal (where in heterosexual contexts, the man is assumed to be the one who gazes).

The insistence on the distinctness of lesbian gender from heterosexual gendering has been critiqued for its lack of attention to the complexity of lesbian desire, particularly in its lack of attention to FEMININITY, and for its utopianism. Theorists such as Nestle have thus argued both that lesbian femininity needs further elaboration, and that we should be wary of celebrating butch/femme relationships uncritically (Nestle 1987). (**Clare Hemmings**)

Further reading

Munt (1998b).

Lesbian mother(s)   Lesbian women become mothers either through heterosexual intercourse in prior relationships with men, through adoption, or through the use of ARTIFICIAL INSEMINATION or other reproductive technologies such as IVF (Saffron 1994). Generally speaking, in lesbian partnerships which are involved in the raising of a child, one of the women is the BIOLOGICAL PARENT, and the other is a SOCIAL PARENT. However, IVF offers the opportunity for two women to invest physically in a PREGNANCY, with eggs being collected from one, and fertilized embryos being implanted in the other. The nascent, although illegal in the United Kingdom and highly controversial, reproductive cloning technologies offer the future possibility of 'gynogenetic' reproduction to women, where a child has two genetic mothers and no genetic father (Sourbut 1996). Where only one woman is genetically related to a child, the partner who fulfils the role of social parent to that child has very limited rights in relation to that child, particularly where couples separate.

Lesbian motherhood poses a particular challenge to the dominant social order, since it embodies both normative (mother) and counter-normative (lesbian) femininity. From this perspective, lesbian motherhood differs from gay fatherhood, in that while reproduction is constructed within the dominant discourse as fundamental to proper womanhood, MASCULINITY is defined more in terms of potency and virility than actual biological parenthood. Importantly, even in the conventional, heterosexual nuclear FAMILY, it is not unusual for one parent to have no genetic relation to the child(ren) of that household, and as such, lesbian motherhood can simply be seen as a reproduction of other accepted family structures. However, the conventional nuclear family is HETEROPATRIARCHAL in structure, and therefore, lesbian motherhood can be seen to constitute a fundamental challenge to the normative institution of the family (see Laird 1999). (**Karen Throsby**)

Lesbian separatism   See SEPARATISM.

Lesbians who have sex with men   A recently coined term, usually applied to lesbians who have sex with men for pleasure – i.e. excluding lesbians who have sex with men under duress (e.g. married but unable to COME OUT), or professionally as SEX WORKERS. In contrast to bisexual, the term refers to women whose affiliations are with the lesbian community, and whose identity is primarily marked by lesbian culture, but who may find that occasional sexual acts with men have a much lower importance in their lives than their social, political, emotional and sexual interactions with other women, much like BI DYKE. However, it may also serve as a means of avoiding using the term 'bisexual' for those who feel it is a less credible political identity (Eadie 1996). One of its earliest appearances in an article by Finkler in 1983, validates the importance of pleasure, honesty and self-discovery as key components of lesbian feminist politics, and suggests that this must also validate sex and relationships with men; at the same time, she explores the discomfort that a lesbian may feel about unexpectedly acquiring HETEROSEXUAL PRIVILEGE when she is given public validation for her relationship with a male lover that she has never been granted with her female lovers (Finkler and Chater 1995). Critics of the term have read this as the colonization of lesbian culture by heterosexual practices – often via gay male culture, which has been interpreted as undermining lesbian culture out of jealousy at women's independence from men. Thus Jeffreys (1993: 142–83) uncharitably suggests lesbians may have sex with gay men because of the continual social message that gay men are inherently sexually exciting in a way that lesbians supposedly are not. (**Jo Eadie**)

Lesbigay   A colloquial abbreviation for 'lesbian, gay and bisexual', often used particularly to indicate that an event or institution welcomes bisexuals. The term was the culmination of a long and often bitter debate through the 1980s over whether bisexuality had a place as part of a shared lesbian, gay *and* bisexual community, or was a distinct community which should organize itself more properly separately (see Hemmings 2002: Chapter 2). In some cases this resulted in bisexuals being excluded from lesbian and gay PRIDE marches, social spaces, and campaigns. The AIDS CRISIS, and subsequent rise of QUEER politics, served to bring together the needs of bisexuals more sharply with those of lesbians and gay men. Although the term gained general currency, some lesbians and gay men felt that they still did not want to share space with bisexuals, but might have no choice, if for instance, the only local pride event or club had elected to brand itself 'lesbigay'– while some bisexuals would argue that there was often only ever a token acceptance, which might not, for instance, extend to male–female sexual or romantic expression between bisexuals in supposedly 'lesbigay' venues. The term has now been superseded by LGBT, which adds 'TRANS' or 'TRANSGENDER' to the list of groups included. This shift is merely one of a number that have been points of tension within post-1960s sexual politics, as different groups have sought to make and break allegiances. Early 'gay rights' marches for instance assumed that the rights of both male and female homosexuals and bisexuals – including some trans people – were covered by the term 'gay', but in fact lesbians argued that their distinctive political demands were being occluded by the term (Faderman 1991: 210–13). (Jo Eadie)

LGBT   A recently coined acronym for 'lesbian, gay, bisexual and transgendered', used to describe social and political events which welcome all those identities. It replaces LESBIGAY, a term which excluded TRANSGENDERED people. Following the sexual liberation movements of the 1960s, as a previously underground network of same-sex venues became a more visible COMMUNITY, one persistent debate has been over who is included and what to call it. Lesbians, bisexuals, and transgendered people have argued that the term 'gay' has been given primacy at the expense of other groups active in a community comprised of many different sexual identities. LGBT reflects a current sense that all four groups play an equal role – although bisexuals and trans people might point out that their position in the list reflects a view on the part of lesbians and gay men that they are something of a late addition. As an indicator of the shifts in the construction of sexual communities, LGBTQI is currently emerging as a replacement that includes those identifying as QUEER and INTERSEXED.

To some extent these terms query the ETHNIC MODEL of sexuality which assumes a single homogenous community, and can be seen as a consequence of the queer movement of the 1990s – one book, for instance, titles itself *Queer Studies: A Lesbian, Gay, Bisexual and Transgender Anthology* (Beemyn and Eliason 1996). But it also assumes that all those groups have found a common ground, although it does so by glossing over hostilities that still exist – it is not uncommon to hear older gay men, in particular, complain about the constantly shifting terms within 'their' community, and for the term to be cited resentfully as an example of 'political correctness'. Certainly, organizations using the term are often more accepting of some forms of trans subjectivity – most obviously gay male DRAG – than others, such as heterosexual male TRANSVESTITES. LGBT should be conceived as a shared umbrella, rather than indicating that the needs and agendas of its component groups have become unified. (Jo Eadie)

Liberation   To liberate is to free. In the context of sexuality, the term refers to collective efforts for sexual and gender liberation, modelled in many ways on the civil rights movement, that gained sufficient numbers and public visibility to be recognized as constituting social movements during the 1960s and 1970s in the United States and Europe. This period has also been described as a 'sexual revolution', a time in some ways epitomized by the 1967 'Summer of Love', but these are ongoing struggles composed of many strands. The term 'women's liberation' is generally used to describe a second wave of FEMINISM aimed at securing rights for women equal to those afforded men. A significant emphasis of this movement has focused on sexual autonomy, including access to CONTRACEPTION and ABORTION (Morgan 1970). Gay liberation refers to a movement to end various forms of legal, economic, and social oppression and discrimination against gays and lesbians (Altman and Weeks 1993). Men's liberation groups in the 1970s to early 1990s challenged the limitations of gender roles for men, sometimes in support of feminist demands for change, at other times finding inspiration in older, mythic representations of manhood (Stoltenberg 1989). Liberatory movements by people with disabilities (Davis 1997: Part IV), TRANSGENDERED people (Feinberg 1996), and people practising SM both confront social inequities and STIGMAS they face and assert their rights for sexual freedom of expression. Conversely, we might query whether, as Reich (1972) believed, sexual REPRESSION is an evil functioning to reproduce oppressive regimes of power. Foucault's work presents a strong counterargument, insisting that sexual repression is a myth (see REPRESSIVE HYPOTHESIS) that persuades us to engage in ritual performances of CONFESSION that are powerful shapers of our sexuality, evoking both shame and fascination (Foucault 1990). 'Liberation' efforts only enmesh us further in such dynamics of confession, and he suggests that it is now liberation from which we need liberating. (**Karen Lovaas**)

Libidinal economy   'Libidinal economy' can be rephrased as 'economy of DESIRE'. 'Libidinal' is an adjective derived from LIBIDO, a term used by Freud to refer to overpowering desire. 'Libidinal economy' signifies an intersection of desire and economy. For instance, SEX TOURISM manifests the confluence of sex and money. Nonetheless, the association of libido with economy is not always taken for granted. Decades ago, especially for rigorous academics, the two terms were allocated to two discrete realms: PSYCHOANALYSIS, founded by Freud, took care of libido; while political economy, where Karl Marx loomed large, was in charge of economy. Although both Freud and Marx were widely read among intellectuals, few bridges were established between the two theorists. When the subject of desire was broached, it was often confined to the individual level rather than in a wider social context; when economy was discussed, the focus was on the society at large rather than the individual. The former was incarcerated in private, while the latter was pushed to the public. However, in his *Libidinal Economy*, the French philosopher Jean-François Lyotard (1993) argues that the 'libidinal', namely the erotic and emotional flows, play a major role in the 'economy', by which he means metaphorically, *all* regulating systems at large. In all everyday exchanges – financial, social, intellectual, political –there is an element of desire and bodily arousal. To revise the prevalent political economy, Lyotard suggests that this libidinal energy should be released, rather than suppressed, in these economies. He does not think libidinal economy is opposed to financial economy; rather, he contends that the two economies are intermingled and libidinal economy can bloom *inside* other economies. Although Lyotard draws on the tropes of heterosexuality, his libidinal politics is useful to those who want to empower NON-HETEROSEXUAL lives by releasing variegated libidinal energy into the status quo (see for instance Grosz 1994). (**Ta-wei Chi**)

Libido   In popular usage, libido refers to the sexuality or general sex drive of an individual. In PSYCHOANALYTIC theory, libido is the term used to describe psychic energy that is bound up with the sexual instinct. In Freud's work on libido, it is figured as a reservoir of sexual DRIVES that is formed as a result of the way that infantile sexuality is managed during the formative stages of development. The libido is often equated with Eros, the life drive and this indicates the extent to which the libido is thought to shape the individual or ego. For Freud, 'we call by that name the energy, regarded as a quantitative magnitude (though not at present actually measurable), of those instincts which have to do with all that may be comprised under the word "love"' (1921: 90). Libidinal attachments are not always consciously sexual, although Freud suggests that they are always unconsciously sexual. (**Caroline Bainbridge**)

Lifestyle politics   A term which began to be used during the 1980s to describe new social movements such as FEMINISM, gay and lesbian campaigns, environmental, anti-global and peace movements. Lifestyle politics reflects a shift from the traditional allegiance to political parties and represents a politics which is based less on class issues and more on issues which reflect personal choices and values. The development of lifestyle politics can be linked to growing affluence over recent decades. Some activists view lifestyle politics negatively and believe it shifts focus away from a more engaged street politics, although examples such as the boycotting of HOMOPHOBIC businesses reflect how it can generate specific campaigns. The focus upon lifestyle politics within sociology can be seen to be representative of the 'cultural turn' within the discipline, whereby theorists began to move away from the traditional analysis of identity as determined by class status. Rather, consumption patterns and lifestyle choices began to be viewed as symbols of active identity construction. In this way, factors such as fashion, sexuality, music and body management were viewed as markers of individual and collective identities, which held greater contemporary significance than traditional class indicators such as voting behaviour and occupation. Further, these areas have been seen as explicitly political as they offer resistance to hegemonic cultural practices. While some theorists argued that social class was no longer significant in contemporary identity formation, others such as Bourdieu (1984) explored class identity through the lens of lifestyle and consumption.

For Bourdieu, cultural tastes and consumption choices have replaced economic and occupational factors as markers of social and cultural difference. Such a focus on cultural symbols has been critiqued by other sociologists who argue that economic and occupational inequalities remain the determining factors that restrict the lifestyle choices of those who are materially deprived. (**Sally Hines**)

Further reading

Field (1995).

Lipstick lesbian   A term first appearing in the 1990s and with two overlapping meanings. Firstly, it is used either in a neutral or condemnatory way, to refer to lesbians who choose a FEMININE style – and may be used playfully by such lesbians to describe themselves (for instance, in contact ads). Secondly it refers to a set of images produced by heterosexual culture – also called LESBIAN CHIC – which represent ultra-feminine lesbians in films and advertising campaigns. Its initial usage may have referred more particularly to economically successful lesbians – that is, lesbians whose economic success obliged them to adopt the dress and behaviour codes of high finance and upper management (Groocock 1994: 109). It is a highly charged term because it seems to reference the colonization of lesbian culture by heterosexual standards of behaviour – often directed by advertisers seeking new imagery to titillate a straight audience. Thus POLITICIAL LESBIANS may use it critically to refer to lesbians who are perceived to have 'sold out' by imitating heterosexual femininity rather than adopting their preferred ANDROGYNOUS styles – as such it is part of an older conflict between certain strands of lesbian feminism, and FEMME identification. But both the disapproval towards, and the eroticized consumption of, the apparent shock-values of the image of lesbian femininity attests to the persistence of the older model of sexual INVERSION, in which the lesbian is assumed to be 'really' a man trapped in a woman's body, expected to dress accordingly. If this image had not continued, lesbians in lipstick would perhaps be less worth remarking on. Debate continues over whether the lipstick lesbian ever existed in any significant numbers, or was an invention of heterosexual marketing (Groocock 1994), but the term has taken root and become linked to lesbians for whom, as Faderman (1991: 292) notes, the diversification of lesbian identities creates a broader community. (**Jo Eadie**)

M

Male circumcision   Male circumcision involves the partial or total removal of the foreskin (or prepuce) covering the glans or head of the PENIS (between 33 per cent and

50 per cent of the total penile skin). References to this practice date back to ancient Egypt and it came to be adopted by some ancient religious communities including the Jews and Muslims who circumcise male children in accordance with Abraham's covenant with God. Numerous indigenous tribes also employ circumcision at puberty to signify ritual entry into adult status.

From the eighteenth century, new medical discourses of sexuality identified the foreskin as a potential site for disease (phimosis, when the foreskin is too tight to be retracted, can lead to the build up of smegma, or 'dick cheese' – an ABJECT bodily substance). In the nineteenth century increasing EROTOPHOBIA and paranoia about MASTURBATION, which was thought to lead to physical 'degeneracy', led to the advocacy of both male and FEMALE CIRCUMCISION as a 'cure' for this supposedly dangerous condition. From the late nineteenth century, removal of the foreskin in infancy was often recommended by the medical establishment and in the United States in particular, the practice became widespread. Today, circumcision is the most common surgical procedure performed in that country (on around 60 per cent of all male infants) although it is considerably less common in Canada, the United Kingdom and throughout Europe. For many men, possessing a 'cut' or 'uncut' penis has become an important signifier of desirability and self-esteem. In recent years there has been a shift in public opinion and male circumcision is beginning to be seen as having minimal, if any health benefits and as an erotophobic practice, akin to mutilation. Some men who were circumcised in infancy, have begun to campaign against the practice and have gone so far as to have foreskins recreated through COSMETIC SURGERY. (**Mark McLelland**)

Further reading

Gollaher (2000)

Male lesbian   Defined from a rather clinical perspective by Gilmartin (1987: 125) as a heterosexual man who wishes he had been born female (or who envies the social position granted to women), but who would still be emotionally and sexually attracted to women even if he *had* been born female. For some men, identifying as a male lesbian is a way of validating a desire for women while avoiding the hegemonic identity of STRAIGHT. Thus, male lesbians differ from *both* male transsexuals and male homosexuals in expressing no emotional or sexual interest in men (Gilmartin 1987: 126). A male lesbian may or may not be a TRANSVESTITE. A well-known self-identified male lesbian and transvestite is British comedian Eddie Izzard. Izzard states: 'It's just that I seem to fancy women but I am a transvestite and I would like to be a woman'. In the area of American pop culture, the character of Riley Finn, on the television show *Buffy the Vampire Slayer*, has been both Buffy's boyfriend and a rumoured male lesbian. Stryker (2001) examines the phenomenon of the proliferation of queer paperbacks from the 1940s–1960s, including *The Male Lesbian*. Perhaps the best theoretically-oriented discussion of 'the male lesbian' concept is by Zita (1998). Zita argues that the term 'male lesbian' is often taken to be an oxymoron; however, male lesbians become real possibilities given the loosening of sex/gender/sexuality constraints afforded by POSTMODERN theorizing. At the same time, Zita argues that the materiality of male and female bodies underscores the suspicion that SELF-IDENTIFIED male lesbians often experience (especially from woman-born/female lesbians), since the identity may be a way of trying to avoid acknowledging HETEROSEXUAL PRIVILEGE. A synonym sometimes used for 'male lesbian' is 'lez boy'. (**Mary Bloodsworth-Lugo**)

Male rape   A form of male-on-male SEXUAL ABUSE, this phenomenon has only been criminalized in the United Kingdom since 1994 (CJPOA 1994), and remains unrecognized by law in many other countries. It may happen in childhood or adulthood; invisibility of public awareness compounds personal suffering of the victims. A difficulty exists in precise definitions of RAPE; for example, a female who procures non-consensual intercourse with a male is not accused of rape (Coxell, King *et al.* 1999). This derives from traditional BINARY roles of gender, sexualized attributes and functions. Despite paucity of data, evidence can be found in the histories of ancient civilizations and colonized peoples (Krishnaswamy 2002); then, as now, male rape is usually perpetrated by heterosexuals, irrespective of the victim's SEXUAL ORIENTATION, and represents an exercise of abusive power. This is particularly so in all-male environments, such as military (e.g. captors in war) and penal systems. In some HOMOSOCIAL environments the perpetual threat of rape becomes an established way of enforcing hierarchies amongst men The victim of rape may suffer further silence in cultures where women are treated as inferior to men: the inference being that a man who is raped has lost his MASCULINITY and effectively has a woman's status. All victims of rape, female and male, may experience characteristic feelings; however, with a defamation of the individual's 'manhood' – 'weakness' at not repelling the event, or an assumed preference for male–male sex (Ericsson 2000) – male rape has its own distinctive STIGMAS. Violation may also take place under other circumstances, such as within an existing gay relationship, with brutal violence, gang rape, or DATE RAPE and with or without the use of disabling substances such as ROHYPNOL. Sexual infections may form a recurrent or permanent reminder of the event. Attitudes of authorities frequently deter victims from seeking help, and there can be an additional silence in countries where homosexuality is criminalized, as admitting to being raped is tantamount to admitting to criminal behaviour. 'Rape scenes' may also be part of an individual's erotic FANTASY, and have nothing to do with the actual non-consensual attack on or by another. (**David Evans**)

Further reading

Mezey and King (2000).

Marriage   An institutionalized arrangement which confers on both members of a couple – usually, but not in all contexts, a man and a woman – claims over each other, and which presumes long-term, MONOGAMOUS, reproductive co-habitation. Marriage is closely associated with reproduction and the formation of the nuclear FAMILY, and exhortations to reproduce are often part of religious marriage ceremonies. Marriages can be authorized in either a religious or a civil context, and are terminated either by the death of one partner, or through DIVORCE. Marriage confers advantages at the level of the state which are denied to those who are cohabiting outside of marriage, such as tax benefits, next-of-kin and inheritance rights, spousal visa rights and pension rights. In some countries, gay couples can register civil unions which confer the same rights as marriage (Lehmann 2001). Although MONOGAMY is prescribed within marriage for both parties, with adultery a legitimate form of evidence required to illustrate the irretrievable breakdown of a marriage in petitions for DIVORCE, traditions of POLYAMOROUS marriage exist both outside the West, and as alternative traditions within Western culture.

Marriage is productive of, and produced by, a set of gendered power relations (Yalom 2001). These power relations are illustrated by the gendered division of labour in the household, where domestic labour and other caring responsibilities are still performed predominantly by women, whether or not they also work outside of the home. More seriously, until recently in the West, marriage was understood as conferring upon men unlimited sexual access to their wives, leaving women little legal protection against RAPE by their husbands. However, in spite of the changes in the law, it still remains difficult to achieve a conviction for rape within marriage, except in cases where the couple were already living separately at the time of the rape. (**Karen Throsby**)

Further reading

Dryden (1999).

Masculinity   Recent academic debates have problematized predominant notions of 'masculinity' and their influence on the politics and practices of sexuality. The idea that masculinity represents a unified personal or social condition is increasingly rejected in favour of a plurality of masculinities which vary culturally, socially and historically. If masculinity is understood as a social variable then it need not even necessarily apply only to men, and FEMALE MASCULINITY becomes a possibility. Masculinities are generally relational and implicated in binary logics. For example, the sense of oneself as masculine often involves SELF-DEFINITION in concert with or in opposition to others, with masculinity defined against that which it is not, i.e. femininity. While multiple masculinities exist in any given context, hegemonic forms of masculinity are also evident (Connell 1987). These are generally heterosexual masculinities, and they occasion greater social power than gay masculinities. Gay men have responded to this in part by creating hypermasculine styles such as the CLONE and the leatherman, which challenge the idea that masculinity is synonymous with heterosexuality. The relationships between gay and straight masculinities are complex, and some argue that the HOMOPHOBIA involved in rejecting male homosexuality acts to discipline all men (e.g. Plummer 1999). This discipline is necessary in part because the symbolic boundary between male homosexuality and HOMOSOCIALITY is blurry and prone to slippage.

Tensions between dominance and ambiguity also play out within the practice of male heterosexuality. Holland *et al.* (1993) argue that heterosexual INTIMACY may represent a site of power and control for men on the one hand and vulnerability on the other. While many men define sexual pleasure in terms of male needs and desires, and seek to emerge from their sexual and emotional relationships with women as 'gladiators' rather than 'wimps', they are also prone to vulnerability. This may result from the possibility of failure or the negative sanctions placed upon voicing emotions when talking about sex with other men. In this way, masculinities can be regarded as potentially unstable PERFORMANCES, subject to cultural anxieties, expectations and prohibitions which individuals may accommodate or resist. (**Chris Brickell**)

Further reading

Whitehead and Barrett (2001).

Masochism   See SM.

Masquerade   See IMITATION; LESBIAN BOY.

Masturbation   Masturbation, whether alone or with company (see CIRCLE JERK), is potentially the most universally practised act of sexual pleasuring. It is witnessed in infancy and can continue throughout life, performed for reasons ranging from desire and gratification, through stress reduction or anger release, to sperm donation. It may be a prelude to, or substitute for, sexual intercourse, and is the safest form of sex whilst FANTASIZING about practices or scenarios that would not otherwise be performed due to their sexual, practical or moral taboos or dangers. However, there is barely a time or culture when for reasons of religion, psychiatry, EROTOPHOBIA, or censorial morality, masturbation has not been condemned. Mental institutions for 'masturbators' only truly receded in the West in the early 1900s, yet in 1994, US Surgeon General Jocelyn Elder was sacked for saying that masturbation is 'part of human sexuality and . . . perhaps should be taught' (Frankel 1994). Many cultures still treat discussion of masturbation, let alone the practice of it, as taboo, particularly so for women: clitoridectomy and FGM (Female Genital Mutilation) are, in part, direct endeavours to prevent the pleasures of clitoral stimulation and masturbation (Rich 1986). In some European languages, to call a person an 'onanista' is literally to call them a 'wanker'. However, Onanism, or 'the sin of Onan' is particular to Judaism, Christianity and Islam, and refers to the acts of a man, Onan, and his practice of COITUS INTERRUPTUS (the 'withdrawal method'): Genesis 38 says 'he repeatedly spilled his seed on the ground'. Numerous parents still tell children not to do it (Ussher and Baker 1993), as they consider it 'dirty' or 'wrong', or, worse still, they perpetuate myths that 'it will drop off' or 'you will go blind'. As long as such a safe and potentially fulfilling sexual activity is stigmatized as taboo, many people cannot incorporate it into their repertoire of sexual pleasures. (**David Evans**)

Further reading

Laqueur (2003).

Medieval sexuality (500–1500) Medieval ideas about sex and sexuality were greatly influenced by the CLASSICAL tradition. In Western Europe the most influential author was the early Christian Saint Augustine of Hippo (354 ACE–430 ACE). Augustine addressed marriage and sexuality, two themes often paired in Classical and medieval scholarship, in a variety of works. Augustine's, *On the good of marriage*, stated that a Christian marriage could be fruitful and positive if three goods, namely procreation, fidelity, and the sacramental bond, were fostered. Procreation, which in the medieval tradition denied any possibility of CONTRACEPTION, was the purpose of marital sexuality. Fidelity and the sacramental bond were the values of 'natural companionship' and the divine presence within the marital union respectively (Clark 1996). Augustine also popularized the hierarchical categorization of women, from best to least good, as VIRGINS, widows and wives. Thus, women were classified on the basis of their sexual activity.

Medieval law dealing with sex and sexuality took shape during the early Christian era, though the Church could not enforce those laws until the later medieval period. The great number of proscriptions in place for people who wished to engage in sexual intercourse was astounding. Sexual customs, as Brundage (1987) shows, depended variously on saints' days, women's physiological cycles, and numerous other factors including clothing, time of day, and, of course, the partner. These proscriptions however did not completely end non-marital sex even in the later medieval period. Countless records of men and women appearing before Church courts for adultery and fornication (sex between unmarried people) survive from the medieval period.

Penalties for breaking laws and customs relating to sex and sexuality included fines. RAPE in Anglo-Saxon England, for example, usually bore a monetary compensation. The status of the woman was the gauge on which the compensation was set. Rape of a high status woman generally required more compensation than that of a woman of lower status (Fell 1984: 62). Cases of rape and other illicit sexual acts, such as fornication and adultery, were fixed in a complex range of fines in King Aelfred's laws (Fell 1984: 62–3). While Christian influences may have reached much of Europe in the early medieval period, pre-Christian attitudes towards sex and sexuality may be seen in the Old Norse sagas. Jochens (1996) points out that the sagas often portray men actively and violently pursuing women sexually. Furthermore, rape and male aggression could suggest that 'marriage by capture' was if not a social norm of settled Norse society then at least practised occasionally (Jochens 1996: 370–71).

Illicit sexual behaviour often appears in medieval sources, whether law codes or court cases, and has thus been the focus of many studies. Medieval attitudes towards PROSTITUTION focus more on the sexual promiscuity than the actual monetary exchange. Three trends emerge, argues Karras, in the history of prostitution; complete outlawry, regulation and taxation, and institutionalization (1996: 243–4). One example of the possible regulations focuses on the appearance and clothing of prostitutes. As Karras (1996: 247) notes, prostitutes were often ordered to wear specific styles and identifiable clothing. As the Church viewed monogamous heterosexual sex within marriage as the only licit avenue for sexual relations, prostitution, adultery, and fornication, as well as homosexual relations appear in Church writings as sins and crimes against nature.

Johansson and Percy (1996) point out that HOMOPHOBIC attitudes appeared as early as St Paul and flourished throughout the medieval period. HOMOSEXUALITY becomes an extremely difficult subject to study as the evidence is almost wholly negative and from the official Church hierarchy point of view. As Salisbury (1996: 81–2) argues, gender and sexuality were defined by medieval authors on the basis of genitalia; 'two genders – two sexes – was the natural state'. HERMAPHRODITES, for example, would be taken as no more that 'monstrosities' (Salisbury 1996: 82). Homosexuality and other variances were viewed in the medieval period as, simply put, abnormalities.

While medieval femininity and women's history generally, has been thoroughly examined since the 1970s (Stuard 1987) the burgeoning field of medieval masculinity has attracted a good deal of attention in the last few years. Several collections of essays are invaluable in studying how men viewed sex and identified themselves by their sexuality (Hadley: 1999). Medieval ideas about sexuality were not uninformed about biology or physiology. Sexual intercourse, while central to procreation and family development, was also viewed, for example, as a method to maintain the body's health. Cadden (1996: 57–8) points out that regular sexual activity, 'like sleeping and waking, like exercise, like eating and drinking', was viewed as central to the body's normal and healthy functioning. Medical knowledge also extended to CONTRACEPTION and ABORTION. (**Andrew Cranmer**)

Further reading

Bullough and Brundage (1996).

Ménage-à-trois   A sexual union involving three people, or 'threesome'. It refers both to a casual sexual encounter and to a formal long-term three-person sexual relationship, often called a TRIAD. It is a staple of PORNOGRAPHY most usually represented as heterosexual, with either two women and a man, or two men and a woman. In the former case, the two women are also attracted to each other, whereas in pornographic representations of the latter, the two men either simultaneously penetrate the woman (vaginally and orally, or vaginally and anally), or they take turns. These representations often play down homosexual contact between the men, but may allow a covert HOMOEROTICISM. Lesbian *ménages-à-trois* are also represented in pornography, often for the heterosexual pornographic market. In pornographic stories and in letters to pornographic magazines, the *ménage-à-trois* often comprises a heterosexual couple who become involved with either another woman or another man, as an extension of their own sexualities. The third party is often treated as a toy to be used rather than as an integral part of the relationship. In this limited representation it is an event in the life of a STRAIGHT couple, rather than a more challenging sexual practice in its own right. Thus while a threesome is held out as a titillating sexual option, monogamous heterosexuality retains its place within the normative framework. In fact, as SEX RADICAL and POLYAMOROUS writings show, the *ménage-à-trois* may be the preferred sexual encounter of many, and may be either a consensual and egalitarian occasional practice, or come to constitute a viable long-term sexual relationship, comprising participants of any genders and/or sexualities (see Lano and Parry 1995). (**Ivan Crozier** and **Jo Eadie**)

Menopause   Menopause is conventionally described as the time when MENSTRUATION permanently ceases as the ovaries cease to produce the monthly ovum and the cyclic supply of ovarian oestrogen is significantly reduced. However, the cyclic release of oestrogen and progesterone often begins to change some years before the end of menstruation. Thus, menopause also refers to the much longer period of a changing cycle, the stopping of menstruation and the symptoms associated with menopause such as hot flushes and sweats. This much longer interval of physiological and emotional transitions is also called the climacteric and occurs some time between 35 and 60 years and is a continuing process of physiological modifications (Boston Women's Health Book Collective 1998).

Women's bodies have historically been perceived as potentially dangerous and some of the debilitating effects of menopause have been linked to 'female poisons' (Furman 1995). The medical profession in the nineteenth century reluctantly took on menopause as a topic worthwhile of investigation but eventually its medicalization conceived menopause as a crucial stage in reaching healthy old age through proper conduct. Pathologized by the medical profession, menopause was included in the Diagnostic and Statistical Manual of Mental Disorders as 'involutional melancholia' until 1980 (Furman 1995) and famously Freud and others characterized menopausal women as 'quarrelsome, and obstinate, petty and stingy, sadistic, and anal-erotic' (Komesaroff *et al.* 1997). With regard to sexuality, menopause presents women with numerous stereotypes such as 'being over the hill', based on the idea that female sexuality is only validated through reproductive HETEROSEXUALITY. This conception has a far reaching socio-cultural impact and points to a difficult relationship between femininity, ageing, sexuality, HRT and BODY POLITICS. (**Natalia Gerodetti**)

Menstruation   A woman's cyclical process of discharging blood and dead cells (menses) from the uterus through the VAGINA from puberty until MENOPAUSE. Universally, this process is symbolic of women's health and fertility. However, according to feminist critics, key issues of power, authority, and silence demonstrate ways in which medicine has claimed the right to speak about women's bodies and regulate their functions (Murray 1998). Examples of regulation include old 'cures,' such as foot-baths, wrapping sheets, and the more disquieting rituals of leeches and applying hot bricks to the navel to induce perspiration (Van De Walle and Renne 2001). A common cultural construction of menstruation inscribes it as taboo, while patriarchally encouraged SHAME silences women's experiences of menstruation, which is still referred to as 'the curse'. In nineteenth-century Western societies menstruation was viewed as pathological: the zoologist and anti-suffragist Walter Heape wrote of menstruation 'leaving behind a ragged wreck of tissue, torn glands, ruptured vessels, jagged edges of stroma ... hardly possible to heal satisfactorily without the aid of surgical treatment' (Martin 1992: 35). In Cambridgeshire, in the early twentieth century, menstruating women were not allowed to touch milk, fresh meat, or pork, because there was concern that such products would go bad (ibid.: 97). In some areas in West Africa there are still 'menstrual huts' that segregate menstruating women from others, and bar them from various sacred religious duties (Price 1984). In contrast, the North American Oglala Plains Indians had a positive view of menstruation, and the Yurok Indians contended that at the time of menstruation, a woman was thought to have heightened powers and 'should not be wasted in mundane tasks and social distractions, nor should ... concentration be broken by concerns with the opposite sex' (Martin, 1987: 236; 129). Menstruation is thus open to a range of cultural attributions of meaning, and feminism has sought to rewrite its STIGMA. Martin, for instance, explores predominantly Western cultural attitudes surrounding menstruation that place it in a private realm marked 'home and family', and juxtaposes this against some women's resistance to this domestic relegation. (**Alison Smith**)

Further reading

Houppert (1999); the online Museum of Menstruation, http://www.mum.org.

Men-who-have-sex-with-men   The term 'Men-who-have-sex-with-men' (MWHSWM or MSM) has been used to describe all participants in same-sex male relationships, regardless of SELF-DEFINITION in terms of sexuality. Adopted in sexual health promotion circles for its supposed inclusivity, it was thought that the use of sexual IDENTITY categorizations (gay, bisexual, straight) in SAFE(R) SEX promotion might repel those who refused a NON-HETEROSEXUAL identity on the basis of their sexual practices. In fact, according to Edward King (1993), this may have amounted to yet more 'degaying' of the AIDS crisis (see SAFE(R) SEX; AIDS CRISIS), and indeed, its 'enthusiastic adoption' in the statutory sector (i.e. government-funded and accountable) was partly due to conservative governments' wish not to be seen to 'promote' homosexuality (ibid., 203). Furthermore, in using a term not used by gay men themselves, many gay and bisexual men felt precisely *dis*included, perceiving a prioritization of the needs of heterosexually-identified men who covertly had sex with other men (ibid., 204). In summation, it might be concluded that the term 'gives the misleading impression that this is a homogenous group with the same needs, obstacles, and potential' (Peter Scott, quoted in King 1993: 205). (**Alex Evans**)

Minoritizing/universalizing 'Minoritizing' is a term coined by Eve Kosofsky Sedgwick in *Epistemology of the Closet* (1991) to refer to ways of understanding same-sex passion that conceive of it as something enjoyed only by a specific portion of the population. The view that there is a GAY GENE, for example, and the seemingly logical extrapolation that those with it are gay and those without it are not, affords a minoritized model of sexuality. Minoritizing models stand in contradistinction to universalizing models. Universalizing ways of understanding same-sex desire see it as being relevant, in a host of ways, to people of various sexualities. In popular terms, for instance, the notion that everyone enjoys 'a bisexual potential' would represent a universalizing view – as would Gore Vidal's (in)famous statement to the effect that there is no such thing as a homosexual person, only persons who engage in homosexual acts (Garber 1995: 42). On this universalizing view, homosexual activity is something in which anyone may engage; and it no longer makes sense to try to divide society into GAY and STRAIGHT spheres. As Sedgwick observes, both minoritizing and universalizing ways of thinking about same-sex passion have circulated, contradictorily, in Western culture throughout the last hundred years or thereabouts, and continue to do so today. However, such contradictions do not diminish these terms' worth as analytic tools. Rather these terms help commentators preserve a sensitivity to the diverse, contested, often fraught, and always heavily freighted structures of feeling surrounding sex and sexuality extant in various cultures at particular historical moments. (**Chris West**)

Mistress Sometimes used as an affectionate term for a DOMINATRIX, but more colloquially a woman in a long-term relationship with a married man who remains in his marital relationship. A mistress may bear the man a second set of children, or may be herself married and have her own children. The mistress may be financially dependent on her partner, especially if children result from the relationship, however the ever-growing economic independence of women may render this situation more and more unusual. These types of relationships usually entail a substantial amount of emotional involvement. The first cases citing 'VIRTUAL SEX' affairs on the Internet as grounds for divorce arose recently, and were deemed valid in spite of the purely emotional nature of the liaisons (King and Hayes 1999). In France the *cinq à sept* tradition is well established, while in Japan, the term for a mistress is *nigo-san*, meaning sweetheart or second wife. Historically the mistress was a prominent figure; royal circles abounded with such ladies while the upper class (especially that of seventeenth-century France) employed mistresses in the interests of the lady of the house (midwives believed that intercourse curdled the milk). The position of mistress should not be confused with those of concubine, PROSTITUTE or courtesan. The latter especially is hard to define in relation to mistress, but one essential difference is that the courtesan may have several lovers at once while the mistress is expected to remain faithful to her partner, who may have other sexual partners outside his marriage. Inherent in this is the DOUBLE STANDARD which governs the relationship: there is no male equivalent to the mistress. Despite the often clandestine nature of the partnership legal recognition of mistresses has been considered especially with regard to property rights (Anonymous 1999). (**Linda Kiernan**)

Further reading

James and Kedgley (1973); King and Jordan (1999).

Modern sexuality   Modernity, the large social period running from the seventeenth century to the present day – essentially the period of the rise of capitalism – has seen a range of different sexual norms and moralities come and go, but certain defining features persist across it as this larger economic shift plays out in distinctive ways in the areas of race, class, and gender. As it broke up the agrarian family structures that came before it, the modern period enabled new living arrangements to emerge – most notably that of high concentrations of unmarried people living in cities, which provided the basis for the modern gay and lesbian COMMUNITIES (Sinfield 1998: 160). The newer family structures became concentrated in smaller households, seeing the gradual decline of the extended FAMILY and the arrival of the nuclear family. While working-class families saw a more equal division of labour necessitated by economic need, with most women taking paid employment, the bourgeoisie created a more polarized BINARY world in which the domestic sphere was held to be the sole province of women. Consequently women were regarded as the embodiment of sanctified domestic values of sexual restraint, whose role was to civilize the sexual instincts of men (Segal 1992: 74–85) – a model that persists in contemporary SOCIOBIOLOGY. However, as burgeoning economic growth in the second half of the twentieth century required an ever greater workforce, this division has been eroded in favour of a more egalitarian division of labour, and with that a notion of men and women having similar sexual appetites. These changes in turn resulted in the need for more effective forms of CONTRACEPTION, culminating in the 1960s with the PILL. FEMINISM has engaged with these changes in a range of ways, but one particular tension has been between whether to hold onto a nineteenth-century notion of women as having a distinctive morality derived from SEXUAL DIFFERENCE, or to take charge of the social changes by which women might take up many of the practices previously restricted to men – such as consuming PORNOGRAPHY. These tensions are often referred to as the SEX WARS.

With the rise of a bourgeoisie dedicated to entrepreneurship, the new middle classes emphasized the importance of restraint and self-control as values both in the business world and sexually. Yet parallel to this world of bourgeois respectability, new technologies allowed for greater circulation of pornography, while the rapid growth of an urban underclass made PROSTITUTION an economic necessity for ever more women. Inspired by medical and eugenic initiatives, an alliance between science and morality sought to regulate these practices in the form of SOCIAL PURITY movements. Just as the white bourgeoisie demonized its racial others, so too it constructed working-class culture as a place of dangerously unfettered sexuality, with fears of a growing – and racially mixed – working class manifesting as calls for sterilization (Doyle 1994: 10–34). The scientific study of sexual diversity – or *SCIENTIA SEXUALIS* – gave rise to SEXOLOGY, whose cataloguing of different sexual 'types' had the ambivalent result of making sexual minorities both more visible and therefore more able to organize politically, but also more amenable to punishment or 'treatment'. But as the nineteenth-century culture of economic restraint gave way to the consumer culture of the twentieth century, hedonism has in effect become the norm (Turner 1996) and calls for restraint in the name of FAMILY VALUES, although still exerting ruthless constraint (for instance, over the sexuality of adolescent girls) appear increasingly anachronistic, particularly since the secularism of modern culture has undermined the legitimacy of religious teachings as a source of sexual morality.

For the West, the colonial period saw the mobilization of fantasies about fundamental racial sexual differences that legitimized Western superiority (Bleys 1996): that oriental countries were the home of a fantastic but listless sexual decadence; that native peoples in Africa and the Americas were in the grip of unregulated sexual desire; and that all non-Western races were prone to homosexuality – beliefs that still structure pornographic scenarios and the expectations of contemporary SEX TOURISM. Thus INTERRACIAL SEX became the site of charged power relations: on the one hand white culture constructed its racial others as possessing heightened sexual allure (specialist all-black brothels, for instance, operated in eighteenth-century London) and as the imagined site of the sexual values that they were in the process of banishing from their own world. Yet at the same time, white people conducted a prolonged sexual terrorism: routine sexual violence against black women (Omolade 1983) remains taken less seriously by white authorities, while violence against black men is often conducted in the name of the sexual protection of white women (for instance, in the case of lynching in the United States). Being to a large extent excluded from bourgeois social structures – whether as unpaid slaves prior to emancipation or as part of the growing poorly paid working class afterwards – black cultures were well positioned to resist some of the social purity drives and evolve instead a more playful language for sexual conduct that does not subscribe to the white bourgeoisie's self-regulation (Gates 1995). This co-existed with the opposite tendency: a stress on a heightened sexual self-restraint and responsibility, in order to mark their difference from the exploitation and double-standards of their white sexual oppressors (Omolade 1983).

In all three areas – race, class and gender – there is visible a pull to regulate sexual desire, but also a set of ambivalent fears and desires towards forms of sexual otherness. These two tendencies of the modern find their epitome in PSYCHOANALYSIS. Obsessed with the ABJECT fantasies of modern sexual culture, psychoanalysis finds them in the dreams of every one of us and – depending on its school of origin – seeks either to cure them, or to enable the patient to live comfortably with them. But this project also established the basis of a new understanding of sexual diversity as an inevitable part of human subjectivity. This would combine with the emergent forms of liberal democracy which characterize the modern period, to create a new SEXUAL POLITICS in which sexuality became seen as an individual right, not to be restrained by the state through CENSORSHIP. In effect, it is this notion that sexual diversity is a given of human experience, that paves the way for the rapid proliferation of POSTMODERN sexualities. (See also EARLY MODERN SEXUALITY.) (**Jo Eadie**)

Further reading

Weeks (1985).

Money shot   Also called the 'cum shot', this is the moment in a hard core PORNOGRAPHIC film where a male performer visibly EJACULATES. It earned its nickname because this is both the moment needed to ensure audiences will pay, and because male performers are paid extra to provide it (Williams 1990: 95). Performers are often required to pull out and ejaculate on the face or body of another performer, in order to ensure the verisimilitude of the sex acts taking place. Patton (1996: 3) notes that in an industry which has generally taken high risks regarding HIV transmission, this has been an unintentional form of SAFE(R) SEX. Williams (1990) argues that the money shot provides a point of IDENTIFICATION for male viewers, who see their own sexual (masturbatory) pleasure mirrored in the scene. She suggests it is also part of the broader tendency of hard core pornography to purport to have conveyed the 'truth' of sex to its viewer. Although the overriding importance of the cum shot has been read as proof of the inherent PHALLOCENTRISM of pornography (Cornell 2000a: 5), it should be remembered that pornography also ensures that female ORGASMS are made visible for the viewer by noise and writhing. While this seemingly equivalent moment remains more contentious since it is easier to fake, male performers may also be deriving little pleasure from ejaculation on demand, which may became painful and pleasureless. (**Jo Eadie**)

Monogamy   In anthropological terms, monogamy refers to the practice of having only one spouse, as opposed to polygamy, which refers to being married to more than one person at a time. Having multiple concurrent marriage partners is endorsed in some cultures and religions, but is largely a criminal offence (bigamy) in the West. Common usage of the term monogamy refers not specifically to MARRIAGE, but to any intimate relationship between two people and which excludes the intimate involvement with others outside of that relationship. Monogamy is normatively prescribed in contemporary Western society, and is seen as foundational to the institution of the FAMILY. NON-MONOGAMY (as opposed to SERIAL MONOGAMY) is constructed within this dominant discourse as deviant, although openly non-monogamous relationships in which partners are free to pursue other intimate relationships can offer a context for developing sexual identities outside of that normative framework. For example, someone identifying as bisexual, may choose to simultaneously pursue intimate relationships with both same-sex and opposite-sex partners. In the heterosexual context, the failure to sustain monogamy in a relationship which is founded upon the exclusion of intimate relationships with others is judged in profoundly gendered terms. Consequently, female infidelity tends to be evaluated far more harshly than that of men (see MISTRESS), who are presumed within the dominant discourse to have only limited control over their sexual urges. This is a view that is endorsed by SOCIOBIOLOGISTS, for example, who view men as inherently driven to secure their genetic survival by mating with multiple females (Fisher 1992; Ridley 1993). Infidelity within marriage by either partner would constitute grounds for DIVORCE in the United Kingdom, although this varies across national, cultural and religious contexts. Infidelity has also been cited effectively as provocation in cases where men have killed their wives. (**Karen Throsby**)

Monosexual   Used in contrast to bisexual to refer to those who are exclusively attracted to members of one sex – i.e. those who would be placed at 0 or 6 on the KINSEY SCALE. Within bisexual politics, the term has been useful in drawing attention to the shared assumptions of heterosexual and homosexual culture that bisexual love and desire are impossible or undesirable – often referred to as COMPULSORY MONOSEXUALITY. Yet as Blumenfeld and Hemmings (1996) argue, this is to ignore the structural differences in the social relations of men and women, both gay and straight, vis-à-vis bisexuals. It does not seem helpful to use a term which appears to suggest that lesbians have as much power as STRAIGHT men in setting anti-bisexual social agendas. Furthermore, it occludes the differences in the types of BIPHOBIA which bisexuals face from different monosexual communities. Moreover, it seems strange that a community which prides itself on seeing beyond either/or logic should use a term which so depends on BINARY thinking. (**Jo Eadie**)

Mouth   See DENTAL DAM; FELTCHING; KISSING; RIMMING; ORAL SEX.

MSM   See MEN WHO HAVE SEX WITH MEN.

MtF   A term meaning male–to–female. The term describes people who were born with male physical characteristics, but whose gender IDENTIFICATION or expression is female. The term commonly describes TRANSSEXUALS, who take female hormones and/or have surgery to modify their bodies. However, the term may also include TRANSVESTITES, CROSS-DRESSERS or DRAG QUEENS who express their female gender identification in ways which are not dependent upon body modification practices, for example by wearing female clothes. An MtF may also identify as a TRANSWOMAN, or simply as female.

MtFs have a long history in the West, which stretches back to Ancient Greece. The first recorded case of male–to–female gender reassignment surgery took place in Germany in 1931. In 1953 there was huge media publicity when an American ex-service officer Christine Jorgensen returned to the United States following gender reassignment surgery. Today MtFs are a vocal campaigning group within the TRANSGENDER movement and are increasingly represented in popular culture. As with individuals who identify as TRANSGENDER or FtM, there are different reasons articulated for female gender identification or expression. Those who identify as transsexual, often report a female identity from childhood, while transvestites, cross-dressers or drag queens may choose to express a female gender only at certain times. MtFs have been the subject of hostile criticism from many feminist writers and activists. The publication of Janice Raymond's book *The Transsexual Empire* (1979) represented a radical feminist attack on transwomen, which affected the dominant feminist position on transsexualism throughout the 1980s. Raymond argued from a SOBIOLOGICAL perspective that gender was determined by chromosomes and early socialization, and thus could not be altered. From this perspective, transwomen were perceived as fundamentally male. In her key article 'The empire strikes back: a posttranssexual manifesto' (1991) trans writer Sandy Stone challenged Raymond's position, arguing that trans women had often been forced to adopt a conventional account of gender in order to qualify for gender reassignment surgery, and urging their critics to recognize the more subversive gender ambiguities that appear in transgender experiences. Her arguments were influential upon a new wave of feminist critics who argued for the inclusion of MtF in feminist politics and culture. (**Sally Hines**)

Mummification   See SM.

N

Narcissism   A term for pathological self-love popularized by Freud (1914a). The term is derived from the CLASSICAL myth of Narcissus, who fell in love with his own reflection. It is often used negatively of FEMININITY – Beauvoir (1953) for instance claims that women become narcissists in order to find the validation which a patriarchal society refuses to give them, but as a result become only more dependent on male approval. Freud argues that since the entire body has an erotic charge, we cannot help but feel some degree of narcissism as we experience the AUTOEROTIC pleasure of exploring our own bodies. This in turn forms the basis of Lacan's (1977a) contention that we can only construct our identities by investing in a physical image of ourselves as whole and complete – a process which on the one hand involves a sexual embracing of our own bodies, but on the other a channelling of our desires into a single, and inflexible, ideal self. Early SEXOLOGISTS viewed narcissism as a part of the aetiology of homosexuality, as it was thought that many homosexual men were in love with themselves rather than with women, and so formed sexual relationships that closer approximated this self-love. As Fraser (1999: 89–90) points out, narcissism is still used HOMOPHOBICALLY today, to justify the assertion that heterosexual relationships involve more of a challenge, by interacting with the difference of another human being, whereas homosexual relationships are read merely as a way of seeking confirmation of one's own self. Bersani (1995) has inverted this charge, by arguing that all oppressed groups – and QUEER communities in particular – can only survive in a hostile world by finding others like themselves (see HOMONESS). Narcissism has thus become an important term within QUEER THEORY for describing a healing self-acceptance which undoes INTERNALIZED OPPRESSION and enables marginalized peoples to celebrate their difference from the social order, precisely by loving others in their own image. (**Ivan Crozier** and **Jo Eadie**)

Narrative   Narratives have been bestowed with different understandings and importance in different disciplines. In sociology, narratives are seen as the popular stories, myths, legends, which bestow legitimacy on social institutions, while grand narratives or metanarratives are generalized, overarching conceptions of social and political life. While much narrative analysis is preoccupied with formal properties of narratives, the importance of stories and story telling has also been stressed for processes of IDENTITY construction. Both collective and individual identities are continuously reconstituted and performed through available narrative forms. Story telling is integral to narratives which have proliferated to an extent where it has been proposed that the production, reading and consumption of stories have provoked a 'narrative turn' in social thought. Story telling has been used by social movements and therapies to create history, coherence and identity. With regard to sexuality, Plummer (1995) proposes the idea that sexual story telling, or personal experience narratives of the intimate, is part of the elaborate symbolic system of social life. Stories can be conservative and preservative by helping to structure the moral life of the individual and the collective, or radical in their implications. For instance, since the 1970s COMING OUT stories, sexual abuse survivor stories or RAPE stories, albeit different in content, have broken the silence about certain sexual experiences thereby being part of a wider social process shifting understandings of sexualities and SEXUAL POLITICS. Stories are part of the process of ordering and organizing, yet they are equally tightly connected to disorder, since there can be a proliferation of conflicting narratives – for instance, in feminist debates over how much weight can be given to positive stories of HETEROSEXUAL relationships in the face of the large number of stories of violence and abuse (see SEX WARS). While sexual narratives are part of sexual story telling, story-telling processes expand from a mere focus on narrative as they overflow to the social and political conditions that generate some stories and not others, and which make it harder for some groups to have their narratives heard publicly (for instance, SEX WORKERS). (**Natalia Gerodetti**)

Negotiation   Negotiation over the type of sex that one is to have is often absent in situations that have a heavily pre-formatted sexual SCRIPT – such as heterosexual intercourse – leaving people unable to negotiate SAFE(R) SEX practices, or pregnancy-prevention, for instance. Within SM communities, negotiation has been developed into a sophisticated art, and is a prerequisite for any form of consensual play in which parties involved reach an agreement between/among participants. Negotiation requires self-awareness, honesty and a willingness to communicate. Most SM practitioners embrace the SM 'motto' 'Safe, Sane and Consensual'. Negotiation centres around issues of CONSENT and health, and involves asking questions regarding physical and mental health, as well as physical and mental limitations. Negotiation should also involve discussing underlying motivations and desires to play, as well as what everyone involved will need for aftercare (e.g. physical and/or mental comfort after a SCENE). Whether embodying a written contract or an oral agreement, negotiation often involves designing a scene, or assigning SAFEWORDS, ROLES and/or FANTASIES. Negotiating creates a safe space where participants voice their likes and dislikes for the imminent play. Roles are partially postponed during negotiation so that every participant, even the most submissive, receives ample space to have input. Although the goal of negotiation is to delineate what is to come, there is room left for creativity and spontaneity. Negotiation may continue after a scene in terms of discussing what was and was not successful. Within the debates of the SEX WARS, SM negotiation is a useful counter-argument to the claim that SM involves a lack of power and control; the prevalence of negotiation in scenes may in fact make SM sex more egalitarian and more consensual than VANILLA sex in which there are so many unacknowledged expectations and habits. (**Caroline J. McKenzie**)

Nipples   These erectile hubs of erogenous flesh are frequently so 'genderized' as to leave their full sexual potentiality relatively untouched. In many cultures, women have to cover them up, have them treated primarily as instruments of nurture – breast feeding – or else have them exposed for the erotic gratification of (predominantly male) onlookers; in some, though not all, cultures, men can bare their chests in various public arenas with impunity, but STRAIGHT men resist eroticization of their nipples since it seems to feminize them – hence the greater comfort with their eroticization in gay culture. These contradictory attitudes frequently mean that nipples, especially male nipples, miss out on aesthetic and erogenous use in sex: 'you mean men have feeling in their nipples too?' (Anderson and Berman 2002). Nipples are also increasingly being used for PIERCING, and the insertion of various forms of jewellery. SEX TOYS for playing with nipples may range from personal, household and sex-shop accoutrements – feathers, ice cubes, or clothes pegs – to the heavier experiences in SM sex, such as whips, hot candle wax and clamps. Although infections of the nipples are rare, 'heavy' nipple play, 'tit torture' or any activity that gets another person's semen or blood onto broken skin, can carry risks of infection; if the skin is broken, then theoretically it is a route of transmission for hepatitis B virus or HIV. (**David Evans**)

Non-heterosexual   An umbrella term, used primarily within the social sciences, for the range of identities, orientations, relationships and behaviours that do not conform to the dominant, 'normal' and 'natural' form of COMPULSORY HETEROSEXUALITY. 'Non-heterosexual' covers a wide range of sexualities – including SITUATIONAL HOMOSEXUALITY, MEN-WHO-HAVE-SEX-WITH-MEN, and BISEXUALITY, as well as the best known non-heterosexual identities: lesbian and gay. To speak of 'non-heterosexual' says little about the diverse character and meanings of these diverse sexualities, but it does expose the central political dichotomy between heterosexuality as the 'norm' and other forms of sexuality as in some way diminished or DEVIANT. As such, the term 'non-heterosexual' is a meaningless generalization except in its use in a political critique of the dominant social construction of heterosexuality itself, in the same way as 'black' is used as a critique of white racial hegemony. (**Paul Reynolds**)

Further reading

Weeks *et al.* (2001).

Non-monogamy   Non-monogamy refers to non-exclusive sexual relationships. In its strictest sense, the term denotes having more than one spouse (polygamy), which includes polygyny (more than one wife) and polyandry (more than one husband). In its broader sense, non-monogamy – like MONOGAMY – does not necessarily imply a legal MARRIAGE and may be practised by heterosexuals, homosexuals, or bisexuals. Throughout history non-monogamy has been common across cultures (Ember *et al.* 1992). Polygyny continues to be practised in many societies in the Middle East and

Africa. Polyandry is much less common, practised in some societies in Nepal, India and China (sometimes with two or more brothers marrying the same woman). In the United States, plural marriage was practised by members of the Mormon religion until it was officially banned in 1890. (Some US mormons still practise it, albeit ille gally.) Today, polygamy (or bigamy) is a crime in the United States, the United Kingdom, and throughout Europe. Adultery (sex in which at least one partner is mar ried to someone else) is also illegal in many jurisdictions. Although not sanctioned by Western governments or religions, extramarital sexual relationships have always been common, in particular the tradition of men having concubines or 'MISTRESSES' or visit ing prostitutes. In the twentieth century non-monogamy was promoted by various sex radical, FEMINIST, and QUEER activists who rejected what they saw as the patriarchal and proprietary nature of compulsory monogamous marriage. Over the past two decades a conscious identity and movement has arisen around POLYAMORY, the practice of consensual, responsible non-monogamy (Anapol 1997). Polyamorists distinguish their lifestyle from adultery, 'cheating', or non-monogamous relationships conducted without the knowledge or consent of a primary partner. Some polyamorous people embrace POLYFIDELITY, or relationships that include more than two people but are sexu ally exclusive outside that group. (**Liz Highleyman**)

Further reading

Lano and Parry (1995).

Normalization   Normalization refers to the process by which some SEXUAL PRACTICE and ORIENTATIONS are accepted as legitimate and unthreatening within a society. Positively, it refers to the process of social change by which previously marginal or STIG MATIZED identities and practices become acceptable – such as 'the normalization of homosexuality' that has happened over the late twentieth century. Classic examples are HIV and AIDS; both have been 'exceptionalized' illnesses (Sontag 1990), but in parts of the world, through the sheer numbers of those affected by HIV or the successful lobbying for fair and equal treatments, HIV and AIDS are moving away from 'exceptionalized' status towards a normalized one. This is even more evident in affluent countries that supply 'combination therapies' to manage disease progression (Steffen 2000). More negatively, the term refers to ASSIMILATION – the process by which marginal groups are tamed or transformed so as to become more acceptable to the *status quo*. This is fre quently the case when subcultures move from invisibilized or ostracized elements of 'normal' societal life, to acceptable minorities within. Notice how the term 'queer' was often used in Western cultures solely for its HOMOPHOBIC abusive affect. Normalization has transformed this term into anything from a reclaimed title of self-affirmation to a respectable discipline in the social sciences, QUEER THEORY. Paradoxically, QUEER in this sense is definitely not about being 'normal': queer challenges normalization (see STRAIGHT ACTING and ANTI-GAY) in that it is de facto assumed exceptional, or, derogatively, perverted and deviant (see GENDERQUEER). It is always an exception from the 'norm', whatever the latter is taken to represent. Normalization may therefore include moves that conform queerness to majoritarian images of normalcy (Warner 1999). The term can also be used to refer to the process by which certain sexual identities are singled out over others and held out as the 'normal' or approved option – 'the normalization of heterosexuality' for instance, refers to processes like wedding ceremonies and adoption rights, which make heterosexuality seem the norm by its being constantly promoted and reinforced. In all its meanings, normalization is therefore one explanation of the transition from stigmatizing separation to inclusive incorporation. However, until all genders and consensual sexualities merit equal civil rights and freedoms from discrimination, and until HIV disease is totally destigmatized, then the process of 'normalization' remains arbitrarily incomplete. (**David Evans**)

Further reading

Warner (1999).

Nudity   The state of being naked has long been considered shameful, and such attitudes are still observable in instances of public bathing – although nude bathing in the sea was considered normal until the mid-nineteenth century (Bell and Holliday 2000), today even topless bathing is considered unacceptable in many countries. Supporters of the right to the expression of nudity – called naturists – espouse the view that the body is natural, and that there is nothing shameful in its display in public. Naturists actively repudiate charges of EXHIBITIONISM, and play down the sexual aspects of nudity – often by emphasizing it as an activity for the heterosexual nuclear FAMILY. Yet running parallel with this, a SEX RADICAL tradition – drawing on LIBERATION movements – advocates more self-consciously erotic use of outdoor spaces, challenging society to accept the sexuality of nudity rather than downplaying it (ibid.).

Nudity enjoys a long history in art. While other forms of SEXUALIZATION were being challenged in the nineteenth century, the fact that classical art represents the body unclothed allowed artists to portray naked people in classical allegories and other ancient scenes. Neade (1992) argues that the female nude became the central topic of Western art, celebrating a VOYEURISTIC male gaze that sought to possess the female body. Since the eroticism of this tradition was downplayed, scandal was usually avoided; nudity is thus an area where a covert eroticism is smuggled under the claims of 'sensuality' or 'physical beauty', which ensure that a sexual aim can always be plausibly denied. This proved important for emergent gay subcultures: in the 1950s and 1960s, certain bodybuilding magazines used the claim of showing physical achievement to circulate gay softcore PORNOGRAPHY; notably different from mainstream bodybuilding magazines in the eroticism of their poses, they also offered photographs for private sale (Dutton 1995: 240–50). Photography has traditionally been seen as a more explicitly sexual field than painting – and photographed nudes were often associated with the OBSCENE. In post-Second World War America, it was photographic clubs that formulated the form that is now most often associated with pornography: the tableau o the naked woman. It was soon marketed by the likes of Hugh Hefner (*Playboy*) and Larry Flint (*Hustler*) in America. These magazines have pushed the boundaries o acceptable nudity in relatively soft pornography from exposing women's pubic hair, to the current close up of the vagina being held open by the model (a practice known as 'fingertipping'). (**Ivan Crozier** and **Jo Eadie**).

Object-choice   This term describes the selection of a person or a particular type o person as a love-object. In the PSYCHOANALYTIC account, adult object-choice is regarded a being shaped by infantile object-choice. There are two modes of object-choice in thi account. Firstly, object-choice may be anaclitic (Freud 1912). In this mode, the objec selected is based on the model of parental figures who have looked after the subject providing her/him with nourishment, care and protection. In Freud's account, thi type of object-choice is driven by our self-preservative instincts. The subject will seel out an object who resembles an image of the parental figure, for example, by choosing a woman who will provide food or a man who will provide protection. Freud argue that male object-choice is often in this mode. The second type is NARCISSISTIC (Freud 1914a). In this model, the subject bases her/his selection of a love-object on the rela tionship s/he has with her/himself. In other words, in the narcissistic mode, objec choice does not forge a new kind of object-relation, but, rather, bases object-relation on the relationship with the self. Freud suggests that women are predominantly narcis sistic in their object-choice. He also argues that this mode of object-choice is usually present in homosexual relationships. In the narcissistic mode, a person may love someone because s/he resembles what s/he is, has been or would like to be. It is impor tant to note that modes of object-choice can shift and alter, and it is possible for both anaclitic and narcissistic elements to be present in one's object-choice. In order to understand object-choice more fully, it would seem necessary to scrutinize the effect of SEXUAL ORIENTATION on how object-choices are made. The Freudian account offers only a limited scope for how this may be done. (See also DEVELOPMENTAL NARRATIVE; KLEIN SEXUAL ORIENTATION GRID; SEXUAL DIMORPHISM.) (**Caroline Bainbridge**)

Objectification   Objectification is the derogatory process of dehumanizing a person or persons to an object. This is most commonly associated with the objectification o women by and for the consumption of heterosexual, patriarchal men (as part of HETEROPATRIARCHAL cultures and cultural practices). Female objectification was one issue that helped re-launch the FEMINIST movement in the United States of America in the late 1960s when protesters argued that the Miss America pageant in Atlantic City was 'sexist and degrading and that it represented wider patriarchal social attitudes which positioned women as objects of exploitation' (Corrigan and Meredyth 1991: 53–4). Female objectification remains a central concern for feminists who have, sometimes controversially, 'pointed to the connections between beauty, female objectifications, rape, violence, PORNOGRAPHY and other forms of female subordination' (Corrigan and Meredyth 1991: 54).

Women have also been implicated in this demeaning process. In psychology 'objectification theory' suggests that women are socialized to objectify *themselves* (see Slater and Tiggemann 2002). This occurs when women internalize and adopt the perspective of others to view themselves. Female 'self-objectification' has been linked to poor body image and, in some cases, eating disorders (ibid.). Feminists such as Naomi Wolf have attempted to address these and similar issues by advocating an approach to fashion, body image, and gender that is more 'playful' and, crucially, inconsequential (1993: 290). Wolf argues, '[a] woman wins by giving herself and other women permission . . . to do whatever we choose . . . A woman wins when she feels that what each woman does with her own body – unforced, uncoerced – is her own business' (ibid.). Men are also increasingly objectified in mainstream cultures and media, though certainly not to the same extent as women and, arguably, not with the same consequences or implications. (**Kelly McWilliam**)

Obscenity   A legal term used to define sexual speech considered to be outside the free speech protection normally granted in constitutional democracies (as opposed to PORNOGRAPHY, a broader term referring to the depiction of sex) (Wolfson 1997: 103ff.). Obscenity has been used as a regulatory category to allow CENSORSHIP of materials allegedly dangerous to young people and to the moral standards of society. Whereas before the nineteenth century, obscenity often encompassed not only sexually explicit materials but also heretical and seditious speech, by the nineteenth century obscenity became a separate legal category in Britain and North America. After 1860, Regina v. Hicklin became widely accepted as the standard in both Britain and North America for determining what was obscene: everything harmful to children or that might produce sexual thoughts in children and encourage MASTURBATION (Heins 2001: 3–36). Hicklin gradually came under attack as courts ruled that adults should not be limited to a standard of reading based on the needs and limitations of children. Challenges to the censorship of important literary works were central to the dismantling of the Hicklin standard, including the *Naked Lunch* (1966) case in the United States (Allyn 2000: 57; 68–70) and *Lady Chatterley's Lover* in the United Kingdom (1960) (Hall 2000: 168–9). In Miller v. California (1973), the United States Supreme Court established a three-point test for obscenity, defining it as that which appealed to prurient interests, was devoid of serious scientific, literary, artistic, or political value and was patently offensive to (local) community standards (Heins 2001: 85–7). Legal scholars and historians have pointed out the ambiguity and subjectivity of all three of these points (Strossen 52–4). Traditional understandings of obscenity have been further complicated in recent years by the redefinition of community and community standards necessitated by the Internet, as well as its challenge to the boundary between PUBLIC AND PRIVATE. (**Gary Schmidt**)

Oedipus complex   For Freud, the Oedipus complex is the origin of sexuality and refers to the set of incestuous wishes and desires that a child unconsciously experiences towards its parents. Freud's ideas centre on the experience of the little boy, who begins unconsciously to DESIRE the mother. However, in desiring the mother, he is threatened with castration by the father – the boy fears that the father will castrate him because of his desire for the mother. This element of the Oedipus complex is known as the CAS-TRATION COMPLEX and is crucial to the dissolution of the Oedipal conflict in the Freudian account. Eventually the boy begins to reject the mother as an object of desire and begins to transfer his identification to the father instead. The implications for masculinity and male heterosexuality are obvious here – Freud argues that the little boy believes that if he starts to act like his father, one day he will be like him, with his own object of desire (woman). Once the boy identifies with the father, the previous period of desire for the mother and rivalry with the father is repressed.

The experience of little girls is much more complicated. On noticing that boys have a penis and they do not, girls are supposed to become aware of the 'fact' of their castration. The little girl considers her lack of penis to constitute a wrong perpetrated against her which is unfair and for which she seeks compensation. The little girl has several options available to her. Firstly, she can DISAVOW her lack of penis, insisting that she does have one. Freud argues that this results in psychosis in later life. Alternatively, the little girl may become fixated on the idea of acquiring a penis. Finally, she may accept the 'fact' of her castration, resigning herself to a status inferior to that of the little boy (see PENIS ENVY). According to Freud, the latter is the route to normative sexuality, and the girl transforms her desire for the mother into hatred for her; libidinal desire is then transferred to the father as an object of affection. Freud does not attribute much potential for dissolution of the Oedipus complex in girls. As a result girls are deemed to be less able to resolve Oedipal conflicts and establish a strong superego. This led Freud to surmise that women are somehow less moral than men, using their feelings and instincts to form judgements in place of a fully-developed sense of moral justice.

There are several problematic elements associated with Freud's ideas about this complex. There is an unquestioning acceptance of the rights of the father over those of the mother and/or child, leading to suggestions that the Freudian schema is a profoundly patriarchal and PHALLOCENTRIC one, and also a disavowal of the importance of the mother. Freud's account of the development of sexuality reifies HETERONORMATIVE notions of desire and fails to offer convincing theories of the development of homosexual and bisexual modes of desire. Against this, Kristeva (1980) and Irigaray (1985a; 1985b), have emphasized the persistence of the mother–daughter PRE-OEDIPAL attachments as a fundamental connection which permanently frustrates the girl's attainment of Oedipal heterosexuality. (**Caroline Bainbridge**)

Further reading

Freud (1908).

Onanism   See COITUS INTERRUPTUS; EARLY MODERN SEXUALITY; MASTURBATION.

Oral sex   The use of a mouth on genitals; known by many names including cunnilingus, muff-diving, fanny licking or RAINBOW KISSING when performed on females, and *fellatio*, cock-sucking or blowjob, when performed on males. RIMMING (FELTCHING) is oral sex on the anus. Oral sex falls anywhere between tender/'VANILLA' sex to within the repertoire of domination and submission (BDSM). In SM and PORNOGRAPHY, it is frequently (though not exclusively) associated with male domination over women or other men. Oral sex challenges traditional sexual notions of 'active' and 'passive', where these terms allude to inserter and insertee, in that the person performing the act may be more active than the one receiving it, while the sexual position '69' includes a complementarity of partners performing mutual oral sex. 'Cock-sucker', 'muff diver' or their equivalents are sometimes used pejoratively to indicate sexual voracity (e.g. 'slut'), or derogatively as a form of HOMOPHOBIA. Conversely, the terms may represent a desired sexual persona and have been reclaimed as positive and affectionate markers of lesbian and gay identity. The institutionalization of heterosexuality means that sexual intercourse is socially located in gendered power relationships which frequently treats oral sex as 'FOREPLAY'. However, oral sex can form a significant part of the sexual experience for those practising alternatives to vaginal or anal intercourse (King 1993). Although evidence of oral sex exists over thousands of years (Love 2002), some cultures proscribe it, because it is non-procreative. Like many others practices, it is embellished with STIGMAS, myths and taboos, particularly in regards to cunnilingus. The more a society condemns non-reproductive sex (EROTOPHOBIA), the more likely it is to criminalize or pathologize oral sex. Concerns are frequently expressed about the safety of oral sex, from sexual infections; epidemiological evidence shows that 'low risk isn't no risk', but in relation to HIV infection, it is usually of far less risk than unprotected anal or vaginal intercourse (see DENTAL DAM). (**David Evans**)

Further reading

Roberts *et al.* (1996).

Orgasm Orgasm has come to represent authenticity in sexual relations because it is assumed to indicate an 'uncontrollable' sexual response – or JOUISSANCE. For this reason graphic descriptions and representations of men EJACULATING onto women are prevalent in contemporary pornography (see MONEY SHOT), while women are expected to perform loudly to prove that orgasm is occurring. Travers argues that as a result of this pressure on partners to orgasm 'enough' or 'visibly' – a pressure that has been added to in recent years with the 'discovery' of FEMALE EJACULATION – it has become impossible to distinguish in any simple fashion between so-called 'fake' and so-called 'real' orgasms, since 'a faked orgasm is often more real than a real one' (1993: 137), by virtue of its furnishing the expected 'proof'. Prior to the late eighteenth century, it was considered that women as well as men had to experience orgasm in order to reproduce although by the nineteenth century this had been replaced by the view that women's sexual pleasure was merely incidental (Laqueur 1990), legitimizing brutal surgery to control women's supposedly unnecessary – and therefore PERVERSE – desires for orgasm (see FGM). Nevertheless, a number of late nineteenth- and early twentieth-century doctors and sexual reformers, including Mary Putnam Jacobi, Havelock Ellis, and Marie Stopes, stressed that sexual satisfaction ought to include women achieving orgasm. A view associated with Sigmund Freud states that there were two types of orgasm in women: the vaginal and the clitoral. In the Freudian milieu, the clitoral orgasm was the immature masturbatory orgasm, while the more mature woman would orgasm through penetration, thus validating heterosexual intercourse over other sexual activities. However, as Haraway (1990) points out, with the advent of second-wave FEMINISM the female orgasm became the symbol of freedom from the expectation that women's primary role was as mothers. In particular, the debate over clitoral versus vaginal orgasm acquires a political resonance, in that the clitoral orgasm can be read as more obviously independent of heterosexual intercourse, and therefore used to legitimate women's sexual agency beyond the confines of COMPULSORY HETROSEXUALITY and the COITAL IMPERATIVE. (**Ivan Crozier** and **Jo Eadie**)

Outing 'The identification of gay and lesbian public figures trying to remain in the closet' (Signorile 1994: ix). This strategy is strongly associated, in the United States with gay journalist Michelangelo Signorile and the direct action group Queer Nation In Britain the most prominent advocates of outing were activist and writer Peter Tatchell and the direct action group FROCS (Faggots Rooting Out Closeted Sexuality). The argument for outing closeted public figures arose and gained much impetus from a new level of militancy and anger among gay people, itself occasioned by the increased HOMOPHOBIA evident in and licensed by the responses of the Reagan–Bush administrations (in the United States) to the crisis posed by HIV and AIDS, and by the repressive tendencies of the Thatcher governments (in Britain). Signorile argued that 'truthful discussion of the lives of [closeted] homosexual public figures [w]as legitimate and significant [given] the larger aim to give courage to mil lions of gay people who stay in the CLOSET out of fear and shame' (Signorile: ix). However he recognized one pitfall of outing (one he admits to having partaken in, hence perpetuated, himself) was that it made 'the revelation of homosexuality into a punishment' (xv). One might argue, indeed, that on account of this, outing helped sustain the dispensation of power which privileged (and privileges) hetero- over homosexuality. It gains its force in direct proportion to the strength of HOMOPHOBIA, and thus replicates the dynamics it ostensibly seeks to challenge. A further criticism of outing is that, ultimately, it ignores the limitations of IDENTITY politics: it supposes a unity of interests among gay people (which closeted gay public figures, especially politicians, may betray), ignoring the importance of other factors such as class position, ethnicity, or general ideological affiliation in determining identity. We might link this to more recent objections made to the notion of 'COMING OUT' as a model for sexual subjectivity. (**Chris West**)

P

Packing   In Anglo-American contexts, the practice of placing items in underwear to create the appearance and feel of a bulging crotch. It refers both to items worn that might be used in sexual encounters – such as a STRAP-ON (Bright, 1990) – and to those worn purely for show. While not gender and/or sexuality specific per se, packing is primarily a cultural and bodily practice of FTMS and bi or lesbian FEMALE MASCULINITIES. Besides 'packing hard', Heine (2002) notes the practice of 'packing soft'. Packing soft can be obtained with relative low-tech procedures such as the use of socks held in place by jockstraps or underwear. In contemporary DRAG KING and FtM cultures, packing is often obtained by stuffing hair gel into a CONDOM that is then tied at the end. Alternatively, 'packing soft' involves the use of a flexible DILDO or other custom made prosthesis. While among BUTCHES, DRAG KINGS and FtMs, packing is often a routine accessory for the PERFORMANCE of a non-aroused embodied masculinity, it can also amount to a highly sexualized activity for the 'packer' as much as for those doing the 'groping'. (**Silvia Posocco**)

Paedophilia   Paedophilia is adult sexual love or desire directed towards children and can be used of adult men or women who are in sexual relations with children of either sex. It is often used interchangeably with PEDERASTY which more properly refers to homosexual relations between an adult male and a boy. The age at which INTER-GENERATIONAL SEX between an adult and a child can be considered paedophilia is a moot point, given the wide disparity in AGE OF CONSENT laws across cultures and time periods. Paedophilia, when defined as a mental disorder, generally refers to an adult's predisposition to seek out prepubescent sexual partners (usually understood to be below the age of 13). However, given the disparity in age of consent laws, in some jurisdictions adults may be prosecuted for statutory rape of a minor even when sexually involved with 16 or 17 year olds. This is a particular problem for gay men, since the age of consent for male homosexual sex has tended to be higher than that for heterosexual sex.

Historically, most societies have not made such a strict division between adult sexuality and childhood innocence as exists today. In the past it was not uncommon for nursemaids to masturbate infants to stop them crying. Cramped living quarters and shared beds meant that children were not sheltered from adult sexual expression and children were considered ready to take on the burdens of marriage and reproduction when they reached puberty (however due to lower nutrition this tended to be somewhat later than is common in modern societies). Given that women have fewer reproductive years than men, there was a tendency for girls to be married off very young to men who were much older. It was not until the Victorian period in the West, when both childhood and ADOLESCENCE began to be conceived of as distinct from adulthood, that there developed the notion of protecting the innocence of children, particularly girls. However, as Kinkaid (1993) argues, the construction of girls as innocent went hand-in-hand with their increasing fetishization and exploitation. Child PROSTITUTION and SEXUAL ABUSE are of particular concern in the modern world with the increase in SEX TOURISM to developing countries. Also, the Internet is playing an increasing role in the production and dissemination of child PORNOGRAPHY. (**Mark McLelland**)

Further reading

Kincaid (1998).

Pansexual From the Greek *pan*, meaning 'all' or 'every'. According to David Cauldwell, a pioneer of sexuality theory, a pansexual person is someone 'who indulges, to a greater or lesser degree, in all discovered forms of sexual expression' (2001: 2). Pansexual is also sometimes referred to as POMOSEXUAL. Pansexualism may be differentiated from bisexuality in that it refers to sexual attraction to and/or loving not only women and men, but transgendered people, as well as the expression of a sexuality with maximum FLUIDITY towards objects, forms and contexts (see POLYMORPHOUS PERVERSITY). In theory, pansexualism questions fundamental assumptions that ground notions of 'sex', 'gender' and 'sexuality'. Pansexualism thus rejects terms such as 'heterosexual', 'homosexual' and 'bisexual' in favour of much more transient impermanent notions of pleasures without labels. Sometimes associated with BDSM whilst other pansexual people emphasize 'all safe-sane-consensual expression of adult sexuality' (Goodwin 2002: 1). (See also LIBERATION.) (**Myra Hird**)

Paraphilia   A clinical term that is defined as 'a condition in which a person's sexual arousal and gratification depend on fantasizing about and engaging in sexual behaviour that is atypical and extreme ... distinguished by a preoccupation with the object or behaviour to the point of being dependent on that object or behaviour for sexual gratification' (Wylde Wear 2003). It is principally used by psychologists and psychiatrists to describe conditions that do not conform to 'normal' notions of sexual behaviour that privilege genital heterosexual intercourse. It represents a tradition that emerged in early psychology, PSYCHOANALYSIS and SEXOLOGY for categorizing 'abnormal' behaviours (Porter and Hall 1995). Krafft-Ebing's *Psychopathia Sexualis*, is a typical progenitor to the study of paraphilia (Bland and Doan, 1998), though the term was first used for this purpose by the psychologist John Money (Money, 1998). It is currently used in exploring a range of sexual behaviours, ranging from the commonly known – FETISHISM, TRANSVESTISM, VOYEURISM, EXHIBITIONISM and SADO-MASOCHISM – to the more esoteric: dendophilia (sexual arousal from trees), emetophilia (sexual attraction to vomit) or plushophilia (sexual attraction to soft toys). There is some justification for studying what might be regarded as abnormal behaviours: where, like PAEDOPHILIA or BESTIALITY, they are deemed to be illegitimate through ethical consensus in society; forms of sexual arousal that might produce health problems or might signify mental health problems, such as apotemnophilia (arousal by amputation) or necrophilia (attraction to corpses); or in sex therapy, where a sexual fixation is having a destructive impact on a person's relationships. However, the problem with the term 'paraphilia' is that it is impregnated with medico-moral pathology, identifying diverse sexual practices as 'deviant' and 'dangerous'. Whilst it is now recognized that the labelling of a paraphilia is inherently cultural, the scientific basis of the language of paraphilia provides an authoritative categorization that pathologizes sexual difference in identity, orientation and behaviour. Hence sado-masochistic sexuality is reduced to a harmful paraphilia, ignoring its discourses of pleasure, desire, CONSENT and subject autonomy. This value-loading towards HETERONORMATIVITY assumes that paraphilias will always be intrinsically pathological, and the challenge for contemporary sexology is to produce more culturally sensitive categories in a form more open to contestation and debate. (**Paul Reynolds**)

Parody   In its literary sense parody can be described as first imitating and then changing the style and subject-matter of another work. Most of the specific characteristics of parody, including its creation of comic incongruity between the original and the parody, and the way in which its comedy can laugh both at and with its target, may be traced to the way in which the parodist makes the object of the parody a part of the parody's structure. Sexual theorists have become interested in parody because of the wide number of parodic sexual subcultures that exist and the way that these call into question the apparent authenticity and superiority of heterosexual culture. Understanding parody as a form of IMITATION or mimicry necessitates something preexisting, or 'authentic', which rather than being seen as given is called into question through the very practice of parody. Thus, IDENTITY, Butler (1990) argues, is constituted by rules of repetition. Yet it is precisely within these practices of repetitive signifying that a subversion of identity becomes possible through acts such as parody, thereby questioning the authenticity of the 'original' and dissolving the distinction between the naturalized original and the mimetic copy. The 'original' is itself constituted as the pastiche-effect of parodic practices. The parodic repetition thus exposes the illusion of naturalized identities such as gender or sexuality. The naturalness of MASCULINITY and FEMININITY, for instance, can be questioned through parodic performances by DRAG QUEENS or DRAG KINGS. However, while practices of identity such as FEMALE MASCULINITY (Halberstam 1998) or CLONES as a form of gay male hypermasculinity can be interpreted as parody, it should be remembered that they are not necessarily experienced as such by their practitioners. (**Natalia Gerodetti**)

Passing   Passing refers to subjects who transverse social IDENTIFICATIONS to purposely adopt, or inadvertently be assigned, identities other than those conferred to them by socially enforced categorizations. Passing may therefore apply to any social taxonomy, including 'SEX', gender, sexuality, 'race', ethnicity, class and religion (Sánchez and Schlossberg 2001).

Theorizations of social practices related to passing arise in the context of analyses of US slave narratives and Harlem Renaissance literature (see Gates 1987). In the texts in question, African-American subjects who pass as white are said to expose the processes though which blackness and whiteness are socially fabricated. Further, as transgression of racialized social orderings often enables progression across hierarchies of gender, sexuality and class, the intimate relation between negotiations of social taxonomies and access to power and privilege is also exposed. Passing is nevertheless dependent upon normative claims to authenticity, and hence ostracism or violence may befall those deemed at any stage to be 'inauthentic' (Ahmed 1999). As argued by Butler (1993), whether passing entails any VOLUNTARISM on the part of subjects engaged in purposeful manipulations of social identities is open to question, as any transgression occurs within a highly regulatory terrain.

Ahmed (1999: 101) notes that passing is consistently predicated upon and enabled by assumptions concerning the readability of the body and the VISIBILITY of identity. It is the existence of socially, historically and culturally specific scopic regimes and related social taxonomies that creates the conditions of possibility for passing to occur. Thus, for subjects to pass as a 'female', 'white', and/or 'straight', there has to be a presumption of ontologies of the subject and of difference grounded in ESSENTIALISM. When understood in these terms, rather than a mimetic ability of the subject to adopt identities of choice, passing appears as a technique that is 'exclusive and exclusionary' (Ahmed 2002: 108), in that some subjects may not be able to pass (ibid., 101), and some identities may be predicated on grounds other than visibility. For instance, some formulations of bisexuality note that certain signs are traditionally likely to be read as 'lesbian' or 'gay', hence leading to accusations that bisexuals are trying to pass when attempting to construct a public bi identity (Walker 1993). (**Silvia Posocco**)

Further reading

Sánchez and Schlossberg (2001).

Pederasty   Pederasty refers to homosexual desire or love between an adult male and a boy and is sometimes used interchangeably with PAEDOPHILIA, a more general term, which refers to the sexual love felt by either an adult man or woman for children of either sex. Pederasty has been a very common mode of homosexual interaction across time and cultures. In the Western tradition, ancient Greek civilization was notable for its acceptance of homosexual love between an adult male known as an *erastes* and a *paides*, or a boy in the early stages of puberty (Dover 1979) from which the term pederasty is derived (see CLASSICAL SEXUALITY). Japan, too, in the Tokugawa period (1600 to 1856) had a well-attested tradition of pederasty between adult samurai known as *nenja* and their youthful retainers or *wakashu* (Leupp 1995). In some tribal societies, such as the Sambia studied by Herdt (1984), pederastic relationships between men and boys were an obligatory part of male initiation rites. However, in all these cases, the relationships between the adults and the youths were considered temporary and did not confer a fixed 'homosexual' status on either party. Unlike in some ancient and tribal societies where pederasty was an acceptable relationship with its own etiquette and rules of conduct, in the modern world it has come to be almost universally despised as one of the most heinous of sexual crimes. Organizations such as the North American Man/Boy Love Association, while condemning child SEXUAL ABUSE, have tried to rehabilitate the practice through appeal to its widespread appeal throughout history, although gay organizations tend to distance themselves from NAMBLA because of the extreme STIGMA now associated with both pederasty and paedophilia. (**Mark McLelland**)

Penetration   See ANUS; COITAL IMPERATIVE; DAISY CHAIN; FOREPLAY; ERECTION; IMPOTENCE; PENIS; RAPE; SEXUAL PRACTICE; STRAP-ON; TRIBADISM; VAGINA; VIAGRA.

Penis   Butler (1993: 59–91) argues that the body is constructed through a process of 'imaginary anatomy', whereby powerful fantasies are attached to body parts. She cites as one example the belief that that sensitive, fleshy, and often small, organ, the penis is really that all-powerful symbol, the PHALLUS. Men may thus invest in the organ an extraordinary range of beliefs and emotions, including that its size defines their worth and that its hardness is a measure of their MASCULINITY (see IMPOTENCE). Hence male culture – both gay and straight – evinces an anxious watching of the penises of other men, in order to make comparisons (Dutton 1995: 235–6). So invested are we in the notion that the penis is the foundation of masculinity, that it was once believed that if a woman's CLITORIS became too engorged its possessor would turn into a man by sheer dint of its size (Laqueur 1990). And yet there is an ambivalence about the large penis. While routinely celebrated in porn as the epitome of masculinity, it is also an object of fear and suspicion, a tendency so widespread that it appears both in CLASSICAL Greece, where despised barbarians and satyrs are depicted with engorged penises (Dutton 1994: 40–4) and in contemporary racism, where the black male's supposed penis size is taken as a signifier of an animalistic desire. Lying beneath this ambivalence is the often expressed male fear that the penis controls its owner: that men are compelled into sexual acts and relationships not of their choosing, but under the sway of the organ. This in turn legitimates an often-used discourse around RAPE, which claims that men cannot control the pull of the penis. Feminism has insisted that men must challenge these meanings, in order to reduce the violence that they imply and learn 'dephallusized relations with women' (Pronger 1998: 77). In terms of SEXUAL PRACTICE, this may involve developing new pleasures – the feminized pleasures of NIPPLES or being anally penetrated, for instance (see STRAP ON) – or a more playful surrendering of the power of the penis to being teased and tickled. A further implication of Butler's argument is that since anatomy is always partly imaginary, it is not only biological males who can feel that a penis is part of their body. Rubin describes how FTM transsexuals can feel that they have an authentic penis, 'grown too from testosterone' (1998: 320) – but also notes that the relatively less effective technology for the surgical construction of a penis over a VAGINA suggests a residual sexism within the medical establishment that is reluctant to give away the power of the penis. (**Jo Eadie**)

Further reading

Friedman (2001).

Penis envy   The theory that women have 'penis envy' was formulated by Freud in his lecture 'On Femininity' (1933). The theory is key to an understanding of Freud's ideas about women's psychological development. He believed that a little girl's path to a healthy and socially acceptable psychological development is more tortuous and difficult than a little boy's. This for two reasons: to become a well-adjusted woman, a little girl has to change both the object of her affection, and the site of her sexual pleasure. For the little boy raised in a nuclear family, the first object of affection is the mother, whose gender is the same as the little boy's future spouse. The little girl also loves her mother, but will have to love a man when she grows up. The boy experiences pleasure by playing with his penis, and will use his penis in heterosexual intercourse as an adult. The girl enjoys playing with her CLITORIS, but will have to settle for vaginal intercourse when she grows up. Ironically, Freud's reasoning seems to imply that the healthiest thing for a girl would be to become a lesbian, who is free to love women (of her mother's gender), and to enjoy clitoral orgasms. But, since sexualities other than heterosexual were considered mental illnesses in Freud's time, Freud suggests that, as she grows up, the little girl develops penis envy, which resolves society's problems and women's psychological dilemmas. A woman who has penis envy will renounce men's privilege and access, and will transfer her desire for them onto the desire to have a baby boy, who will possess the envied organ.

Freud's theory might have applied to some of his patients, especially middle-class women in early twentieth-century Vienna, who bargained their freedom against the benefits of a good marriage, and accepted to live in the shadow of a man. However, Freud's theory mistakenly universalizes the specificity of their situation. It conflates a woman's desire to possess a penis with her desire to share in the privileges a penis afforded, including access to education and the professions, control over one's estate, liberty to travel and enjoy sex, ability to give one's family name to one's children, and jurisdiction over one's body and person. It is understandable that women might have wanted these privileges, but claiming that they would want a penis dangling between their legs is another story. Freud claimed that femininity is a riddle, but never asked women to help him solve it; as he told women in his audience at the lecture, 'you are yourselves the problem' (113).

Psychoanalytical FEMINISM grappled with this issue in the context of the nascent second-wave of the feminist movement in France. Torok's (1992) confutation of Freud's theory claims that it reflects his own PHALLOCENTRISM rather than any female characteristic. Cixous (1973) represented a woman's body as an integrated whole, devoid of the 'appendage' that makes men feel vulnerable. (**Serena Anderlini-D'Onofrio**)

Further reading

Mitchell (1974: Chapter 8).

Performance   An actualization or demonstration of (gendered) IDENTITY in order to connect with other(s) sexually or socially or communicate dramatically a particular message. All identity hinges on some degree of physical and linguistic performance: unlike mere expressiveness, performance implies an audience and an intended message. Performance implies a self-consciousness of the production of this message as well as a possible pleasure. It is both more general and personal in application than the ritual enactments of carnival or other culturally-posited practices; the latter connote a certain participation in a collective through ritualized acts with potentially subversive and constitutive signification. Performance in sexual acts connotes proficiency, ERECTION, ability to achieve ORGASM or other pleasurable states (e.g. EJACULATION, FEMALE EJACULATION, EROGENOUS ZONES). Performance in terms of gender (see PERFORMATIVITY) is an intentional act expressing gender based on the understanding of gender-identified behaviour. Ideally such acts have political implications in that they question the validity or dependability of established sex/gender roles. Thus, the DRAG QUEEN or DRAG KING provides an excellent example of the tragi-celebratory potential of performance to articulate an identity based on social and cultural codes and presuppositions about biological or essentialized sexual identity and the breaking or subversion of these. Also compare BUTCH, CAMP, CROSS-DRESSING, CRUISING, FANTASY, FEMME, FLANEUR/FLANEUSE. Since the 1980s, gender performance has been keenly explored in theory (e.g. Butler 1990, 1999; Jagose 1996). (**Susan K. Mooney**)

Further reading

Parker and Sedgwick (1995).

Performativity   The potential for change and diversity based on the power of PERFOR-MANCE to convey gendered identity according to the self-conscious, stylized expression of the subject. J. L. Austin (1962), in the context of speech act theory and his classic *How To Do Things with Words*, coined this term. For Austin, performativity exceeds 'expressiveness' or 'mimicry': it implies authorial intention and creates a new relation or set of relations. A performative is a sign that contributes to identity and to an action or the development of a relation between the subject and other(s). One of Austin's examples of a performative speech act is that of a minister performatively stating: 'I pronounce you man and wife'. Like all signifying speech acts, performatives depend on the participants understanding particular social contexts in order to accept, reject, or subvert the potential value of these. Austin recognizes the possible misapprehensions of such acts as well as ironic variations of performative acts. Butler (1990) has extended Austin's semiotic performativity to that of the field of gender identity: she asserts that all gendered identity is performative in that gender is acquired socially and culturally. It can thus be learnt, expressed, parodied, or re-interpreted by anyone regardless of sex and gender. In QUEER THEORY, performative can be considered virtually constitutive of queerness, in that queer identity rejects an innate ESSENTIALISM and rather is highly conscious of its acts which perform gender or develop a gendered relation (Jagose 1996; Parker and Sedgewick 1995). See, for example, CAMP, GENDER BLEND-ING, FEMININITY, GENDERFUCK, LESBIAN GENDER, QUEER.

At first blush, performativity seems to complement Freud's basic concept of POLY-MORPHOUS PERVERSITY, i.e. that everyone's sexuality derives from the organization of drives which are not at first connected to a particular gendered sexuality. However, performativity emphasizes the supposed agency of the subject to select identity; given such privileging of the notion of a fully-conscious, autonomous self, the experience of the unconscious is not prioritized. Performativity asserts a political agenda against gender norms, and BINARY conceptions of sexuality. In contrast to the SEXUAL POLITICS of the mid-twentieth century (whose aim was the achievement of civil and human rights) performativity posits itself as non-essentializing or 'free-floating'. The potential tautology occurs when performativity reiterates expressions of norms, thus confirming the power of these to signify in ways that organize our social being, and also ignoring the unconscious forces that also contribute to our sexual and gendered ways of being. At its worst, performativity can be viewed as a desire to mimic established power through over-valuation of the subject. (**Susan K. Mooney**)

Further reading

Parker and Sedgwick (1995).

Perverse dynamic   Coined by Dollimore (1991), who argues that modern culture defines various sexual acts and desires as perverse or unnatural. Once these acts are specified as perverse, a wide range of social mechanisms come into effect to monitor groups and individuals for signs of these transgressions, and to punish or educate them into changing. However Dollimore suggests that as a result, we come to experience PERVERSION as a potential that exists inside us all, and contrary to the attempts to render certain desires or practices unthinkable, they in fact become our obsession, gaining visibility and power through the processes that attempt to marginalize them. The 'perverse dynamic' refers to the paradoxical effect of this forbidding: the culture which tries to expel certain behaviours, in fact makes those behaviours essential to the social and psychic life of all its members. This model may therefore be seen as closely related to Foucault's notion of perverse implantation (1990: 36–49), in which professionals concerned with sexual hygiene encourage us to see ourselves as having sexual problems which we must identify and then attempt to cure, leading to a CONFESSIONAL SOCIETY in which so-called DEVIANCE gains visibility. (**Jo Eadie**)

Perversion   A term from nineteenth-century SEXOLOGY and PSYCHOANALYSIS for all forms of DESIRE and SEXUAL PRACTICE that differ from a designated norm – now largely replaced by the term PARAPHILIA. With growing liberalization, certain activities once regarded as perversions have now become legitimate SEXUAL ORIENTATIONS (e.g. homosexuality) while others remain STIGMATIZED. Politically, the concept of the perversion has a policing function: like the idea of DEVIANCE, it defines those activities that fall outside social respectability in order to discourage them. The correlation of this is that 'if only the "perverted" is forbidden, then anything not forbidden becomes compulsory' (Carol 1993: 153): we are all expected to take part in reproductive, penetrative, heterosexual intercourse.

In the psychoanalytic account, perversion is an attempt to deny CASTRATION: that is to deny that there is a SEXUAL DIFFERENCE between men and women. The seeking of pleasure other than in heterosexual penetration is seen as a way of avoiding recognition of this difference: the male MASOCHIST, for instance, is said to be avoiding recognizing his DOMINATRIX as a woman (Kaplan 1993). Conversely, sexology views perversion as having a wider range of possible origins – sometimes genetic, sometimes a response to childhood trauma, sometimes merely curiosity. Practitioners within both disciplines take different attitudes to the social place of perversions: some regarding them as benign sexual variations, others more concerned with cure and treatment. The term has been reclaimed by the SEX RADICAL movement as an ironic term for socially stigmatized pleasures. One crucial difference between these usages is that where psychoanalysis and sexology view perversion as compulsive, sex radicals are more likely to argue that their perverse sexual practice is playful and chosen (Adams 1996: 27–48).

In his highly influential account of the history of perversion, Foucault (1990) argues that these differences are less significant than the combined overall effect of the various professions who suddenly took an interest in sexual phenomena. He suggests that while their aim was to outlaw, punish, and cure these sexual activities, the effect of this attention was firstly to make perversions more visible and stable within the social order; secondly to make more people likely to suspect themselves of a perverse potential (see PERVERSE DYNAMIC); and finally to enable perversion to become the basis of an IDENTITY and of campaigns for rights and SEXUAL CITIZENSHIP. (**Jo Eadie**)

Further reading

Dollimore (1990).

Phallic mother   The phallic mother is a PRE-OEDIPAL construct of FANTASY embodying a synthesis of all facets of infantile psychosexual development. In Freud's account of infantile development, all children experience a phallic stage in which they believe themselves to possess a PENIS regardless of their sex. It is during this phase that children formulate the fantasy of the phallic mother who is deemed either to be endowed with an external PHALLUS or phallic attribute or to have somehow preserved the male's phallus inside her. In considering the PSYCHOANALYTIC account, it is important to remember that the child is not yet fully aware of the fact of gender and/or SEXUAL DIFFERENCE. The phallic mother is construed as an omnipotent figure positioned to be able to grant the child her/his every wish and to function as its object of desire. The child also fantasizes that the phallic mother desires her/him as a sexual object. The plenitude associated with this period is shattered by the onset of the OEDIPUS COMPLEX because the child suddenly becomes aware of sexual difference and is no longer able to maintain the fantasy of the maternal phallus. At this point, the omnipotence associated with the phallic mother is displaced onto the father figure and the mother comes to be regarded as 'CASTRATED'. However, the archaic memory of the relation with the phallic mother comes to constitute our ultimate desire insofar as we seek to regress to the blissful state of union with her. The phallic mother is also associated with the perceived threat of the female genitalia to masculine power and male sexuality and she can easily become a persecutory figure of anxiety. A return to the state of fusion with the phallic mother thus occupies a paradoxical position in the psychoanalytic account of heterosexual male DESIRE. Men aspire to this state as much as women do, but such fusion would entail the surrender of masculinity itself and also a willingness to incorporate the mother's desire for the father. The struggle against such a fantasy can be seen as underpinning the exhibition of HOMOPHOBIA. (**Caroline Bainbridge**)

Further reading

Creed (1993).

Phallocentrism   A term that is used to describe the promotion of the masculine as the root of power, meaning and value in culture, ideology and society. The term is associated with patriarchal power, and, following the perspective set out in the work of French psychoanalyst Jacques Lacan, it can be understood as relating to the dominant law of the father that characterizes patriarchal society. In Lacan's (1977b) account, the PHALLUS is the signifier of power, meaning and DESIRE. His idea is based on Freud's (1908) observations about the role of the PENIS in the formation of sexual identity. Given that the boy has a penis and the girl does not, Lacan builds on Freud's ideas to suggest that the phallus is the key term by which we should understand the relative positions and values of masculinity and femininity. Lacan argues that the phallus is not the same as the the the penis in Freud's account. Rather, it is a linguistic signifier of the cultural value of the penis. Lacan asserts his view that no-one actually possesses the phallus, since it is only ever a symbol. However, because men seem to have the phallus, they become dominant. Women, on the other hand, are seen to lack the phallus and are consequently situated as other in relation to a masculine norm. Phallocentrism, then, alludes to any aspect of patriarchal society and culture which regards men and masculine characteristics as central and normative. In such a system, women and the feminine come to be seen as marginal and of less value.

Phallocentrism is a monolithic system in which the phallus is privileged as the key signifier of sexuality and power and in which presence is valued over absence. The term is also applied outside the realm of PSYCHOANALYSIS. For example, the stress on the penis and EJACULATION as central to sex at the expense of other aspects of the male body (e.g. anal sex, nipples) can be seen as phallocentric. Similarly, obsession with penis size as the signifier of sexual prowess and the desexualization of lesbian sex which occurs because men assume that sex that does not involve a penis can't be 'real' sex at all are further examples. (**Caroline Bainbridge**)

Phallus   The phallus is an image of the male reproductive organ existing in culture with a symbolic significance. It is related to the anatomical concept of the PENIS. Phallic rituals have existed since antiquity, as in the Dionysian festivals.

The concept has been widely used and developed in PSYCHOANALYSIS. Lacan (1977b) started off with Freud's idea that women have PENIS ENVY, and, having realized they cannot get a penis, desire a male child who has it. Lacan moved Freud's idea from the physical/psychological level to the socio-symbolic level. For both Freud and

Lacan, woman represents the absence of a penis, therefore a lack, or the image of a castrated man. The phallus is a mirror image of the penis that symbolizes the fear of castration; it is also the symbol of this lack. Therefore, to enjoy the phallus one must not 'be it'. Since the mother desires the phallus, the little boy tries to be it to satisfy her. Being the phallus makes one unable to exchange it, and exchanging the phallus makes one a player in the network of exchanges that constitutes socio-symbolic power. In this view, having a penis does not automatically enable one to exchange the phallus. A BUTCH LESBIAN who fucks her partner with a DILDO is a subject in the exchange, whereas the little boy who tries to be the phallus for his mother is not (see Reich 1999).

The concept of the phallus has also entered critical theory via PHALLOCENTRISM and phallogocentrism. Both concepts were used in Derridean deconstruction to point to the centrality of the phallus in modern cultural discourse. The second term emphasized the connection between the phallus and logos, or the word 'logic'. It indicated that discourse is inflected in the masculine even as we think of it as neutral, non-gendered. (**Serena Anderlini-D'Onofrio**)

Piercing   As one of the many practices associated with contemporary trends in body modification, piercing involves the deliberate anchoring of physical objects in and through the SKIN. While piercing has long been a touchstone of tribal cultures and the rites of passage specific to them, it has only been in the last 30 years that the Western piercing scene has 'exploded from an obscure, partially illegal, underground activity – specifically associated with the gay, FETISH, and modern primitive subcultures – into a major cultural phenomenon affecting the mainstream' (Housk 2002: 7). Evidence of the West's widespread embrace of body piercing abounds in popular culture and everyday life: piercing is now commonly used to enhance both the body's aesthetics and the sensations emanating from the body's EROGENOUS ZONES. It should be noted, however, that piercing – as both a process and an artefact – remains bound up in the elaboration of culturally marginalized sexualities. In the gay male community, for instance, ear piercing was from the 1960s to the 1980s considered a major signifier of homosexual identity and solidarity (Housk 2002: 9). And, as Green (1999) shows, piercing is still viewed by gays and lesbians as an important way to resist the REPRESSIONS and erasures of HETERONORMATIVITY. In these contexts, then, piercing produces the QUEER body as recognizable and distinct, and functions as a sort of embodied challenge to the West's prevailing codes of sexual conduct. Piercing is also a vital component of both homosexual and heterosexual sadomasochistic (SM) rituals. Here piercing enables a sensual exploration of pleasure and pain and, ultimately, discloses the pierced partner as completely given over to or owned by his or her dominant partner (Housk 2002). In general terms, piercing can be seen as a multifaceted pursuit that is at once psychological and physiological, superficial and profound. While it can, for some people, function as little more than an accessory, for others, piercing constitutes a full-scale attempt at reclaiming corporeal experience and expanding the boundaries of the embodied self. (**Marc Lafrance**)

Further reading

Featherstone (2000).

pill, The   A birth-control drug containing a combination of oestrogen and/or progestin (progesterone), also known as oral CONTRACEPTIVES. The pill works mainly by preventing ovulation, however it also causes cervical mucus to thicken, preventing the easy passage of sperm to the cervix and alters the lining of the womb so that even if a fertilized egg arrived, implantation would be highly unlikely. Side effects such as weight-gain, nausea, headaches, decreased libido and depression have been attributed to using an unsuitable pill brand or type – although some feminists argue that the safety of the contraceptive pill for women has yet to be guaranteed (Clarke 2000). In 1960 the FDA approved its use on the public market in America which was followed a year later by its introduction in Europe. Its popularity grew fast (despite condemnation by the Catholic Church); within ten years over 12 million women were using the drug. Women could now control their own contraception independent of the sexual act, no longer depending on their partners to take precautions. Occurring alongside the widespread legalization of ABORTION, the pill is often taken to have facilitated new sexual and economic freedoms, while disengaging sex from its reproductive framework and reframing it as a RECREATIONAL activity (Segal 1994: 8–12). However Watkins (1998) suggests that the arrival of the pill merely coincided with a revolution in attitudes to sex that were already underway.

While it remains the most widely used form of contraception in the developed world it has led to questions about exactly how much freedom it bestows on women. Has it burdened women with sole responsibility for something they would rather share with a partner? Since the pill offers no protection against STDs, has it actually exacerbated the frequency of their transmission leading to the situation where both barrier method and pill should be used (see SAFE(R) SEX)? Has it encouraged men to regard women as sexually available? Attempts to redress this male–female imbalance with regard to contraception and protection from STDs are currently in trial stages with the development of the male pill. (**Linda Kiernan**)

Further reading

Marks (2001).

Pimp   The term 'pimp' is hardly ever used among people who work in the SEX INDUSTRY. It is a term coined by outsiders and researchers to refer to those who exploit or manage the labour of sex workers. Note that the term 'pimp' is, in theoretical terms, unhelpful because it collapses too many types of people – or 'third parties' – into one stigmatized category. This reduces the opportunity to understand the important and different influences that these actors may have on the life and working conditions of sex workers. Most sex workers rely on the support of third parties in their work – many third parties are crucial to the protection and safety of sex workers and to the provision of SEX WORK itself (Pheterson 1993: 55–7). In countries where sex work is criminalized it becomes an underground activity which may and often does attract criminal elements. Many sex workers, since they cannot count on the protection of the police, have to rely on the protection of 'pimps' – against abusers and even police harassment. However, some third parties, since they are not regulated by the law, can and do exploit sex workers. The latter have usually no legal mechanism to address exploitation. A good BROTHEL owner or 'pimp' is one who provides good working conditions and pay, just like any other good employer. There is nothing inherently exploitative about sex work, but its status and sex workers' lack of civil and industrial rights offer few mechanisms to limit the behaviour of bad employers. Relationships vary greatly between sex workers, their employers and other third parties, including even those defined as 'traffickers' (Bindman 1997): slavery is at one end of the continuum and very good business arrangements are at the other. Stereotypes, simple labels and moralistic analyses can obscure the multiple realities within sex work. 'Pimping' is outlawed in countries where PROSTITUTION is either prohibited or criminalized. In the United Kingdom, for instance, legislation states that anyone 'living off the immoral earnings of prostitution' can be prosecuted. The legislation has been criticized as it impedes sex workers from having a normal family life – since partners and grown-up children are vulnerable to such prosecution. (**Ana Lopes**)

Further reading

Kempado and Doezma (1998).

Plastic sexuality   Coined by Giddens (1992a), 'plastic sexuality' refers to sexuality 'freed' from the needs of reproduction: sexuality, or more accurately SEXUAL PRACTICE, becomes an avenue of self-expression and self-realization, rather than being closely tied to propagation. Birth control and CONTRACEPTION occupy a key position in Giddens's argument, principally as means to unlock women's sexual pleasure; he thus points to the sexual revolution as a turning point in the remaking of 'PURE RELATIONSHIPS'. In linking sexuality with self-identity, Giddens also pays homage to Sigmund Freud, crediting PSYCHOANALYSIS with the 'discovery' of plastic sexuality. Other key figures for Giddens in this context include Marcuse and Reich, both of whom present visions of non-repressive societies in which Giddens spies traces of plastic sexuality – sexuality used for personal and interpersonal pleasure, as part of what Giddens calls 'the radical democratization of the personal' (1992a: 182). Moreover, plastic sexuality can be equated with the movement away from the COITAL IMPERATIVE: away from the ideal of sex as penis–vagina intercourse, and from the rule of the PHALLUS. Although he relies solely on anecdotal reportage to access data, Giddens discusses homosexuality in the light of plastic sexuality, too; and at times points towards lesbian and gay relationships as models – especially given what he sees as their complete separation of sex from reproduction. The key point to his discussion, however, is to explore the reshaping of sexual intimacy in the light of other personal and social transformations – and to attempt to understand the relationship of a phenomenon like plastic sexuality to these broader processes. (**David Bell**)

Pleasure and danger   See SEX (II); SEX WARS.

Polari   Also spelt Palare, Palari, Parlare, Palarie, a secret form of language, mainly spoken by gay men, DRAG QUEENS and lesbians in the United Kingdom in the twentieth century. Derived from numerous lexicons associated with stigmatized subcultures (PROSTITUTES, beggars, travelling actors and seafarers), Polari most likely evolved out of Parlyaree, a form of slang used by some members of the above groups, which itself was influenced by Elizabethan Cant, Italian (Hancock 1984: 395) and other European languages. Over the first half of the twentieth century, Polari became established as a form of theatrical language, used in music halls and later the West End revue theatres of London (some heterosexual entertainers also used it). Other influences on Polari at different times have included rhyming slang (popularly associated with the East End of London), back slang (the practice of saying a word as if it is spelt backwards), were Yiddish, American Airforce slang and the slang of 1960s drug users (Burton 1985: 40). In addition to this, gay men and lesbians added numerous words associated with homosexuality. Popular lexical items include: *bona* (nice), *eek/ecaf* (face) *riah* (hair), *lallies* (legs), *vada* (see/look), *nanti* (no/none/don't), *ajax* (next to), *troll* (walk), *naff* (tasteless), *cod* (awful) and *fantabulosa* (great).

For many people, Polari functioned as a lexicon of evaluation, allowing its users to gossip about the sexual attractiveness and availability of other people while they were still present. Adjectives for example, tended to contain evaluative loadings, rather than being neutral descriptors. Polari allowed people to cautiously express their sexual identities, or to be outrageously and openly CAMP. While Polari is usually classed as a lexicon rather than a language, there is some evidence to suggest that adept speakers employed a telegraphic style of grammar, which made it different from English (Baker 2002). It is certainly the case that different varieties of Polari existed at different times.

Polari was popularized and publicized by the BBC Radio comedy programme *Round the Horne* (1964–9) where it was spoken by two camp characters called Julian and Sandy (Lucas 1997: 87). By the 1970s, perhaps as a result of media over-exposure, the partial decriminalization of homosexuality in 1967, and a move away from camp identities within the gay scene, Polari gradually declined in usage. By the 1990s, a small revival of interest in Polari had recast it as an important piece of British gay her-itage. (**Paul Baker**)

Further reading

Baker (2002).

Political lesbianism   A movement and identity that emerged from 1970s FEMINISM and the rise of SEPARATISM as a challenge to the organization of women's lives by men. A political lesbian declares her independence from the HETEROPATRIARCHAL world of mas-culine values, and chooses as a political statement to bond herself to other women instead. As such, she is 'lesbian' in the sense that she values the primacy of emotional, social and political bonds between women and has taken a conscious decision to exclude male control, intimidation and violence from her life. It may also be a decision to explore sexual love with other women, but need not be so – although even for women not sexually attracted to other women, it is often the case that political les-bianism may lead to desire, coming out of the experiences of intimacy created by shared social and political action. It thus testifies to the SOCIAL CONSTRUCTION of sexual-ity, which changes as new social possibilities emerge, in this case the culture of WOMAN-IDENTIFIED WOMEN which made 'elective' lesbianism feasible (Faderman 1991: 204–9). Although crucial for freeing many women from the restrictive bonds of heterosexual-ity, political lesbianism has remained controversial. Firstly, some heterosexual and bisexual women have queried whether this identity holds itself up as the superior form of political identity over those of other feminists: for instance, there has been much debate over whether Ti-Grace Atkinson's famous slogan was: 'feminism is the theory, lesbianism is the practice' – implying that all feminists *must* choose lesbianism – or 'feminism is a theory, lesbianism is a practice' (Hutchins and Ka'ahumanu (eds) 1990: xxiv). Secondly, some lesbians have objected to political lesbianism on the grounds that it DESEXUALIZES lesbianism and APPROPRIATES an authentically sexual lesbian identity for the benefit of straight women (Jeffreys 1993: 77–8). (**Jo Eadie**)

Polyamory   Polyamory is a state of being, an awareness, and/or a lifestyle that involves mutually acknowledged, simultaneous relationships of a romantic and/or sexual nature between more than two persons (Bloomquist 2000; Loving More 2002a). As a lifestyle, polyamory came to prominence in the 1980s and 1990s, when, especially in the Western United States, many NON-MONOGAMOUS sexual players came together to found polyamorous communities. Later on, similar groups were estab-lished in a variety of US and non-US regions (Loving More 2002b). Historically, polyamory has been practised in cultures governed by polygamy, a person's ability to have more than one spouse. Polygamy includes varieties like polygyny, a person's abil-ity to have more than one wife, and polyandry, a person's ability to have more than one husband. The first has been common in many Islamic societies, the second in pre-colonial, indigenous, and pre-historic societies. In contrast to POSTMODERN polyamory, in these older social orders, polygamy was a social norm and not a personal choice (Bloomquist 2000). Various cultural influences and developments have made the recent growth of polyamorous communities possible. They include: New-Age spirituality, with its emphasis on taking into one's hands one's relationship with the sacred, and with its disregard for religious doctrine; New Paganism and Wiccan religions, with their rejection of monotheism and openness to polytheistic belief systems and pantheistic spiritualities; the FEMINIST movement, with its emphasis on disclosure, equality, and consent; the bisexual movement, with its awareness of bisexual behaviour in both gay and straight communities; and, finally, the AIDS crisis, with its accompanying fear of infection from sexually-transmitted lethal pathogens, and its attendant SAFE(R) SEX ethics. Polyamorous people can be exclusively lesbian, gay, or bisexual, yet their efforts to get past the limitations of MONOGAMY erode set BINARISMS, including the myth that being part of a closed dyad is the only authentic form of love. Polyamory can be seen as a new word for non-monogamy that turns a negative into a positive, thus honouring people's capability to share and multiply their love and honest an consensual ways, regardless of prevalent social norms, and in full awareness of a partner's need for safety and emotional centeredness. (**Serena Anderlini-D'Onofrio**)

Further reading

Anapol (1997).

Polyfidelity   Polyfidelity is a form of POLYAMORY in which a group of people are emotionally and/or sexually faithful to one another. The group who shares emotional and/or sexual involvements is called an expanded family. Its members have multiple sexual partners, but their sexual activity is either completely restricted to members of the group, or permitted with outsiders only with the approval of other group members. Expanded families can be organized in group marriages, TRIADS, dyads, and other kinds of open or closed arrangements: group marriages involve a number of partners in the same type of group commitment; triads involve three members; dyads involve two members who practise NON-MONOGAMY. In each case, members choose various degrees of openness to outside partners. For example, two members in a given expanded family may establish a primary, secondary or tertiary relationship between themselves. Primary relationships involve a high degree of commitment, as in marriage. Secondary relationships can be close and ongoing, but the degree of commitment is lower. Tertiary relationships can be emotional and/or sexual, with a minimum degree of involvement. Polyfidelity describes the degree of commitment in the relationship among members in an expanded family group. While members may agree on engaging in secondary and/or tertiary relationships with persons not part of the group, they also agree to be primarily involved with group members only (Bloomquist, 2000; Loving More, 2002c). (Serena Anderlini-D'Onofrio)

Polymorphous perversity In PSYCHOANALYTIC thought, this term describes the relatively unorganized state of sexual and libidinal drives and desires in a human being. It is usually used in the context of infantile sexuality to describe the ways in which children in particular are prone to direct their libidinal energies at any object that may be used to provide pleasure. In the Freudian account, sexual pleasure is defined as any pleasure experienced on or through the body, and is not limited to genital pleasure (Freud 1905b). The polymorphously perverse child actively seeks pleasure as it is not yet subject to the constraints of REPRESSION. Polymorphous perversity is thought to evolve as a child moves through various psychosexual stages of development, such as the oral, anal and phallic phases. In the oral stage, for example, pleasure is taken from sucking and biting. In the anal stage, there is an emphasis on the control of the sphincter, leading to pleasure in control and in the sensations of the anal region of the body. It is possible to become fixated on any one of these stages, and all the pleasures associated with these stages persist into adult sexuality. Fixation, however, is usually interpreted as leading to PARAPHILIAC sexualities. Polymorphous perversity is also important in the context of PANSEXUALITY, where the term is used positively in alternative sexual communities to describe a more liberated mode of adult sexuality. (**Caroline Bainbridge**)

Pomosexual Both as a noun and as an adjective, 'pomosexual' means 'postmodern sexual', describing a new contemporary experience of sexual identity. Queen and Schimel (1997) are so encouraged by this concept that they advocate the power of pomosexuals to cross the boundaries of sex, gender, and sexuality – leading for instance, to MALE LESBIANS. Postmodernism problematizes many notions often taken for granted, such as IDENTITY and intentionality. It is often assumed that identities are stable (for instance, men are considered to be always male) and that people can control their intentions, or egos (for instance, a certain woman has the intention to be a STONE BUTCH). Yet in the light of pomosexuality, neither identity nor ego is stable. Since identity and intention, two coordinates in life, are destabilized, life seems to be threatened. Nonetheless, a life without secured identity and intention might be closer to our everyday experience – how do you know that your soccer coach is not a transsexual person in the CLOSET? The claims of the pomosexuals animate the imagination of new identities, as if identities were masquerade costumes that people can freely try on and take off. However, this supposition is predicated upon the belief that people can control their intentions: 'I' intend to become a stone butch – how can we guarantee that 'I' and my intention are not as transient as the identities? In the pomosexual age, the identities and the intentions are similarly out of control. Hence the pomosexual paradox: before my ego wants to choose identities, my ego might fall apart as identities do. (**Ta-wei Chi**)

Pornography   Formally, pornography can be defined as representations of sexual activity or sexualized bodies. Yet this immediately raises questions. How much skin needs to be shown before an image is pornographic? What counts as sexual activity – a lingering kiss or a love-bite? Are certain works of so-called 'high culture' pornographic when RAPE occurs in them, or when there is NUDITY in a painting? Can medical material be pornographic? Some vagueness of definition suits the state, since it allows charges of OBSCENITY to be brought for political ends, and in current scares over Internet child pornography it is clear how far the strong feelings aroused by the term are used to justify new laws and policies (for instance, the monitoring of e-mail by employers).

One key contemporary distinction is between hard and soft core. Hard core pornography records 'real' sex acts taking place: instances of ORAL SEX, MASTURBATION, penetration and ejaculation (see MONEY SHOT), with clear representations of the genitals. Soft core is defined by its absence of those feature: bodies are partially exposed, and no actual sex occurs. While many countries outlaw hard core material, soft core porn has effectively been legalized across most of the world, often by claiming to be part of the more respectable category EROTICA. Soft core imagery has become a staple of global media, to the point where it has ceased to be a meaningful category, bearing out Dworkin's (1981) contention that hegemonic representations of women are all fundamentally pornographic.

The debates around pornography within SEXUAL POLITICS can be understood as a series of questions – on which campaigners take different, and more or less rigid positions (see SEX WARS). A partial list of these follows. In a world structured by misogyny, can there be representations of sex which do not demean women? Can performers make free choices to enter pornography as a legitimate employment or does the SEX INDUSTRY make use of economic and psychological vulnerability to coerce them (Cornell 2000a: 8–9)? Is it safe to give the state the right to censor sexual material, particularly since much anti-pornography legislation has been part of governmental attempts to clamp down on SAFE(R) SEX material or public representations of gay and lesbian sex (Patton 1996: 118–38)? Are there innumerable pornographies, each with their own rules, agendas, and styles (Barker 2000), or is there behind these superficial differences one single theme: the humiliation of women and the OBJECTIFICATION of the female body (Dworkin 1981)? Should pornography be analysed in terms of the wide ranging interpretations that its viewers put on it (Strossen 1995), or in terms of its underlying thematic: sex is an act of control (Dworkin 1981)? Can gay and lesbian pornographies embody different attitudes or do they repeat the same conventions as HETEROSEXUAL pornography (Williams 1990: Chapter 8)? Does pornography play a key role in shaping male and female sexuality, or is it merely an effect of deeper social inequalities (Russell 2000)? (**Jo Eadie**)

Further reading

Cornell (2000b).

Post-gay   Post-gay is a term that comes with a built-in presupposition: that all identities – including, therefore, gay IDENTITY – are SOCIALLY CONSTRUCTED, historically contingent categories. Post-gay, then, signals that the historic moment that belonged to gay is passing. A corollary of this is the recognition that gay is an inadequate term for understanding all expressions of same-sex passion. Although not the first to deploy the term, Sinfield (1998) argues that 'gay' is a historical phenomenon born of the increasing strength of homosexual subcultures in North America and North-Western Europe. As such, gay denotes a Western, metropolitan identity (1998: 6–7) that pertains in a particular period. Sinfield analyses four current challenges (posed by racial minorities, the Queer movement, bisexuals, and men who have sex with men/women who have sex with women); explores how, from each of these quarters, gay has seemed inadequate; and argues that the depth of these inadequacies, hence the strength of the criticisms of gay that arise from them, demands 'a reconsideration of our post-Stonewall identities' (1998: 14). Sinfield differentiates his argument from that articulated in the controversial collection of essays, *Anti-Gay* (Simpson 1996) (see ANTI-GAY). For others, such as Scheide (2002) post-gay primarily signifies the belief that understanding individuals in terms of their sexual identity is inherently limiting and, therefore, politically undesirable (see also HETEROFLEXIBLE, BICURIOUS). He sees 'the first principle of post-gayness [as] the notion that homosexuals should be able to define their identities by something other than sexual preference' (2002: 2). While the phenomenon described by Scheide and the position taken by Simpson announce (albeit to varying degrees) the end of an allegiance to gay subculture, Sinfield's argument is that 'a more intelligent and critical subculture' (1998: 16) is needed. (**Chris West**)

Postmodern sexuality   This latest, contemporary phase of the social change of sexuality can best be thought of as an intensification of the features that define the period of MODERN SEXUALITY. Following Foucault's (1990) claim that existing power structures depend on our placing sexuality at the centre of our subjectivity, we can see how the triumph of consumer culture encourages us to think of our sexualities in the same way we think of our purchases: temporary sources of individual pleasure. Postmodern society is marked by faster changes in the types of careers, relationships and fashions in which its citizens engage, and rapid changes in our sense of who and what we can be lead to greater FLUIDITY in our sexualities also (Edwards 1994: 142). From the collapse of the ideal of lifelong MONOGAMY, to the marketing of SM paraphernalia as a new accessory in sex shops, we are encouraged to think of our sex lives as places of constant change and innovation. As a result, formerly clear forms of sexual IDENTITY become less secure and the concept of a lifelong SEXUAL ORIENTATION becomes less meaningful. In its place, sexuality becomes like a marketplace in which new practices and identities are explored and discarded at will. This change in turn loosens the assumed fixity of old identities allowing for new forms of HYBRIDITY such as the oxymoronic identities LESBIAN BOY and MALE LESBIAN (Zita 1998).

In terms of sexual theory, this is accompanied by the decline of ESSENTIALIST positions and the rise to prominence of SOCIAL CONSTRUCTIONIST accounts, in which all aspects of sex and gender are viewed as created by temporary social formations, and therefore open to change as society changes. Consequently, SEXUAL LIBERATION movements have shifted their emphasis away from calling for the social legitimacy of alternative sexualities, and towards calling for a social recognition that sexuality itself must be understood firstly as an inalienable individual right, hence entailing new modes of SEXUAL CITIZENSHIP (Bell and Binnie 2000); and secondly that existing social structures are inadequate for delivering this since they are tainted by rigid sexual assumptions, that pervade every aspect of the organization of the workplace, schools, and government policy (Warner 1999) – a position epitomized by QUEER THEORY.

The liberation of sex from procreation, that began with modern improvements in CONTRACEPTION means that sex is no longer a 'natural act' (Tiefer 1995) limited by 'natural' rules, but is instead a place of free choice and imagination – phrases which reveal how much postmodern sexuality is influenced by the logics of the free market economy which shapes it. Transsexuality has been cited as only the most obvious instance of this change. While some TRANS THEORISTS have welcomed this argument that transsexuality is the emblem of the postmodern (Stone 1991), others have suggested that it trivializes what is a deeply felt and innate gender identity by making it appear merely cosmetic (Prosser 1998). This in turn raises the question of whether the postmodern account of sexuality is in fact accurate: are our identities and our bodies less secure or less deeply felt? And if they are, is this necessarily liberating or might it be a terrifying prospect? To give only two examples, the rise of forms of VIRTUAL SEX has enabled the global sex trade to flourish, and the citizens of poorer countries – particularly women – become drawn into a marketplace where sexual services are sold globally on the Internet. Similarly, new sexual health crises – particularly the AIDS CRISIS – are reminders that sexual pleasure is not simply part of a hedonistic lifestyle choice, but puts our mortal bodies on the line. Postmodern sex thus remains caught up in relations of power which protect some social groups from the worst effects of these changes, while leaving others ever more vulnerable (Sinfield 1998: 198) – contrast, for instance, the West's treatment of AIDS through expensive drug regimes with the lack of treatment available across Africa. The fears around sexuality that the modern period inaugurated have intensified to the point that Kroker and Kroker (1987) have coined the term 'panic sex' to describe the shared feeling that sexuality is too unstable to provide us with a secure sense of self, or a refuge from the more mundane areas of our lives. Many groups respond to these changes by an attempt to reassert sexual values from earlier periods, such as the resurgence of a Christian promotion of VIRGINITY and the New Right's call for FAMILY VALUES – resistant counter-movements attempting to halt these postmodern changes, whose hostility has become a symptom of a newly polarized sexual landscape. (**Jo Eadie**)

Further reading

Queen and Schimel (1997).

Pregnancy   Pregnancies tend to be divided into the welcomed and the disapproved those pregnancies which occur in the confines of married, heterosexual relationships to women in approved social groups (in terms of race, class, age, and disability) are approved, and all others are not. Pregnancies straddle the PUBLIC/PRIVATE distinction They are thought of as private domestic events, yet subject to public policing, since society is considered to have an interest in the foetuses pregnant women bear Theoretical work on pregnancy began with a focus on questions about foetuses (questions about ABORTION, in particular). Feminist work investigates why pregnancy is thought to be primarily about foetuses and seeks to focus on women's experiences during pregnancy. A great deal of feminist thought has been devoted to critiquing the medicalization of pregnancy and birth (Martin 1987). Psychoanalytic (Kristeva 1982) and phenomenological approaches (Young 1984) have been used to investigate women's experiences of pregnancy. Some feminist moral theorizing about pregnancy draws upon an ethics of care tradition and focuses as much or more on women's experiences of pregnancy as on questions about foetal rights or foetal personhood. Work in sociology and anthropology examines such topics as how new diagnostic techniques alter women's experiences of pregnancy, and how women give meaning to pregnancy loss, in a culture that discourages discussion of the topic. Huntley (2000) argues that women's sexuality in pregnancy is similarly relatively unexplored, in part because of the pervasive influence of the Madonna/WHORE dichotomy, such that women are not supposed to be sexual in their role as mothers (see Longhurst 1998) Gender identity becomes very salient in pregnancy, with some experiencing GENDER EUPHORIA and others (especially female-to-male TRANSSEXUALS) experiencing GENDER DYSPHORIA. (**Amy Mullin**)

Premodern sexuality   A general term used to indicate the period leading up to the European industrial revolution of the eighteenth century. Viewed by some as comprising both the MEDIEVAL and the EARLY MODERN periods (roughly 500 AD to 1700 AD) premodern may also include, though less commonly, the CLASSICAL period. Boswell (1995: xix), for example, uses premodern to describe the time between the Greco-Roman world and industrial Europe, and implies that premodern and non-industrial societies have similar sexual moralities. The idea of a premodern sexuality suggests continuity over time rather than the traditionally studied compartmentalized stages of Classical, medieval, or early modern history. Murray (1996: xii–xiii) argues that intellectual, economic, and political developments throughout history lessen the value of broad temporal studies for those historical disciplines, though the history of sexuality does benefit from such an approach. The idea of continuity then has recently come into favour among, most notably, social historians. Studies covering two or more periods of history, such as Boswell's (1995) study of 'same-sex unions', skilfully utilize the idea of a premodern period. Of course, geographical variations from North America or Europe to Africa or Asia, means that the actual period covered by the term premodern depends on particular cultures and societies. Hanley's (1997) *Everyday Things in Premodern Japan*, for instance, examines Japanese material culture between the seventeenth and nineteenth centuries. The term premodern has also been used for any study before industrialization resulting in premodern becoming a less poignant term for broad historical studies. Western (i.e. European and colonial North American) views of sexuality in the premodern period, especially after the rise of the Christian Church, were heavily based on Judeo-Christian teachings. While normative behaviour was defined by male, often CELIBATE, clerics, recent scholarship delves into questions of different sexual orientations and what was viewed by the Christian Church as deviant behaviour (see also MEDIEVAL SEXUALITY; EARLY MODERN SEXUALITY). (Andrew Cranmer)

Pre-oedipal   The pre-oedipal period precedes the onset of the OEDIPUS COMPLEX in the PSYCHOANALYTIC account of psychosexual development. The period is characterized by an all-consuming attachment to the mother-figure which is often seen as blissful but which can easily slip into a terrifying and overwhelming sense that the mother is all-devouring. During this period, children regard the mother figure as a PHALLIC MOTHER. Popular mythologies around the threat constituted by the female genitalia as VAGINA DENTATA can be traced back to this formative stage of psychosexual development.

The pre-oedipal period is regarded as being more prolonged in girls than in boys. The complexity of the relationship to the mother determines the role of the pre-oedipal in defining our sexual identity and preferences. In boys, it is argued that it is much more difficult to distinguish between the pre-oedipal attachment to the mother and the Oedipal version of this, because the object of each is the same. For both sexes, the pre-oedipal relationship with the mother is crucial in the formation of the lost object. After separation from the mother is enacted by the Oedipus complex, subjects struggle to regain a sense of the lost pleasure experienced in this period. In the Lacanian account of psychoanalysis, this pursuit of that which is lost is articulated in terms of DESIRE for the *objet a* which always eludes us, generating an incessant desire for the archaic mother.

Much contemporary French feminist theory seeks to reclaim the pre-oedipal period in order to sketch out a domain for the feminine that resists the constricted parameters of PHALLOCENTRISM. Thinkers such as Kristeva (1980), Irigaray (1985b) and Cixous (1976) seek to show how feminine desire needs to be re-thought in terms of the pre-oedipal period in order to overthrow patriarchal structures of language and DESIRE. Similarly, Benjamin (1988) argues that the father figure also has a role to play in the pre-oedipal scenario, just as the mother figure has an important role in the symbolic order to language. She sets out a clear refusal of the cultural imperative that seeks traditionally to align the pre-oedipal mother with all that is primitive, regressive and dangerous in the formation of sexual identity and preferences. Much of this feminist work has a specifically lesbian element in its stress on the notion that girls begin their lives with a strong attachment to another woman, which may await reactivation in adult sexuality. (**Caroline Bainbridge**)

Prepubescence   See INTERGENERATIONAL SEX; PAEDOPHILIA; POLYMORPHOUS PERVERSITY; PUBIC HAIR.

Pride   Pride is the affirmation of queer sexualities – particularly collective, organized demonstrations of such support – and is part of wider moves for QUEER acceptance and VISIBILITY. (COMING OUT is often considered one of the first displays of individual pride.) Pride festivals are held internationally often in June, in memory of the Stonewall Riots in June 1969. The first known 'pride' marches took place in 1970 in five American cities, including New York where the Stonewall Riots originally occurred. The first British 'pride' march happened in August 1971 in London, and has occurred annually since. Pride events have been the focus of debates – sometimes bitter – over which sexual minorities were welcomed (see Hemmings 2002: Chapter 2): early marches were argued to exclude lesbians by calling themselves 'Gay Pride'. Most pride marches now use 'queer' or 'LGBT' to indicate their equal inclusion of lesbians, gay men, bisexuals and transgendered people. Some of the most common 'pride' symbols include: the rainbow flag, pink and black triangles, and various combinations of gender symbols (see Rainbow Icon Archive 2003). The rainbow flag is arguably the most common, and certainly the only one intentionally designed as a symbol of queer community pride. The rainbow flag was first used at the 1978 San Francisco Gay and Lesbian Freedom Day Parade as a symbol of the unity of local queer communities. It has since grown in popularity, to the extent that it is recognized by the International Congress of Flag Makers as the official flag of the queer COMMUNITY. Since the early 1990s, 'pride' has also become synonymous with the COMMODIFICATION of queer identities. This has been characterized by the 'appropriation of once radical language in advertisements', to the extent that 'pride' has become one of the 'most common words in the names, slogans, and advertisements of companies targeting gay consumers' (Chasin 2000: 133–4). (**Kelly McWilliam**)

Prostitution   Prostitution is defined as exchanging sexual services for money – although many of those who exchange sex for material rewards would not define themselves as prostitutes (Saunders 1998). Sexual services offered may vary with the gender of client and prostitute, but include relief through intercourse, ORAL SEX or using the hand to masturbate the client. Some DOMINATRIXES offer domination services without sexual relief and assume that they are thus not working as prostitutes – but this is legally a grey area. Contrary to stereotypes of certain persons as psychologically or sexually prone to become prostitutes, the main reason why people enter prostitution is economic (Pheterson 1993). For many, prostitution as an economic activity is a viable choice out of a limited range of possibilities, and is therefore comparable to other types of low-status labour. There are many reasons why people seek the services of prostitutes, including: being part of mobile populations where clients are in locations where they do not have time to form established sexual relationships (business travellers, migrant labourers); people seeking sexual experiences that their established partners do not offer (e.g. SM) or which they do not want publicly acknowledged (e.g. CLOSETED gay men unwilling to form a visible same-sex relationship) (Elias *et al.* 1998).

Bindman (1987) recommends that prostitution be redefined as SEX WORK as a preliminary condition for the enjoyment by sex workers of their full human and labour rights, a possibility currently impeded by the fact that prostitution is only totally legal and part of a regulated industry in few places, including Nevada (United States), the Netherlands, and some states of Germany and of Australia. Everywhere else it is either prohibited or criminalized. In the United Kingdom, prostitution itself is legal, but many activities related to it, such as soliciting, advertising or organized prostitution are illegal. For most prostitutes the work involves being part of a community rather than acting as an isolated individual – not least because prostitution is, in general, a stigmatized activity (even where it is legal) and those who practise it have a low status within the mainstream society (Bullough and Bullough 1987). (**Ana Lopes**)

Further reading

Phoenix (1999).

Psychoanalysis   Psychoanalysis is a theory and method of treatment for neurotic illnesses that was developed by Sigmund Freud during the late nineteenth and early twentieth centuries. Freud trained with Charcot in Paris, working with him on HYSTERIA. He subsequently sought to develop a theory of the mind that centred on a notion of the unconscious as central to the organization of all minds, whether healthy or unhealthy. Psychoanalysis is interested in the impact of early childhood development on adult life. It is particularly concerned with the development of sexuality in infancy and on the role of the LIBIDO and FANTASY in formulating our SEXUAL IDENTITIES. Using the mechanism of REPRESSION, the unconscious acts as a kind of storehouse for all our memories and inhibitions relating to our experience of infantile sexuality. As a therapeutic method, psychoanalysis seeks to access the unconscious in order to deal with repressed material which might be hindering adult life at the level of sexual and/or emotional function. In this way, psychoanalysis works to liberate the patient from the constraints of symptoms, anxieties and inhibitions. There are now several schools of psychoanalytic thought and practice including those established by Melanie Klein (known as the Object Relations school) and by Jacques Lacan working in France. Many feminists have taken issue with Freudian ideas, arguing that his ideas are PHALLOCENTRIC (Millet 1969) or that they conform to the HETEROSEXUAL MATRIX (Butler 1990). Other feminists, though, have remained more sympathetic to psychoanalysis, arguing that it is useful in helping to explain the dominant patriarchal ideology of the West (see Mitchell 1974). A number of French feminists remain indebted to psychoanalytic ideas in their efforts to formulate a mode of feminine discourse (Irigaray 1985a 1985b; Kristeva 1980). For Foucault (1990), however, psychoanalysis plays a central role in the Western HYDRAULIC MODEL of sexuality. (**Caroline Bainbridge**)

Further reading

Mitchell (1974).

Pubic hair Since body hair continues to be associated with animality and sexuality within Western culture, there are societal taboos against women having too much body hair and against men for not having enough (Dutton 1995: 304). While there is consequently the fashion of bikini-line waxing for women, not all pubic hair removal is socially acceptable. For example, the explicitly sexual removal of pubic hair is often seen as a PERVERSION. However, sculpting pubic hair for nominally *aesthetic* reasons has become increasingly COMMODIFIED, and to a certain extent, NORMALIZED, being available in an array of salons. Thus institutions retain the privilege of deciding for whom this is a pleasure, and for whom it is a perversion. While wealthy women may pay for pubic hair sculpting, Finger (1997) describes the consequences for DeVonna Cervantes of continuing to dye her pubic hair after she became a paraplegic. Once the rehabilitation staff saw that her pubic hair was pink after catheterizing her, the staff psychiatrist was sent to speak with her. Cervantes, in an almost hour-long debate, convinced the doctor that this was normal behaviour for her. The negative reactions she experienced draws attention to the larger current cultural crisis around the sexuality of disabled people.

The complete removal of pubic hair has traditionally symbolized a regression to prepubescence, and might therefore be seen as enabling a fantasy of sex with a child-like partner (particularly when older men encourage younger women to shave their pubic hair). Yet within consensual sexual situations, the act of allowing another to shave one's pubic hair signifies a great amount of trust. Members of the SM community may include their 'shaved status' when describing their particular proclivities, while shaving or being shaved is often part of a fetishistic practice. Many DRAG KING performers are rumoured to use their girlfriend's pubic hair when making moustaches or goatees, also know as 'flavour savers'. (**Caroline J. McKenzie**)

Public sex Term used to describe particular sexual acts, practices and cultures centred on use of public space. Most commonly associated with gay male culture, the most prominent forms of public sex are COTTAGING – sex in public toilets – and CRUISING scenes based around bathhouses, beaches and parks (Leap 1999). In some locations, elaborate cultures have grown up, catering for distinct sexual proclivities. Lieshout (1997) studied a remote highway rest area in the Netherlands, popular with LEATHERSEX participants. Public sex is the regular target of moral panics, and law enforcement often attempts to police activity on the grounds that it represents a threat to the moral order (Dangerous Bedfellows 1996). Public sex is also at the heart of AIDS-related health promotion activism, based on the premise that MEN-WHO-HAVE SEX-WITH-MEN in this kind of environment get missed by campaigns targeting 'out' gay scenes. Indeed, the stereotypical public sex participant is often seen as CLOSETED and engaging in quick, anonymous sex. In truth, however, public sex continues to have an important role to play in numerous sexual subcultures, and has increasingly been seen as radical or transgressive, especially in light of attempts to regulate it (Califia 1994). Because of its continued demonization – including demonization from within the gay community – public sex remains newsworthy, especially when 'public figures' are caught engaging in it; pop star George Michael's mistaken liaison with an under-cover cop in a Los Angeles toilet being a recent example. Less often discussed forms of public sex include various forms of EXHIBITIONISM and VOYEURISM, such as 'dogging', and more specialized practices such as sadomasochistic kidnapping. Whatever the detail of the scene, all forms of public sex raise critical issues about ownership and use of public space and the SEXUAL POLITICS of the PUBLIC/PRIVATE divide. (**David Bell**)

Further reading

Leap (1999).

Public/private   This contested opposition most commonly refers to the difference between domestic and FAMILY life on the one hand, and political and social life on the other. It also refers to the attempt to create and manage that difference as valid or self-evident, and as the cornerstone of modern, liberal, Western democracies. The public/private distinction has been critiqued from a range of perspectives and disci-plines. Feminist critics suggest that the public/private divide assumes an adult *male citizen* for whom the domestic sphere has typically been a site of freedom from work and political or civic engagement (Pateman 1988). For those who are dependants, or whose work takes place within the home, the 'private sphere' offers no such respite. A more radical reading suggests that the artificial division of the world into public and private works to protect the patriarchal organization of the home, preventing the state intervening in what become known as 'private concerns'. Marital or adult–child vio-lence in the home thus becomes understood as 'domestic' and its victims placed out-side the realm of state protection. In an international framework, marital violence being understood as 'domestic' also has implications for women seeking asylum on that basis, since this defines it not as *political* violence.

Theorists of sexuality have complemented these debates by suggesting that a public/private divide also maintains and presumes HETEROSEXUAL PRIVILEGE. Only when the 'private' in question is normatively heterosexual are its boundaries respected. The state has, and continues to be, more than happy to intervene in our 'private lives' to ascertain the extent of and to punish DEVIANCE (Rahman 2000). Laws proliferate determining who we are allowed to desire, love and live with freely – how old, how many what race or ethnicity, what sex or gender, and which acts. Again, in international contexts, state-to-state variation in legislation on sexuality means that borders are less open to anyone outside a normative Western democratic model of the family. (**Clare Hemmings**)

Pure relationship   According to Giddens (1992a), the pure relationship represents a new kind of SEXUAL CONTRACT. His work looks at love and eroticism in the broader context of changes in self-identity and social life, and describes emerging new forms of relationship. He offers the following succinct definition:

> a situation where a social relation is entered into for its own sake, for what can be derived by each person from a sustained association with another; and which is continued only in so far as it is thought by both parties to deliver enough satisfactions for each individual to stay within it. (Giddens 1992a: 58)

At the heart of this formulation is a loosening of the traditions that previously kept couples together (MARRIAGE, life-long commitment, etc.) and the brokering of a new mutual agreement founded on the absolute equality of both partners. The relationship becomes an extension, therefore, of Giddens's notion of the self as a reflexive project. What this means is that we actively scrutinize and seek to improve ourselves – most obviously by drawing on the rhetoric of self-help – and then similarly apply this logic to our relationships. The couple asks questions constantly, monitoring the relationship: is this still right for me? What reasons do I have for continuing in this relationship? How might my life be arranged otherwise? Giddens stresses that this represents a new consensual and democratic form of private life for the couple. In a similar vein, Beck and Beck-Gernsheim (1995) highlight the problem in contemporary societies caught between tradition and modernization. In both cases, outside forces exert pressures on the couple-form, and it is in the process of adaptation that new forms of relationship can emerge. (See also POLYAMORY, PLASTIC SEXUALITY.) (**David Bell**)

PWA/PLWA   An acronym for 'Person With AIDS' or 'Person Living With AIDS'. First used in 1983 titles for US organizations 'People With AIDS Alliance', and 'PWA Coalition', Shilts (1988) highlights how PWA also became part of a new lexicon of 'AIDSpeak', using destigmatizing terminology to define individuals diagnosed with various AIDS Defining Illnesses (ADIs) or AIDS Indicator Conditions (AICs). 'PWA' is inaccurate for HIV positive people without an AIDS Indicator Condition (Moore 1996), therefore, the terms PWHIV/PLWHIV are also sometimes used. As personal acronyms, the terms were designed to be more empowering than 'AIDS sufferers/patients' and non-stigmatizing or judgmental, unlike 'AIDS victims'. As Watney (1994) states, the person with AIDS is invariably imprisoned within the demeaning category of the 'victim', in which he or she is stripped of all power and control over the actual complex meaning and dignity of an individual's life. The STIGMA and negative judgements which routinely surround people with HIV and AIDS show no real sign of abating even more than 20 years after the syndrome was named, and the terms have still not found currency in the mainstream media. (**David Evans**)

Q

Queer Dictionary definitions of 'queer', which is probably rooted etymologically in the Low German *quer* – 'oblique, crooked'– yields a range of meanings. As a verb it means 'to spoil, thwart or compromise', and as an adjective it means 'not usual or expected', 'eccentric or unconventional', 'suspicious' and 'nauseous or unwell'. These characteristics are inscribed in the noun, defined as an 'offensive term for homosexuals'. Queer became a part of a common pathological vocabulary for the DEVIANT, abnormal and immoral 'other' with the emergence of a MODERN homosexual identity from the late nineteenth century. Queer particularly represented the notion that homosexuality involved pathological forms of femininity in gay men (CAMP) and masculinity in lesbian women (BUTCH). From the 1960s, the term was slowly expropriated by emergent lesbian and gay COMMUNITIES both culturally as a 'catch-all' for NON-HETEROSEXUALS and then politically as a means of turning heterosexist language upon itself and making a positive statement of identity – 'Queer and proud'. Queer became a language for the mobilization of non-heterosexuals against the moral, medical and legal compulsions towards heterosexuality. To be queer was to celebrate difference, typified in the 1980s by the emergence of Queer Nation in the United States as a backlash to Reaganite Republican Conservativism, and the queer politics of OutRage against Thatcherite Conservatism in the United Kingdom. Queer also became a means of extending sexual politics from lesbian and gay rights to questioning or 'querying' the whole notion of fixed sexual identities, uniting those who have this questioning in common, whether lesbian, gay, bisexual, transgendered, heterosexual or of any other SELF-DEFINITION. This to some extent follows the ideas of QUEER THEORY, although queer politics has tended to engage in this 'querying' through a politics of cultural protest, with high media visibility and aesthetically creative cultural forms of political ACTIVISM. (**Paul Reynolds**)

Further reading

Blasius (2001).

Queer theory   Queer theory takes its central features from three sources: French poststructuralist philosophy (particularly the work of Michel Foucault), critical feminist theory and critical literary studies. Queer theory came out of North American lesbian and feminist literary critiques in the late 1980s, notably the work of Eve Sedgwick (1985, 1991) and Judith Butler (1990, 1993), motivated by their frustration that even emancipatory theories such as feminism seemed to assume an implicit heterosexuality and fixity of subject in their approach to SEXUAL POLITICS. Queer theory was first formally represented as a coherent theoretical approach by Butler (1990), when she elaborated a queer critique of gender categories; Butler herself, however, has elsewhere questioned whether she was not in fact engaged in critical feminist writing rather than in producing a separate theory (Osborne 1996: 109–25).

The major surveys of the field (Seidman 1996; Seidman 1997; Turner 2000) agree that queer theory is built upon four central concepts. First, it resists any categorical statements about essences in human subjects. Hence biological, psychological or social categories do not provide legitimate foundations from which the gendered or sexual self can be categorized. Bodies of knowledge such as scientific, legal and moral discourses, that produce fixed identities and behaviours, are not attempts to understand the sexual self but to impose constraint upon it. This analysis applies as much to the development of more positive categories of lesbian and gay identity as it does to the pathological identities formed from medico-moral discourses (see ANTI-GAY). Queer theorists reject these foundations and expose the idiosyncratic historical development of such foundations, revealing the ignorance, interests and prejudices of those who make sexual knowledge (see ESSENTIALISM and SOCIAL CONSTRUCTIONISM). By identifying foundations and essences as discursively constructed, they enable difference to be explored, refusing the BINARY structure of gendered and sexual identities – male/female, masculine/feminine, heterosexual/homosexual – in favour of a FLUID 'zone of possibilities'. Second, queer theory is structured around the primacy of the individual subject. The subject's unique passage is through a 'lifeworld' of categories and identities created by the institutions within which the subject is socialized. These categories divorce the subject from autonomy in their sensuous feelings and expressions, acting as a constraint to their imagination. Queer theorists see the subject as a text inscribed by these dominant discourses, uncover the violence of this process and reject it. Third, queer theory recognizes that the power of foundational categories and the means of their deconstruction lies in their PERFORMATIVITY. Foundational categories such as 'woman' or 'heterosexual' are made meaningful because they are performed and so normalized in everyday behaviour, language or symbols (e.g. dress). Performance makes these categories 'real', and represents their internalization as 'truths'. Queer strategy is to disrupt these categories by performing difference, including seeking desire outside of genitally or identity-focused constructions of sexuality or refusing the 'normal' in dress codes (see DRAG and GENDERFUCK). Performativity is the means by which subjects 'rewrite their text' with their own hand. Finally, queer theory is transgressive. Its politics are intrinsically those of challenging extant bodies of knowledge. Given that queer theory rejects fixity, it is always fluid, becoming rather than being. In a sense, then, it is more accurate to talk of queer theor*ies* or strateg*ies*. Hence, a transgressive performativity of the subject is always immanently critical and disruptive of both established categories *and* queer ruptures of those categories.

Queer theory has been enormously influential in understandings of sexuality in the last decade, but it is not without considerable problems. Jeffreys (2003) has criticized it for engaging in a subject-based strategy that deconstructs gay and lesbian identities whilst failing to provide a concrete means of struggling against HETEROPATRIARCHAL power. Fraser (1998) and Kirsch (2000) have criticized its deconstructive project through the weaknesses of its literary theory and post-structuralist roots – that it represents subjects and their social contexts as 'merely cultural' (Butler 1998), dissolving knowledge into discourse, and therefore fails to address the social and material terms of power. So, for example, queer critiques of transsexuals who seek to change their identity from one gender category to another seem unappreciative of the terms of struggle transsexuals go through. Wilson (1993) has observed that the logic of transgression without an underlying political critique is that the heterosexual patriarch can always claim the ground of the transgressive subject. The transgressive nature of performativity has been challenged by debates around whether 'transgressions' such as CAMP are understood as a politics or an apolitical cultural PARODY (Cleto 1999). Whilst queer theory is undoubtedly an important critical tool, it is difficult to conceive of its political reconstruction of emancipation outside of individuated autonomy. This might say more about the freedoms of the queer theorist in the academy than it does about conceiving freedom from the vagaries of HETERONORMATIVE patriarchal societies. (**Paul Reynolds**)

Further reading

Jagose (1996); Sullivan (2003).

Queerbashing The verbal and physical manifestations of HOMOPHOBIA, including taunting marchers at Gay Pride Parades, advocating the death penalty for LGBT people, assault, violence and harassment. Herek, Cogan and Gillis (2002) suggest that while many attacks fit a commonly perceived pattern – taking place in public places and often involving several assailants – assaults also take place in the home or workplace, and may involve colleagues or family members. In spite of various advancements toward pro-gay successes like gay marriage laws in some states, homophobic religious groups, such as the Westboro Baptist Church of Fred Waldron Phelps Sr argue that the Bible supports the death penalty for gays, and protest at the funerals of people who have died from HIV/AIDS, as well as at those of victims of homophobic hate crimes, famously Matthew Sheppard (1976–98). On 6 October 1998, Sheppard was pistol-whipped, brutally beaten, tied to a fence and left to die by two men in Wyoming,

United States. After spending five days in a coma, Sheppard died on 12 October 1998 His parents, Judy and Dennis Sheppard created a Hate Crimes Prevention Ac (HCPA) in hopes of adding SEXUAL ORIENTATION to current hate crime legislation.

Herek, Cogan and Gillis suggest that queerbashing 'functions as a form of terror- ism, sending a message to all lesbians, gay men and bisexual people that they are no safe if they are visible' (2002: 14). While fear of violence or abuse keeps many mem- bers of the LGBT community in the CLOSET, many out members assert their out statu: by staging 'kiss-ins', which involve same-sex couples kissing in public to raise aware- ness of HOMOPHOBIA, and taking political action, such as campaigning to include anti- gay crimes in hate crime legislation (see Jeness and Broad 1997). However complicating any simple notion of queerbashing as an expression of heterosexua supremacy, queerbashers may include straight-identified men who also have sex with men (MSM) but wish to resist the negative stereotype of gay men as feminine, or some gay-identified groups such as the Gay Skinhead Movement, which had its heyday in the mid-1980s and was centred around the valorization of hyper-masculinity (**Caroline J. McKenzie**)

Further reading

Herek and Berrill (1992).

R

Rainbow kissing   A rainbow kiss involves a woman who is menstruating having unprotected intercourse with a man; after he has ejaculated inside the woman's VAGINA he sucks out the SEMEN and menstrual blood, then kisses the woman, passing the fluid into her mouth. It is a variation on WATERSPORTS, FELTCHING and rainbow showers, in which a menstruating woman urinates on her sexual partner(s). Paglia (1990) see: MENSTRUATION as an ultimate symbol of woman's power over man, through this sign o woman's primordial, cyclic, affiliation with creation and regeneration. Many patriar- chal cultures and religions have turned menstruation into a 'curse', a sign of unclean liness, weakness and something shameful (Owen 1993). Rainbow showers use thi: symbol of womanhood, and encapsulate beliefs that have been disrespectful o women, and piss them out over another in sex. Consensual rainbow kissing symbol izes a unity of female and male, and a return of the power of the menses to their orig inator. This practice thus involves a rejection of stigmatizing myths and a validatio. of menstrual blood as a legitimate sexual fluid. SAFE(R) SEX implications would appl primarily to semen, since menstrual blood is not necessarily as risky as circulating blood for pathogens. (**David Evans**)

Rape   Rape is most commonly understood as SEXUAL ASSAULT by one or more people on the body of another individual without their consent. Writing on rape has been most extensive within feminist and sexuality studies, where concerns about the HETEROSEXIST and misogynist nature of law, family, and social life, are brought together. Perhaps the most lasting intervention concerning rape within FEMINISM has been its theorization as violence against women, rather than as sex (e.g. Brownmiller 1975). Related work argues that rape is simply the extension of heterosexual power relations between men and women. In this line of argument, heterosexual relations codify and fetishize men's power over women, whereby penetrative (penile–vagina) sex between a man and a woman is itself a representation of the violence of rape (Dworkin 1987). Lees (1997) has highlighted the links between the treatment of women in rape trials and their treatment within society more generally, focusing on the use of derogatory terms to describe women and girls who do not conform to a marital, heterosexual model of sexuality. This work has impacted on legislation concerning the definition of rape (away from forced heterosexual penetration), and forced increased legal and social acknowledgement of rape within marriage as both possible and widespread.

Work on rape by black and transnational feminists has taken two primary directions. Firstly, black feminists have argued that the persistent idea of the family or heterosexual relations as the primary site of violence against women only makes sense for white women who do not have to face daily and institutional racism from which the family can offer valuable respite (Bhavnani 2000). Similarly, the dominant form of feminist protest against rape – 'reclaim the night' marches – are challenged for commonly taking routes through black or immigrant neighbourhoods, reproducing strong cultural and historical assumptions that white women have most to fear from black men (Davis 1982). The second direction has been to think about rape in an international rather than national or domestic context. Rape and trafficking of poor women has been highlighted as a dominant feature of globalization, and the role of rape in conflict situations has brought attention to the links between the objectification of women's bodies and fundamentalist nationalism (Moghissi 1999).

Rape is not only something that men do to women. Recent material has focused on rape between women and between men, as well as between children, and between adults and children. While the bodies here may be different, the feminist theorization of rape as power remains key to understanding rape as first and foremost an act of violence and control (see MALE RAPE). (**Clare Hemmings**)

Further reading

Marcus (1992).

Reclaiming See APPROPRIATION; COSMETIC SURGERY; FEMME; FAG; HERMAPHRODITE; HYSTERIA; NORMALIZATION; ORAL SEX; PERVERSION; PRE-OEDIPAL; QUEER; RAPE; VAGINA; WHORE.

Recreational sex Recreational sex is sex performed for the primary purpose of pleasure. Recreational sex is sometimes contrasted with procreative sex, or sex that is performed between a man and a woman with the intention of reproduction. Often, the term is used in a demeaning or denigrating manner to describe sexual activities that are NON-MONOGAMOUS, involve multiple partners, and/or are NON-HETEROSEXUAL. This denigrating use of the phrase suggests that procreative heterosexual activities are natural and healthy, relying upon ESSENTIALIST and/or SOCIO-BIOLOGICAL assumptions about sex and gender in which women are presumed not to desire sex for pleasure and men desire sex for pleasure almost exclusively. QUEER sexuality has attempted to reclaim the term as a SEX-POSITIVE practice, implying that all genders are naturally able to enjoy sexual activities without mandated limits or social constraints. (See also CRUISING and FUCK-BUDDIES.) (**Rachael Groner**)

Red light district The term refers to areas where commercial sex establishments operate. Establishments may include BROTHELS, sex shops, adult video and magazine shops, striptease clubs, table and lap dancing clubs, and adult movie cinemas. In the past, brothel owners used to hang a red light or lantern outside their establishments to indicate the nature of their business to potential costumers. In some areas or streets, there would be a row of red lights outside buildings. Some red light districts are extremely old and famous. Amsterdam's red light district, right at the heart of the old city, is a major tourist attraction; its main defining characteristic is the fact that sex workers exhibit themselves in shop windows. Other famous red light districts include the Reeperbahn in Hamburg, Germany; Patpong in Bangkok, Thailand, and the Sonagatchi in Kolkatta, India (see SEX TOURISM). They vary immensely in terms of type of establishments and workers' conditions. Commercial sex establishments usually attract other businesses such as bars and restaurants, since red light districts are usually lively nocturnal places. Red light districts are often safe places for SEX WORKERS to operate from, since they create a sense of COMMUNITY. In London, local authorities' recent efforts to eradicate commercial sex businesses from the most ancient and famous local red light district, Soho, were met with protest not only from the sex work activists but also from local residents and shop keepers, who recognize that Soho's tradition as a red light district is an important attraction for tourists and business (see also SEX TOURISM). (**Ana Lopes**)

Re-gaying See AIDS CRISIS; SAFE(R) SEX.

Repression Repression is one of the major defence mechanisms operating in the psyche according to PSYCHOANALYTIC theory. It is the mechanism by which unacceptable desires, wishes, thoughts and instincts are made unconscious. Repressed material is mostly that which is forbidden or taboo in the course of normal social interaction including sex, aggression and anti-social behaviour. In this respect, repression is closely bound up with notions of SHAME and EROTOPHOBIA. Repressed ideas are held in the unconscious under pressure and always struggle to get out. They make themselves manifest in dreams or slips of the tongue and also indirectly influence behaviour and experience. Freud suggests that repressed material will always return in some guise or other and reach the conscious mind in a distorted form. This is called the symptom and can encompass any form of unconsciously directed behaviour. For example, Cowie (1997) suggests that straight men may watch pornography because it allows them to experience their own repressed desires to occupy the passive role of the women that they view. In many horror films and gothic novels, the monster embodies the repressed content of a society or individual, hence many of the overtly sexual overtones apparent in such texts (see Creed 1993).

SEXUAL POLITICS could be seen as a concerted attempt to reduce the forces of repression in society in favour of LIBERATION. For Freud (1914b), without repression, we would not be able to perform any socially useful activities. There is an important distinction to be drawn between a general usage of this term to refer to a sexually harmful force and a more psychoanalytic usage which implies that it is a psychically necessary process. In his critique of psychoanalysis, Foucault (1990) suggests that Freud's work on repression is part of the Western HYDRAULIC MODEL of sexuality (see REPRESSIVE HYPOTHESIS). (**Caroline Bainbridge**)

Repressive hypothesis   Like the HYDRAULIC MODEL, a term coined by Foucault (1990) to describe the dominant understanding of sexuality in the MODERN period: sexuality is an essential truth inside us, repressed by the social order. In fact, Foucault argues, this belief is the result of centuries of institutions that have used this claim to regulate our behaviours; the church, eugenics and PSYCHOANALYSIS have conspired to make us think that sexuality is the key to who we are, because that has made us more obedient to their proclamations. The sexual LIBERATION movement mistakenly accepts this underlying position, even as it as tries to turn it on its head: when it urges us to throw off repression, it is in fact leading us to embrace the very beliefs that best suit the modern socio-economic system. From gay pride t-shirts to COSMETIC SURGERY, the increasing SEXUALIZATION of everyday culture has fulfilled Foucault's predictions: the more we think we are free to be sexual, the more we are enslaved to buying the goods and services that we feel we need in order to be true to our sexual selves. Social changes that might seem to generate greater freedom instead impose new regulations upon us. For instance, COMING OUT as lesbian and gay only creates new regulations about the PERFORMANCE of these identities: to be BUTCH or FEMME, TOP or BOTTOM; gay or STRAIGHT – but nothing in between (hence the BIPHOBIA directed against bisexuals). Against Foucault's pessimism we can instead see such identity choices being taken on more creatively.

From the perspective of sexual SCRIPTING, regulated identities are only the starting point for more individualized ways of living. Indeed, it is not clear what Foucault sees as an alternative – except for a utopia in which, he suggests, we no longer have 'sexualities' at all, but simply 'bodies and pleasures' (159). (**Jo Eadie**)

Rimming   Slang for analingus or oro-anal sex, which involves licking and/or sucking an ANUS, or licking a finger or other object that is entering someone's rectum, and forms part of the sexual repertoire of many people (Tomlinson 1999). Gay men in particular have eroticized the anus in an act of resistance against its abjection in Western culture. Many sexual health or genito-urinary (GU) clinics in the West have statistics on male same-sex clients who participate in rimming; these men can then be offered SAFE(R) SEX advice, as well as prophylactic vaccination against hepatitis A and B (HAV, HBV). However, owing to the public taboo in many cultures around discussing anal sex, limited epidemiological evidence and safer sex materials on rimming exist for other groups. The anus is supplied by nerve endings from the same origin as the genitals (S4), so erotic sensations from oral stimulation can be exceptionally intense. Individuals who know the risks associated with rimming might negotiate their acceptable levels of safety/risk. The cleaner the anus being rimmed, the less there might be risks of infectious germs (pathogens) – however, some people thrive on the sweat, tastes and odours. Pathogens can be limited by using barrier protection, such as DENTAL DAMS. However, the anus is never 100 per cent free of germs and rimming might lead to self-limiting diarrhoea. Other pathogens are potentially more serious, especially if shit actually gets in to another person's mouth (see COPROPHILIA). Unfortunately, due to the silence and taboo around discussing anal sex, many people are either unaware of the gratifying sensations that can be gained from rimming, or do it without knowing how to diminish risks to their health. (**David Evans**).

Rohypnol   Rohypnol, the commercial name of Flunitrazepam, is a Benzodiazepine, or central nervous system depressant (Schmidtlein 1998: 1). Rohypnol is addictive, with common effects including drowsiness, muscle relaxation, confusion, decreased blood pressure and memory impairment. Since the early to mid-1990s, Rohypnol has generated considerable media attention – particularly in the United States – as a DATE RAPE drug. This occurs when Rohypnol is slipped into the drink of an unsuspecting individual, who becomes intoxicated, and is SEXUALLY ASSAULTED when sedated, later having little or no memory of the attack (Schwartz and Weaver 1998: 321). It is its after-effect of memory impairment that has complicated legal recourse for the victim, who often cannot identify their attacker (see Riveira and Hart 2000). Researchers continue to explore ways of screening for Rohypnol, with a number of effective options currently available. Rohypnol – produced in 1 and 2 milligram tablet form – can be ingested orally, snorted or injected, and is frequently taken with other drugs, including alcohol and heroin. It is a popular prescription sedative throughout Europe (Schmidtlein

1998: 1), and is used legitimately to treat insomnia, as a preanaesthetic and as a sedative hypnotic. It is legally available in over 60 countries worldwide, although is was banned in the United States in 1996 citing its increasing use as a date rape drug, and was the catalyst for the Drug-Induced Rape Prevention and Punishment Act passed by Congress in 1996 (Schmidtlein 1998: 2). In 1997, Hoffman-La Roche Inc. (the manufacturer of Rohypnol) produced a new version of the drug that dissolves more slowly, is detectable in clear liquid, and leaves a residue in the glass (Schmidtlein 1998: 1), as a means of addressing these concerns. (**Kelly McWilliam**)

Role   A role is a complicated mélange of characteristics that express one's IDENTITY or aspects of one's identity. There is some overlap between role, identity and PERFORMANCE, but we might distinguish them by saying: an identity is experienced as internal and therefore able to exist even without any external expression (e.g. 'I know I am a lesbian, but nobody else knows'); a role is a set of culturally recognized behaviours, props and attitudes, that enable one to take up a certain way of being, whether gladly or reluctantly (e.g. 'I felt I could only be a lesbian by dressing up for the role'); a performance is the making concrete of a role or identity in public (e.g. ' I gave my best butch performance at the club tonight'). Traditional psychological theories have seen roles as rigid social constructs, imposed by community norms, determining behaviour, and leading to emotional distress at the inevitable failure to live up to their prescriptions (Segal 1990: 65–9). But within sexual communities roles are more often seen as self-chosen constructs, adopted because they provide pleasure – such as TOP and BOTTOM in SM communities – and a sense of belonging, often coming out of historical tradition, such as BUTCH-FEMME (Innes and Lloyd 1996: 12). SM roles may be adopted temporarily (e.g. in a SCENE or at a SEX PARTY) or for longer periods (e.g. in a contracted relationship for any given amount of time). Clear-cut roles are often criticized as being limiting and oppressive, or derived from inequalities of status (Jeffreys 1993: 73–5); however, roles may be combined and/or altered to fit one's identity (Duncan 1996) – for example, in the lesbian community one might identify as a BUTCH bottom or be in a butch-on-butch couple (Innes and Lloyd 1996: 23–6) as opposed to a more traditional butch-femme couple. Those who do not have clear-cut roles may be pressured either to chose a primary role or to pick one and 'stick with it' (See SWITCH.) (**Caroline J. McKenzie**)

Romance   See COMMODIFICATION; HONEYMOON.

Rough trade   Gay slang for a male working-class partner for casual sex – often a male PROSTITUTE, hence the term 'trade'. Weeks (1991b) has described a long history of gay sex across class lines, driven by the assumption that working-class men were more open to sex with other men, both because they were viewed as sexually voracious and because they needed the money. Soldiers in particular had a reputation for being a reliable source of rough trade. Weeks argues that rough trade comprises both a 'sexual colonialism' in which working-class men and boys become a source of convenient sex, and a socially safer mode of sex, since occasional sexual contacts with those who lived elsewhere were easier to hide from society than a more sustained relationship. Sinfield (1994: 130–60) suggests that this is rooted in the fact that gay male identity that was formed through a leisure-class sensibility: aestheticism, EFFEMINACY, and wealth. The strength of this class connotation enabled many working-class men to enjoy homosexual practice, without feeling any risk of becoming 'queer' (in its early twentieth-century sense). Prevailing notions of INVERSION meant that gay desire was assumed to be modelled on heterosexual desire: the feminine homosexual needed a masculine partner, one who could only be found outside his class. Consequently the working-class body was read as authentically masculine, so that access to rough trade gives access to 'real men'. The continued popularity of rough trade within gay culture suggests the power of this legacy – even though many men report being QUEERBASHED after such encounters. The supposed MASCULINITY of trade is reflected in SEXUAL PRACTICE, in which the trade man will often take the active role during anal intercourse or oral sex. In this sense there may be a residue of HOMOPHOBIA and INTERNALIZED OPPRESSION, which views rough trade as a compensation for the despised effeminacy of a gay identity. In recent decades the privileging of class as the ground for masculine gay sexuality has been eroded by the incorporation into gay culture of masculine identities as an option for men of all classes – in LEATHERSEX or by STRAIGHT ACTING gay men, for instance. (**Jo Eadie**)

S

Sadism   See SM.

Sadomasochism   See SM.

Safe(r) sex   Safe(r) sex involves the undertaking of sexual practices which remove (in safe sex) or limit (in safer sex) the potential for transmission of HIV/AIDS. The discovery that many were choosing to ignore altogether health advisors who forbade the majority of common sexual acts led to the adoption of a harm-reduction model (Patton 1985; King 1993: Chapter 3), advocating safer sexual activity which only *limited*, rather than eradicated, risks. Always a source of much controversy, safe(r) sex campaigns have emanated from community action, governmental health organizations, and a vigorous voluntary sector. Governmental campaigns initially took a heavily heterosexualized, 'de-gayed' approach, creating a myth that 'AIDS affects everyone equally'. This was highly damaging, however, and activists lobbied for a re-gaying of AIDS which would redirect funds to where they were most needed (see King 1993; Watney 2001: 235–41). In the United Kingdom, attempts to wrest control of AIDS policy from the Governmental Health Education Authority led to gay community campaigns becoming largely formalized into voluntary sector organizations (e.g. Terrence Higgins Trust and Gay Men Fighting AIDS), some becoming so well-funded that they have been accused of becoming an unaccountable 'AIDS industry'. Concomitantly, some have argued that the predominantly HIV negative status of service providers in this sector had led to an emphasis on prevention rather than help for those already affected. Finally, as Patton notes, while safe sex and its promotion may have EROTOPHOBICALLY dissolved central parts of a gay identity, HIV prevention work may have had a confirmatory effect on gay COMMUNITIES overall (Patton 1985: 135). (**Alex Evans**)

Further reading

King (1993).

Safeword A term of SM subcultural slang, usually discussed in NEGOTIATION before a SCENE, which may be considered a part of having and/or giving CONSENT. Safewords are words used in a scene to signal distress or discomfort and a desire to slow or end play immediately; in every scene, everyone directly involved should have a safeword, including TOPS or dominants, who may also become tired or physically/emotionally overwhelmed. Safewords are often used in place of 'stop' or 'no more' because sexual play can involve scenes where 'stop' is not adequate to end play, as it may be a part of the play, and not to be taken literally (e.g. a FANTASY rape scene). Typical safewords include 'green' to continue play, 'yellow' to slow play down, and 'red', which completely ends play. 'Safeword' is also a popular safeword. Play may resume after additional negotiation is completed; however, in some circles, 'red' ends play completely for that scene. Safewords are used to protect and to enable communication between and among people in a scene, and there is no shame in 'safewording'. (**Caroline J. McKenzie**)

Sapphism Often used as a euphemism for LESBIANISM, the term refers to love between women and derives from the female Greek poet Sappho, whose poems celebrated homosexual and bisexual desire. Sappho was from the island of Lesbos, where, several centuries before the Greek golden age, a rather egalitarian society existed, and women were educated in theory and philosophy in the famous *thiasoi*, or schools for women. Sappho was a teacher, and her relationship with some of her female students had erotic connotations engendered by the shared inquiries and process of learning. Sappho wrote nine books of poetry, most of which were destroyed. As a result, the content of her poetry has a mythical aura, and her name has served to indicate erotic practices and desires that were often hidden from social consciousness. In the modern era, the word 'Sapphism' has been used as a generic term to allude to women's erotic and sometimes unfulfilled desire for one another. It connotes the hidden and inner characteristics of this desire, rather than its outer manifestations, more often indicated as lesbianism. In the eighteenth century, Sapphism referred to a type of desire between women common among the educated women of the aristocracy. It was associated with French noblewomen devoted to poetry and literary salons. Sapphism has also been associated with the constitution of a lesbian culture and identity in England in the early twentieth century. The concept of the 'new woman' emerged in the suffrage era through women's struggles to gain access to education and the professions. This development has been traced by Doan (2000), in her work on the famous trials of Radclyffe Hall and her controversial bestseller *The Well of Loneliness* (1928). (**Serena Anderlini-D'Onofrio**)

Scat   See COPROPHILIA.

Scene   A scene is the PERFORMANCE of SADOMASOCHISTIC acts, which have been SCRIPTED through NEGOTIATION to embody participants' FANTASIES. They often involve scenes revolving around ROLES of TOP/BOTTOM, but may also include other FETISHIZED relationships, such as doctor/patient, teacher/student, parent/child (see DADDY), police officer/prisoner, pirate/wench, etc. Scenes may or may not involve uniforms (e.g. military, medical, police) or fetish wear (e.g. LEATHER, denim, rubber, PVC); they may include mise en scène like slings, racks, frames, restraints, FETISH wear, whips, chains, knives, ropes, hoods, scarves, hand/ankle cuffs, etc; and may take place in PUBLIC or PRIVATE. In public, a scene may be obvious, such as at an SM bar, or may be less obviously between two people who are covertly 'in role'. In some cities, the SM community organizes play parties, including scenes where onlookers may or may not be welcomed to participate. The historical precedent set by the Marquis de Sade – known for cruel and unconsensual treatment of servants and prostitutes – implies that scenes have elements of real power inequality. In the more modern sense, play in scenes problematizes real life inequalities, and therefore appears to be egalitarian, negotiated and 'merely playing' at inequality – although McClintock (1993) argues that the scene will inevitably also be shaped by the real inequalities between participants. Scenes provide avenues to explore the complexities and dichotomies of power and other 'taboos', such as NARCISSISM and EXHIBITIONISM. The SM community borrows a strikingly high percentage of its language from theatre, drawing attention to its self-consciousness and artifice (Meyer 1993). In this sense, those in a scene are self-aware and reflective about their practice (Duncan 1996). (**Caroline J. McKenzie**)

Scientia sexualis   A term coined by Foucault (1990) to describe a key feature of MODERN SEXUALITY, the transition from the powers of the church over persons and morals – e.g. in confessing to a priest – to the establishment of so-called 'scientific' psycho-sexual medicine. This concept, the 'science of sex', originated in opposition to sexualized humanity in the erotic arts (*ars erotica*) as set out in SEX MANUALS across the world. Although the phenomenon appeared culturally enlightened, in fact it proved quite the opposite. Whereas the *ars erotica* gloried in the pleasures of sex, the *scientia sexualis* pathologized them. It is principally an amalgam of EROTOPHOBIC superstition, religion, psychiatry, medicine, and associated myopic elements of reproductive and HETERONORMATIVE moral systems. Any SEXUAL PRACTICE or condition considered outside this moral framework, e.g. non-reproductive sex or physical ailments, were first a sin, and later a PERVERSION or (psycho-) pathology, what Krafft-Ebing (1965) termed *psychopathia sexualis*. An early subdivision, SEXOLOGY, also dealt with physical and psychological sexual maladies, but as Grey (1993: 45) says, 'sexual disorders were the playground of assorted quacks with their dubious remedies for venereal disease, impotence and so forth, and many of the remedies were as harmful as the conditions they purported to cure'. (**David Evans**)

Script   The concept of sexual scripts was developed in the 1970s by John Gagnon and William Simon (1973), within a form of sociology known as symbolic interactionism. Gagnon and Simon rejected ESSENTIALISM and the HYDRAULIC MODEL, arguing that there is no such thing as innate sexuality or sex 'drives'. Instead, sexuality is a matter of scripts: social meanings and conventions which individuals learn within social settings and in interaction with others. Our culture specifies appropriate objects and aims for sexual relations and also the times, places, sequences of gesture and utterance involved in sex acts. Scripts vary across cultures and historical periods, and Simon and Gagnon reject PSYCHOANALYSIS as indifferent to these variations.

The theory of sexual scripts is concerned with the relationships between social processes and individual life experiences. While individuals must organize these as they initially develop their sense of a sexual self, their relation to scripts stabilizes once they find a pattern that 'works'. COMING OUT as lesbian or gay, for example, may involve experimenting with the different types of sexual practices, fantasies and improvisations made available within the context of a number of subcultures. When changes occur to socially available scripts, such as when moving between cultures, a reorganization of one's sexual self may be required. A number of more recent writers have recognized the promise of Simon and Gagnon's concept of scripts. Scott and Jackson (2000) have noted how sexuality is scripted in gendered terms, often involving assumptions about active male sexuality and passive female sexuality. Gutterman (2001) has argued that some scripts are branded onto individuals more emphatically than others, allowing us to rewrite dominant sexual scripts to some degree. (**Chris Brickell**)

Seduction   From the Latin *seducere*, to lead aside or astray. Seduction may exist in different degrees, however it is usually defined in the sexual sense as the enticing of a person (traditionally a woman) into sexual intercourse using psychological and emotional rather than physical force. Bribery or promises of marriage may be employed in this respect. In Greek myth seduction was regarded as a serious crime and up until the twentieth century if a man refused to marry his pregnant partner a suit could be issued for the crime (McLaren 1999: 43). The seriousness of the act lay more in its effect on the 'victim's' future prospects for marriage and the financial implications, especially if the act had resulted in PREGNANCY. In contemporary society the act of seduction may sound outdated: women who were traditionally seen as the targets of seduction, are now moving to a more level playing field with men, leading to the situation that any physical sexual coercion is deemed SEXUAL ASSAULT if not rape. However we might make comparisons between seduction and DATE RAPE. This violent meaning of seduction is in contrast with the term's traditional romantic connotations; an identity reinforced by its appearance in literature throughout the centuries (Newman 1988). The concept of seduction has been adapted in the modern world in a number of ways, in courses and self-help literature. Some publications offer techniques in a tongue-in-cheek manner, however others make more serious claims of success for the customer, leading to concerns that seduction's link to rape/date-rape/assault may become inextricable. Although the term reinforces traditional notions of active MASCULIINE desire and passive FEMININITY, it does also highlight the complexities behind what is often assumed to be a straightforward question of determining whether CONSENT has been given in sexual situations. (**Linda Kiernan**)

Self-definition   With respect to gay, lesbian, bisexual, and transgender (LGBT) IDENTITIES and communities, 'self-definition' represents the idea that LGBT individuals have, or should have, the right to name and define themselves. By way of self-definition, the power of naming is given to individuals and COMMUNITIES affected by the labels used to designate them. Self-definition thereby stands in contrast to a history of naming by others – especially those with more social and political power; for instance, medical and religious institutions. Given that much external labelling has been repressive in nature, self-definition is especially significant for (sexual) minorities since it affords an empowerment made possible through identifying *oneself*. Interesting debates have occurred vis-à-vis the concept of self-definition, especially when one's self-definition does not match one's behaviour (that is, behaviour considered typical of a given identity). For example, it could be asked whether a self-professed STRAIGHT man who engages in the tea-room trade (or COTTAGING) is *really* gay or bisexual. Or whether a self-defined lesbian who sleeps with a man is *really* straight or bisexual (see LESBIANS WHO HAVE SEX WITH MEN). On the side of self-definition, Chvany states, 'Even if someone's self-definition contradicts their behaviour, there can be good reason to trust their word on it. Some lesbians and gay men discover bisexual desires after years of exclusively homosexual fulfilment. Should we *require* them to identify as bi?' (1999: 20). At the same time, an individual *may* alter a self-definition precisely to reflect present attractions and behaviours, as in the following example: 'I had been in a sexual relationship with a wonderful woman for one year, and I was identifying as lesbian at the time. I found myself attracted to a man who was interested in me .... We broke up and I began a sexual relationship with the man' (Rust 2000: 163–4). The woman subsequently identified herself as bisexual. (**Mary Bloodsworth-Lugo**)

Semen   The product of male EJACULATION, containing seminal fluid and sperm (although the latter only makes up a small percentage), and emitted during the male ORGASM, or extracted from the TESTICLES for use in IVF. Semen was considered a vital fluid from antiquity to the end of the nineteenth century, and was linked to the (wholly imaginary) nineteenth-century medical condition, spermatorrhoea, a leaking of semen from the penis caused by too much MASTURBATION which it was believed could lead to blindness, exhaustion, and in extreme cases, death. Thus within SOCIAL PURITY campaigns semen was represented as a substance needing to be conserved (Mort 1987: 42–4), a position in keeping with a larger nineteenth-century bourgeois economic and financial language of saving and restraint. While semen has often been the carrier of STDs, its role in the transmission of HIV has changed its connotations radically. Gay male culture has defiantly continued a playful eroticization of semen in the face of a fearful conservative discourse which pictures 'bodily fluids' as impure and seeks to conflate the possibility of dangerous fluids with those groups whom it has seen as dangerous subjects. This may be a part of a larger male discomfort at bodily fluids as theorized by Grosz (1994), who argues that because the male body is stereotypically pictured as solid and self-contained, the capacity for FLUIDITY and leakage represented by semen is a constant anxiety. Much AIDS literature also insists that women must take the active role in insisting on CONDOM use – a position which both forces women into the role of 'the hygenic and moralistic gatekeepers of the world' (Pearl 1990: 188) and yet also recognizes the widespread failure of heterosexually active men to take responsibility for the potential danger their semen now poses. (**Ivan Crozier** and **Jo Eadie**)

Separatism   A political stance of withdrawal and exclusion, originating with 1960s Black Civil Rights activists, but soon after adopted by radical FEMINISTS of the same period, as a means to 'forging identity and gathering strength' (Smith and Smith 1983: 126). 'Vigorously obscured, trivialized, mystified, and outright denied by many feminist apologists' (Frye 1983: 96), separatists are caricatured, even within many feminist communities, as angry, white, middle-class, colour-blind, man-hating, book-burning, anti-sex, lessie feminazis. Feminist detractors – often termed 'coalitionists' – argue that separatism is not a viable political analysis or strategy, as it downplays all but the sexual sources of women's oppression. As one such group, the Combahee River Collective expressed it:

> Although we are feminists and lesbians, we feel solidarity with progressive Black men and do not advocate the fractionalization that white women who are separatist demand. Our situation as Black people necessitates that we have solidarity around the fact of race. (1983: 213)

Many non-separatist feminists believe that lesbian separatists neglect to include any meaningful analysis of race and class in their theory and practice. They also charge white radical lesbians with obscuring women of colour's presence in and influence on the lesbian separatist movement. Many of the critiques of separatism are well placed and have been raised by lesbian-feminists themselves. Gage (1997: 206), for example, acknowledges that lesbians of colour have compelling reasons for questioning the motives of white women in a movement that by definition excludes roughly half of their communities from participation. On the other hand, she points out, lesbian separatists – regardless of colour – have equally compelling reasons for distrusting the motives of coalitionist women, pointing to the prevalence of lesbian invisibility and HOMOPHOBIA in their organizations. Bunch (1972: 2) explains:

> Although there have been innumerable battles over class, race, and nation during the past 3,000 years, none has brought the liberation of women. While these other forms of oppression must be ended, there is no reason to believe that [women's] liberation will come with the smashing of capitalism, racism, or imperialism today.

Instead, Bunch argues, women will be free only by destabilizing patriarchal society. As envisioned by lesbian separatists, political independence includes independence from patriarchal political and social systems – and space. Consciously constructed woman-only space promises girls and womyn-born-womyn a safe environment within which to gather and heal from oppressions they suffer at the hands of boys and men. (Note: male-to-female TRANSSEXUALS are categorically excluded from any separatist definition of 'woman'.) There are, of course, degrees of separatism from temporary women-only events (e.g. concerts and conferences) to lives completely without men (e.g. all-lesbian houses and communes). As to sexual orientation, heterosexual and bisexual separatists exist, though they are clearly few and far between. Just as 'one does not automatically have to be a lesbian to be a radical feminist', notes Winter (1998), one does not automatically have to be a lesbian to be a separatist, 'but the connection is, you will no doubt appreciate, a logical one'. (**Tamarah Cohen**)

Further reading

Hoagland and Penelope (1988).

Serial monogamy   The practice of conducting consecutive relationships which exclude intimate involvement with others for the duration of particular relationships. Serial monogamy may be an outcome of a succession of unsuccessful relationships which were intended, or hoped, to be permanent when entered into, or may be a more deliberate lifestyle choice. Serial monogamy ranges in scope from a limited number of relatively long-lasting relationships, to a large number of very short-lived relationships. The defining feature of serial monogamy is that the relationships take place consecutively, rather than concurrently, and that each relationship is based upon an assumption of monogamy, although not necessarily permanence, for the period of its duration.

Serial monogamy is ambiguously located in relation to dominant discourses, since while it conforms to social norms which proscribe intimate relationships with more than one person consecutively, it reflects a 'failure' to sustain a particular intimate relationship. Serial monogamy is negatively associated in popular discourse with being unreasonably selective about a long-term partner (particularly for women), or being unable, or unwilling, to 'settle down'. For women, serial monogamy is often perceived negatively, since it is seen as risking the postponement of motherhood, or alternatively, of producing FAMILY structures which contravene the normative standards of the patriarchal nuclear family. Serial monogamy contravenes cultural prescriptions against intimate relationships with numerous partners, whether consecutive or concurrent, particularly where relationships are relatively short-lived. This is particularly true for women and girls, who are at far greater risk of being labelled as promiscuous than men and boys, and for whom the label itself carries substantially greater pejorative weight (Holland 1998). SOCIOBIOLOGISTS argue that serial monogamy is the inevitable outcome of (heterosexual) men attempting to live monogamously, since this is seen as running counter to their instinctual desire to achieve genetic survival through mating with as many females as possible (Fisher 1992; Ridley 1993). (See also MONOGAMY and NON-MONOGAMY.) (**Karen Throsby**)

Sex (I)　　The routine first question asked after birth is: which sex is it? Yet SEXUAL DIMOR-PHISM – the notion that humans are naturally divided into two sex categories, male and female, and that these form the basis of social life – has been challenged by scholars in recent decades. The 1970s saw a number of feminist writers develop the distinction between 'sex' and 'gender' posed by psychiatrist Robert Stoller in 1968. It was argued that while 'sex' represented the natural attributes of the categories of male and female, the term 'gender' could be applied to the cultural overlay which created boys and girls, men and women. One famous development of this was Rubin's 'sex gender system': 'a set of arrangements by which the biological raw material of human sex and procreation is shaped by human, social intervention' (Rubin 1975: 165).

During the 1990s the sex/gender distinction came under increasing scrutiny on epistemological and political grounds. Many theorists agreed that the distinction relies upon culturally and historically specific forms of knowledge, particularly the BINARISM of nature v. culture. Beyond this agreement, the critics diverge. Those who prioritize embodiment argue against the division of sexed bodies from the social interventions and individual experiences they engender. Others suggest that the notion of a natural sex category is itself a contradiction in terms. For example, Delphy (1993) argues that the male/female distinction itself comes to possess social meaning only within politically-enforced, hierarchical social relationships between the two categories. A further challenge to the idea of a natural binary between male and female is posed by INTERSEXED individuals – those born with genitalia which are 'ambiguous', varying from stated norms around appearance, function and size. Kessler (1998) argues that these variations reveal that the physical criteria used for attributing sex are not dimorphic. Such variations bring into question the exclusivity of male and female as categories of sex, and may even challenge the division of the population into two sexes on the basis of genitalia. (**Chris Brickell**)

Further reading.

Laqueur (1990).

Sex (II)   In recent years many scholars have argued that the relationships between sexual DESIRES (what we want to do sexually), SEXUAL PRACTICES (what we do do) and IDEN-TITIES (how we identify), and the social meanings of these, are highly complex and contingent to particular contexts. For example, in contemporary Western societies sex between men or between women usually indicates particular identities ('gay', 'lesbian'), while in CLASSICAL Greece it reflected relationships of status, power and subordination. Anthropologists have examined how gendered notions of 'active' and 'passive' sexuality structure the meanings granted to sexual practices in some contemporary cultures (Murray 2000). Foucault's writing has been influential, particularly his rejection of the idea that the nineteenth century saw a REPRESSION of sexuality (Foucault 1990). Instead, he argued that this period saw sexuality incited through an explosion of discourses. Particularly important was SEXOLOGY, through which sexual acts and 'types' were catalogued in minute detail and laden with medico-moral significance. For Foucault, the power expressed through the discourses of sexology and other forms of knowledge is primarily productive of sexuality, not repressive of it. The relationships between sex and power have been highly contested in recent years. The 'pleasure and danger' debate divided those who wished to reclaim the pleasures of sex from the strictures of moral evaluation and the idea that sex poses dangers, particularly for women, and those who argued that inequality remains central to the constitution of sexuality (see SEX WARS). Those adopting the latter view argued that sexual coercion is still significant and the DOUBLE STANDARD continues to privilege male desires over female ones. Therefore, HETEROSEXUALITY ought to be analysed not only as the most respectable form of sexuality, but also as a set of gendered practices (Jackson and Scott 1996). (**Chris Brickell**)

Sex education   See ABJECT; CENSORSHIP; COPROPHILIA; DATE RAPE; EROTOPHOBIA; SEX TOYS; SEXUAL HEALTH.

Sex industry   The sex industry includes a range of practices involving the exchange of sex and/or sexually related goods or services for money: PROSTITUTION establishments, street workers, striptease clubs, peep shows, PORNOGRAPHY publications and production companies, sex shops, and TELEPHONE SEX lines. The distinction between the sex industry and the mainstream entertainment industry is blurring, as erotic imagery is becoming integrated in the mainstream industry (e.g. fashion, films, theatre and music videos). The sex industry is a global industry and its size and visibility differs from country to country. For instance, in structure and size Australia's sex industry is very similar to the religious industry – both employ approximately 20,000 people, both have three or four major groupings with a number of independents in between, and both sell intangibles like 'fantasy', 'desire' and 'hope' along with an extensive 'spin-off' range of products (Patten 1997). Within the industry a handful of people make most of the profits, while because it is STIGMATIZED and very often underground, SEX WORKERS within this industry are often exploited and lack the protection and rights granted in the majority of the mainstream industries. (**Ana Lopes**)

Further reading

Plachy and Ridgeway (1996).

Sex manuals   Most literate cultures have produced manuals detailing those procedures for having sex that were considered both 'proper' and 'natural' according to their respective discursive regimes. Foucault (1990) draws a broad distinction between Eastern cultures which he sees as having developed an *ars erotica* centred on pleasure – the third-century Indian classic the *Kama Sutra* and seventeenth-century Japanese 'pillow books' can be seen as examples of this trend – and Western societies that have focused more upon a SCIENTIA SEXUALIS or a 'scientific' discourse aimed at creating the optimum conditions for procreation. However, this distinction is certainly too broad since many Chinese sex manuals were concerned with establishing the ideal time to have sex based on complex and elaborate Taoist principles (Van Gulik 1961), and Western marriage manuals such as the seventeenth-century *Aristotle's Masterpiece* were clearly concerned with pleasure (Porter and Hall 1995). Significantly, Western manuals from the seventeenth to the nineteenth century were particularly concerned with women's pleasure since female ORGASM was considered conducive to conception. Recent research into sex manuals, drawing upon feminist and postmodernist theories, has stressed their regulatory and disciplinary nature. Manuals have tended to focus on 'good' (procreative) sex as opposed to 'bad' (pleasure for pleasure's sake) sex and have been both HETERONORMATIVE and PHALLOCENTRIC, understanding sex primarily in terms of penetration of the VAGINA by a PENIS. It is only in recent years that sex manuals celebrating erotic practices outside of what Rubin (1984) terms the 'charmed circle' of procreative heterosexual sex have become common. Yet even lesbian and gay sex manuals can be seen as regulatory, subjecting the individual to what Foucault refers to as 'the austere monarchy of sex' (1990: 159), since in these texts sexual fulfilment is unquestionably deemed central to a happy life. (**Mark McLelland**)

Further reading

Melody and Peterson (1999).

Sex parties   Sex parties became popular with the advent of the sexual liberation movement. In these parties some kind of both consensual and not-quite-consensual sexuality is practised. In the early 1970s, sex parties were attended by players willing to experiment with new and unconventional sexual practices; the SEXUAL ORIENTATION of players was secondary. The use of drugs like marijuana, hashish, and LSD was not uncommon. In the late 1970s and early 1980s, sexual parties proliferated and became more specialized. Especially noteworthy are the sex parties for gay men in cities with large gay male populations, like San Francisco, where numerous bath houses were opened. Sex was casual and often anonymous. Players had numerous, sometimes countless partners. The use of sexual stimulants was common, with high use of nitrate inhalants called Poppers. Consent was considered desirable, yet the use of substances often made it a moot point. During the AIDS era, SAFER SEX became a common practice at sex parties and the exchange of body fluids among sexual players was dramatically reduced. The need for protection also made consent a necessity, thus reducing the use of drugs and causing sexual players to relate to one another more personally. This encouraged more women to participate in sex parties, which became especially popular in bisexual communities (see also SWINGING). (**Serena Anderlini-D'Onofrio**)

Sex positive/sex negative   'Sex positive' refers to someone or to a culture within which sex is understood as a source of healthy pleasure (Chapkis 1997). On the other hand, a 'sex negative' culture is generally hostile to sex – or EROTOPHOBIC – advocating restraint and repression and often insisting on a narrowly prescribed set of SEXUAL PRACTICES. Sex positive writers defend open discourse around sexuality and the availability of information on sexual matters. Most sex positive writers argue that sexual liberation is an integral part of women's liberation. They believe that traditional morality represses women by viewing their needs as secondary to those of men. However, the term is also used by advocates of FREE LOVE or SWINGING, who might in some cases reject a feminist critique in favour of a more hedonistic view of sexual LIBERATION.

Within FEMINISM the terms have been deployed as part of the SEX WARS to differentiate between the position that sex is primarily a source of pleasure for women, and the position that it is, under existing social arrangements, primarily a site of oppression. During the so-called 'sex wars', SEX RADICAL writers claimed the term 'sex positive' for themselves, arguing that writers such as Andrea Dworkin and Catherine MacKinnon were 'sex negative' in that they held that heterosexual sex was inescapably degrading, or, like Hoagland and Penelope (1988), argued that only in lesbian sexual practice could women find sexual freedom. For instance, for Dworkin (1987), sexual intercourse is the sanctioned and normalized invasion, violation and abuse of women by men. Sex negative feminism is also accused of arguing against representations of sex: for instance along with MacKinnon (1994) Dworkin has consistently held that PORNOGRAPHY, understood as the 'theory' behind RAPE, is violence towards and objectification of women. However, those who hold these positions present the counter-argument that it is *they* who are sex positive, in that they hold out for a world of truly egalitarian sexual relations, and are critical of existing sexual relations only because they are dominated by male power. (**Ana Lopes**)

Sex radical   A term for those seeking and advocating more egalitarian, experimental and challenging forms of sex – whether as public activists or solely within their personal SEXUAL PRACTICE. Its roots include the FREE LOVE Movement – a grassroots movement of men and women of the late nineteenth century who, discontented with the inherent social, economic and political inequalities of the marriage institution, participated in discussions about the relation between sexuality and women's rights. Originally founded in America, this movement led the foundations for later generations of feminists by placing sex and sexuality at the heart of public debate. One of the pillars of the movement was Moses Harman (1830–1911), publisher of the newspaper *Lucifer: The Light Bearer*. This was one of the few publications that openly promoted CONTRACEPTION as a viable choice for women and called for forced sex within marriage to be considered RAPE. In 1890 Harman was imprisoned on charges of OBSCENITY.

In the context of twentieth-century FEMINISM, 'sex radical' refers to authors who are usually portrayed as positive towards sex, which they understand as a source of pleasure and power for women (Chapkis 1997). Vocal sex radicals include Susie Bright, Pat Califia and Gayle Rubin. Despite their differences, these authors have in common the perception of sex as an instrument of LIBERATION, a means to take control over one's life. They see sexuality as a fertile ground for subversion and sexual liberation as being a fundamental part of women's liberation. Following from this SEX POSITIVE vision, some, like Califia also argue that, likewise, SEX WORK can be liberating for those who perform it. Sex radical feminist writers have, for this reason become allies of the sex workers' rights movement in campaigns for the decriminalization of all types of sex work. (**Ana Lopes**)

Further reading

Califia (1994).

Sex tourism   Sex tourism refers to both domestic and international travels that involve sexual services. Sexual tourism is more often practised by both heterosexual and homosexual men than by women, for men enjoy more economic means and a greater range of excuses to travel than women. In first world countries, middle-class gay men are consumers par excellence, whose expenses on sex tourism can be phenomenal: in the United States, Key West and Palm Springs are famous gay resorts, where travellers have a high expectation of sexual adventures. However, sexually motivated tourists are noticeably more interested in exploring 'exotic' cultures other than their own. In the early twentieth century, privileged tourists from Europe and the United States used to hire young Arab boys in North Africa. André Gide exposes the European obsession with the Arabian bodies in his novels (see Dollimore 1991: 335–8). Today, Bangkok has become the global sex capital for both straight and gay men. Very often, tourists are from former imperialist or neo-imperialist countries, and their destinations are the ex-colonies. For instance, Japanese tourists patronize the sex industries in Taiwan and other South-Eastern countries. In the arena of INTER-RACIAL SEX, 'Orientalism', exchange of money, and unequal power relations are strongly intertwined. Many impoverished countries are perfect destinations for sexual tourism, for there might be looser laws, if any, about SEX WORK, AGE OF CONSENT, and so on. Therefore rich tourists, including those who drawn to PAEDOPHILIA, enjoy more accessible sexual services during their travels than in their home countries. Remarkably, the economically emerging cities, such as Hong Kong, Singapore, Seoul, Taipei, also export their sex tourists, especially gay men. These gay tourists are so attracted by the myth of the gay COMMUNITY in the United States and Europe that they are eager to experience the legendary San Francisco, New York, and Berlin. Thus new modes of sex tourism are being born. (**Ta-wei Chi**)

Further reading

Ryan and Hall (2001).

Sex toys   A general term covering all objects used as part of sexual activity, from those solely designed for the purpose of sex (such as DILDOS), to everyday objects appropriated for sex (such as clothes pegs). Rubin (1984) notes that 'sex with manufactured objects' is a category that falls outside the 'charmed circle' of 'good, normal, natural, blessed sexuality'. It is neither procreative nor natural. In coining the term 'sex toys', SEX RADICALS are therefore detaching sexual activity from its reproductive or moral framework and instead positioning it as RECREATIONAL, and presenting all types of sexual pleasure as equally valid by defining stigmatized items – such as the whips and harnesses of SM – as being no more dangerous than a VIBRATOR. Viewing them as valid sources of potential pleasure, some activists have called for sex toys to be a part of sex education programmes for young people. More critical writers have seen sex toys as part of the COMMODIFICATION of sex, with the production of dangerous and over-priced items (Califia 1994: 209) and the shaping of sexual practice in an oppressive direction by creating sex toys that impose a restrictive view of sex. For instance, Jeffreys (1993: 32–6) argues that dildos perpetuate the COITAL IMPERATIVE by which the female body is defined as hole waiting to be filled, while blow-up dolls may be seen to encourage the OBJECTIFICATION of women by presenting women as passive objects of male sexual pleasure. (**Jo Eadie**)

Sex wars   There have been disputes over the role of sexuality in women's liberation and oppression within 'first-wave' and 'second-wave' FEMINISM, between heterosexual and lesbian feminists, and perhaps particularly sharply within lesbian communities (Healey 1996). By the 1980s, this debate was perceived as a war of positions, known as sex wars, mostly between 'radical feminists' and 'sex radical feminists'. The former are usually portrayed as being hostile to sex, which they understand as the source of women's oppression; and the latter are usually portrayed as positive towards sex, which they understand as a source of pleasure and power for women (Chapkis 1997; see SEX POSITIVE/SEX NEGATIVE). SEX RADICALS defended experimental sexual practices including SM, lesbian BUTCH-FEMME, PORNOGRAPHY and SEX WORK; radical feminists read these practices as instances of INTERNALIZED OPPRESSION, which hindered women's liberation, and stressed instead women's sexual oppression through RAPE, SEXUAL ABUSE and the SEX INDUSTRY. Sometimes referred to as the division between 'pleasure and danger' after the title of Vance's (1984) collection, Duggan and Hunter (1995) argue that this pushed the fight for sexual liberation into a series of isolated and divisive political struggles.

However, the portrayal of the debate as 'sex wars' is an oversimplification that hinders rather than illuminates understanding of the discussion: the case is far more complicated. Crucially, there are important differences of perspective within these two polarized camps. For instance, from the perspective of some radical feminist writers – e.g. Dworkin (1987) – heterosexual intercourse itself must be abolished and PROSTITUTION is seen as only a clearer example of the dynamic of male dominance than other SEXUAL PRACTICES, whereas other writers – such as Barry (1979) – argue that positive sex is based on trust and sharing, and thus that prostitution is not sex, but abuse of sex. In this latter position, sex is misrepresented in prostitution and pornography and this misrepresentation endangers the possibility of positive sex, which is nevertheless held out as an important political ideal. Similarly, in seeking greater freedoms for women, SEX RADICALS do not deny the sexual abuse that women face, but place it in a structural context. For instance, Delacoste and Alexander (1987) argue that it is the STIGMA imposed on sex work that permits violence against sex workers, while Kempadoo and Doezema (1998) argue that it is the marginal position of sex workers that denies them protection from abuse and renders them vulnerable to exploitation. They reject the notion of sex workers as exclusively victims, although they admit their marginality and vulnerability The debate within feminism is an ongoing and complex one. Although sometimes useful, terms such as 'sex wars' may hide the complexities and diversities within the debate and its participants' views. (**Ana Lopes**)

Further reading

Duggan and Hunter (1995); Healey (1996).

Sex work The terms 'sex work' and 'sex worker' were first used by prostitution rights activist Carol Leigh (see Leigh 2003). Publications such as *Sex Work: Writings by Women in the Sex Industry* (Delacoste and Alexander 1987), have established it as the preferred term for economic activities within the SEX INDUSTRY. While some writers use the term sex work as a synonym for PROSTITUTION, those who first used the term intended it to be a general one, including everyone who exchanges sexual services for some form of economic gain. In this sense, activities in the SEX INDUSTRY, such as stripping, lap dancing, PORNOGRAPHY, etc., are included. The term has played a key role in ACTIVISM within the sex industry: it acknowledges the exchange of money for sex and it helps to establish prostitution and other activities in the sex industry as recognized work and economic activities. This term calls attention to the fact that sex workers demand not only human and civil rights, but also labour rights. The sex workers' rights movement aims at reclaiming rights that are generally granted or thought to be due to others but that have been systematically denied to sex workers. The main issues are vulnerability to violence and arrest, unacceptable working conditions such as low pay and health risks, and exclusion from civil and social institutions and systems (Overs 1997). Thus, sex workers' organizations, despite variations, campaign for the repeal of prostitution laws and to end the STIGMA associated with sex work (including the scapegoating of sex workers for AIDS and other STDS). Most writers place the launching of the movement in France in 1975, as local prostitutes occupied a church in Lyons in order to draw public attention to police harassment and the injustice of the existing law prohibiting prostitution. In San Francisco in 1973 Margo St James founded COYOTE (Call Off Your Old Tired Ethics). In Britain, the English Collective of Prostitutes was founded in the mid-1970s and is still active. Numerous sex workers' organizations exist and campaign across the world, from Australia to Delhi to South Africa. Most of them are functioning simultaneously as support groups (Overs 1997). Moreover, some groups within the sex workers' rights movements act as a union, although without official union status. In the United Kingdom a sex workers' organization founded in the year 2000 operates under the name of the International Union of Sex Workers (www.iusw.org), making the point that resistance to exploitation within the global sex industry must be organized at the international level too. (**Ana Lopes**)

Further reading

Kempadoo and Doezema (1998).

Sexology The study of sexuality begun by medical doctors and psychiatrists in the late nineteenth and early twentieth centuries. The last two decades of the nineteenth century saw a multiplication of 'perversions' (Oosterhuis 2000: 44–5), as doctors and psychiatrists such as Richard von Krafft-Ebing, Havelock Ellis, Magnus Hirschfeld and Sigmund Freud began to categorize and look for causes of so-called sexual abnormalities, including homosexuality (alternatively: Uranism, contrary sexual feeling, or INVERSION), EXHIBITIONISM, SADISM, MASOCHISM, PAEDOPHILIA, and FETISHISM. Historians identify two principle strands of sexology: biomedical and PSYCHOANALYTIC. While, for example, Hirschfeld viewed homosexuality as congenital and looked for its causes in endocrinal abnormalities, psychoanalysts like Freud believed 'perversions' to be caused by developmental problems. Later, as the centre of sexology moved from Europe to North America, there was a division between empiricists such as Alfred KINSEY, whose publications are credited by some as being essential to the emergence of the gay liberation movement, and psychoanalysts, who resisted the depathologization of homosexuality (Rosario 2002: 103ff.).

There is disagreement among scholars regarding whether sexology played a stigmatizing role towards sexual 'DEVIANCE' by pathologizing it or fostered social tolerance by removing it from the jurisdiction of morality. Some recent scholars have argued that early sexology was embedded in the racist and sexist discourses of eugenics and closely linked with nationalism and misogyny (Bland and Doan 1998). Others argue that the portrayal of sexology by adherents of SOCIAL CONSTRUCTIONISM overemphasizes the power of the medical/psychiatric community over sexual identity and ignores the role played by sexual minorities in the construction of their own identities (Oosterhuis 2000). Some scholars, such as biologist Simon LeVay, believe that proof of the innateness of homosexuality, such as was pursued by Hirschfeld, will ultimately lead to the recognition of the rights of sexual minorities (see GAY GENE). (**Gary Schmidt**)

Further reading

Bland and Doan (1998).

Sexual abuse   One of a number of overlapping terms coined by FEMINISM, along with SEXUAL ASSAULT and SEXUAL HARASSMENT, to draw attention to the widespread sexual violence by men against women and girls. The term is now used almost exclusively to refer to unwanted sexual attention directed against children, either violent, or coercive, or when apparently consensually obtained by an adult's long-term persuading of a child that they have a sexual interest in that adult (called 'grooming'). It can include sexual looks and speech, as well as physical contact.

Having been put on the agenda by feminism, the growing acknowledgement of the seriousness of abuse has led to an expansion of the original concept: that rates of sexual abuse are high amongst boys as well as girls (estimates of abuse of boys varies from between 1 in 6 (Hopper, 2003) to 1 in 10 (Cawson *et al.* 2000)); that abusers include women as well as men; and that abusers may often be older children as well as adults – most frequently, children who have themselves been abused and who are repeating the behaviour they experienced at the hands of an adult (see Hopper 2003 for a summary of debates over these statistics).

In the name of FAMILY VALUES, calls for protection of children by, for instance, the police publicly identifying known sex offenders, has led to the pulling of sexual abuse out of the political analysis of inequality within which feminism originally framed it. The existence of organized PAEDOPHILE networks which abduct children, such as that which scandalized the Belgian government in the 1990s, are for the most part rare and the prominence given to them in the media serves to divert attention away from the most common locus of sexual abuse: the nuclear family. Given that children are most likely to be abused by their fathers, or other close male relatives (Cawson *et al* 2000), and given that most sexual abuse is performed by heterosexual males (including that against young boys), the media obsession with gay men as potential abusers and with so-called 'stranger danger' (rape and abduction of children by lone paedophiles) should be interpreted as a wholesale social denial of the real risks that children face within the family (Singer 1993: 43). While sexual abuse is often viewed as the acts of monstrous or pathological figures, a more political reading places sexual abuse in the contexts of the wider inequalities which render children powerless to challenge adults' authority over them and which contribute to a climate in which children lack independence and information. The conservative discourses that claim to be 'protecting' childhood therefore consolidate the circumstances that put children at risk (**Jo Eadie**)

Further reading

La Fontaine (1990).

Sexual assault   A range of behaviours in which a person is in some way coerced to have sexual contact with another. The type of force used may be physical or psychological in nature, including the threat of violence. These include RAPE by an intimate acquaintance (DATE RAPE), or stranger rape of an adolescent (statutory rape), and various forms of molestation. A common and important pattern in these offences is that the majority of perpetrators and victims know each other, despite the proliferation of messages encouraging greater fear of strangers. There is significant divergence among statistical estimates of prevalence depending on the definitions and methodologies being used; they are also problematic because of underreporting. While levels of gendered violence appear to differ widely across time and cultures, the preponderance of studies report that most sexual assaults are committed by men against women. Therefore, historically, the research has focused on female victims of sexual assault. In recent years, work is also being done regarding male victims and within the context of gay and lesbian relationships (Mezey and King 2000). Among causative factors analysed in much of the research is a history of sexual violence within the perpetrator's family. However, over the last three decades, the social meaning of sexual assault has evolved from being widely perceived as a private issue to being viewed as a social problem. In large part this is a consequence of feminist activism (Brownmiller 1975).

During this period, more attention has also been paid to the cultural contexts and messages contributing to the pervasiveness of sexual assault, for example, the legacy of the history of women as the property of men (Searles and Berger 1995). (**Karen Lovaas**)

Further reading

Schulhofer (1998).

Sexual capital 'Sexual capital' represents assets based on the possession of prized sexual attributes – a body shape, a look, a sexual technique. If a person flaunts their sexual charisma, she might be considered a person equipped with sexual capital. The notion of capital is derived from political economy, according to which capital is economic, such as money and facilities. This analysis, however, only considers economic assets; it ignores other assets such as education and prestige. Non-economic assets should not be overlooked, for they also decide why some people are more privileged than others. Bourdieu (1984) expands the notion of capital beyond its economic scope, and emphasizes non-economic capital, especially the 'cultural capital', which includes knowledge, arts and so on. A penniless person might be equipped with cultural capital, such as the talent in music, and as a result survive well in a capitalist society, with the support of a music-loving patron. Once the notion of capital is freed from the economic realm, it can refer to other assets in addition to the cultural ones. Sexual capital is such a notion modelled on cultural capital. With sexual capital, a person without economic or cultural capital could earn a living by charming other people. To increase sexual capital, many people are obsessed with weight control, fashion, and the COSMETIC SURGERIES that are claimed to be able to enlarge their penises or breasts. COMMODIFICATION is thus found in these beautified bodies. While sexual capital might result in advantages, it does not guarantee happiness, however. A woman considered sexy among straight men might be less popular in a lesbian community. Moreover, sexual capital can be a double-edged sword. While some people gain power with their sexual capital, others, such as those who work in PROSTITUTION and for PORNOGRAPHY, can be vulnerable to exploitation from the consumers who own economic capital. (**Ta-wei Chi**)

Sexual citizenship Although an age-old social and political concept, the modern notion of citizenship has undergone something of a renaissance since the 1980s, perhaps most notably in so-called liberal democracies such as the United Kingdom and United States. In this context, the discourse of citizenship stresses a balance between rights and duties, and is seen to confer a sense of membership and belonging rooted in common purpose. In the United Kingdom, the Conservative Thatcher–Major governments traded heavily on the rhetoric of citizenship, introducing a Citizen's Charter that outlined individuals' rights and responsibilities (Cooper 1993). Although seen as aligned with the 'New Right' politics of Thatcher–Major and Reagan–Bush, the logic of citizenship has been retained by 'Centre Left' parties such as New Labour in the United Kingdom. It has also been adopted by non-party-political movements, who have sought to use its legal and political power to effect change. Among such groups have been campaigners for 'sexual minorities', who have increasingly utilized the language of citizenship to make claims for inclusiveness and equality under law (Evans 1993). However, what is often labelled sexual citizenship is often more properly seen as a set of rights-claims: the right to marry, the right to serve in the military, the right of access to welfare, and so on (Bell and Binnie 2000). Masked behind this comes a set of implicit duties, most notably the duty to ASSIMILATE. In the campaigns of 'mainstream' gay rights groups such as Stonewall in the United Kingdom, for example, certain fundamental rights are demanded: but the price to pay for those rights is behaving responsibly. This sets up an uncomfortable BINARY between (in this instance) 'good homosexuals' and 'bad homosexuals' – and only the former group can ever claim to be citizens. The effect of this manoeuvre on ACTIVIST strategies can be to surrender some 'rights' for the sake of others. This means that agitating under the banner of sexual citizenship is always going to involve potential compromise. (**David Bell**)

Further reading

Bell and Binnie (2000).

Sexual contract　In the liberal 'social contract' individuals give up the absolute freedom that is their birthright in exchange for the benefits of political society. In her influential book, *The Sexual Contract*, Pateman (1988) argues that a prior contract has already taken place that positions men and women unequally in relation to that absolute freedom. The sexual contract that precedes the social contract is naturalized and thus hidden within theories of the democratic state and makes women's social contractual position ambivalent. Pateman gives a number of examples of this prior contract. In marriage, what appears to be a contract between two free individuals is in fact an exchange between two men, the father and the husband-to-be, as evidenced in a woman's change in name from her father's to her husband's. Her 'consent' is thus real but not free, since to refuse an offer of marriage is not to 'remain free' but to remain her father's property. In PROSTITUTION, what may appear to be consensual economic exchange between two free individuals is similarly compromised by the woman's consent having a direct impact on her value in the above exchange. Pateman's argument has been taken up by Mills in his work on *The Racial Contract* (1997), in which he argues that a racial contract also exists prior to the liberal social contract, positioning non-whites and whites differently in relation to freedom. This is clearest in the context of slavery and colonialism of course, where white men and women literally possess or circumscribe black bodies, but it is also formative in contemporary contexts where access to state institutions is mediated by race. (**Clare Hemmings**)

Sexual difference   The concept of sexual difference came to prominence in the French and Italian FEMINIST discourse of the 1970s, a discourse highly inflected by deconstruction. Sexual difference, or *différence sexuelle*, or *differenza sessuale*, indicates the social, cultural, linguistic, and psychological space that stands between the anatomical and physiological ways in which women and men differ from one another. It further points to the cultural constructions that these differences engender, which are in turn influenced by biological evolutions and technological transformations. Sexual difference indicates the different ways in which feminine and masculine subjectivities are constructed in a given cultural arena. Theories of sexual difference explain these differences as variables subject to cultural change that are neither eternal, nor essential, nor natural. Therefore, the concept of sexual difference encompasses both women's compliance with normative FEMININITY and their potential to challenge it.

Etymologically, the phrase 'sexual difference' comes from a rather misogynist French adage, *vive la différence*, in which *vive* means 'up with' and *différence* is used as a euphemism for a woman's mons or pubic area. In this respect, feminist theories of sexual difference are self-empowering reclamations of derogatory expressions, much in the style of 'black is beautiful' or the more recent 'queer nation'. However, in its relatedness to deconstruction, the French word *différence*, 'difference', is evocative of the neologism *différance*, 'deferment', as indicated in Jacques Derrida's *L'Écriture et la différence* (1978). In this context, sexual difference is a process of ongoing deferment of the equality in difference to which both women and men legitimately aspire.

The concept of sexual difference entered Anglophone and American feminist discourse in the 1980s, with the translations of earlier works by Cixous (1976) and Irigaray (1985a, 1985b), and with widespread interest in Jacques Lacan (1977a) and Derrida (1978). The important voices in this transition are Teresa de Lauretis and Rosi Braidotti, both of whom theorize sexual difference as a paradigm analogous to, yet different from, the American Anglophone concept of gender. Braidotti (1991) and de Lauretis (1990) defend Irigaray and Cixous from accusations of ESSENTIALISM coming from American feminists. In Anglophone feminist discourse, French feminist theory is often perceived as essentialist, namely prepared to accept differences between genders as natural. Braidotti and de Lauretis point out how sexual difference allows a more articulate examination of how physiology, anatomy and cultural formations interact, thus bringing the body and its related discursiveness into the frame of Anglophone feminist debate. (**Serena Anderlini-D'Onofrio**)

Further reading

Schor and Weed (eds)(1994).

Sexual dimorphism   A HETERONORMATIVE concept that posits two stable and mutually exclusive sexes (that is, 'opposite sexes') and that gender roles for men and women are based on biological facts. Laqueur explains sexual dimorphism as being committed to the view that 'the body provides a solid foundation, a causal locus, of the meaning of male and female' (1990: 163). A number of recent scholars, including Laqueur, have maintained that such presumed biological facts (that is, 'the body' or the category 'sex') are more accurately described as sociocultural interpretations of phenomena than natural givens. For example, Butler has asked: 'are the ostensibly natural facts of sex discursively produced by various scientific discourses in the service of other political and social interests?' (1990: 7). The logic of sexual dimorphism poses several consequences for sexuality/gender studies: sexual dimorphism implies that sex and gender are linked naturally and necessarily. Thus, male bodies are expected to adopt 'masculine' traits and female bodies 'feminine' ones. The sexes are established as 'opposites', and the so-called opposite sex is posited as the only 'proper' OBJECT-CHOICE of sexual desire. As a consequence, HOMOSEXUAL desire is conceived as 'unnatural'. Additionally, within the rationale of sexual dimorphism, intersexuality is rendered invisible (that is, INTERSEX babies are born more often than most of us know) and a problem to be fixed (that is, intersexuality has been considered a 'condition' in need of resolution – from a sexually ambiguous body to *either* a male *or* female body). In contrast to the idea of two sexes, Fausto-Sterling (1993) has maintained the existence of at least five. This fact implies that 'nature' has never clearly demarcated a boundary between male and female, despite widespread (mainly Western) views to the contrary (**Mary Bloodsworth-Lugo**)

Sexual harassment Coined by feminists in the 1960s, this form of sexual exploitation comprises unwelcome sexual advances, requests for sexual favours, and other verbal or physical conduct of a sexual nature. It is important to note that while in theory the victim as well as the harasser may be either a man or a woman, the bulk of sexually harassing activity is directed against women by heterosexual men. Documented incidents can be traced back to the 1800s (Jones 1996) and in some cases women's complaints were taken more seriously then than they are today – albeit with reference to notions of 'ungentlemanly conduct' (Jose and Bacchi 1994). Cockburn (1990) notes that women are often expected to collude with the sexualized environment of the workplace, and refusing to do so is regarded by men as making them 'spoilsports'.

Three notable feminist activists – Catherine MacKinnon, Andrea Dworkin, and Susan Brownmiller – have sought to define sexual harassment as a form of sex discrimination resulting from patriarchal practices, and therefore necessarily falling within the remit of anti-discrimination legislation. Arguing that the everyday use of language can be employed in oppressive terms and therefore constitutes sexual harassment, MacKinnon (1994) claims that speech constitutes a mode of violence and should be legally regulated in a similar manner to physical acts such as SEXUAL ABUSE or RAPE, and 23 industrialized countries currently have specific laws regarding sexual harassment (Wyatt 2000). While her critics have expressed concern that MacKinnon's position infantilizes women, it has also been opposed by SOCIOBIOLOGY, which has claimed that men are biologically programmed to be sexual aggressors and that sexual behaviour in the workplace is merely symptomatic of a biological inheritance. Others have suggested that harassment is better tackled as a problem of individual interactions and that men are less responsive to challenges if the incident is framed as a problem of patriarchal oppression (see Jose and Bacchi 1994). (**Alison Smith**)

Further reading

MacKinnon (1979).

Sexual health   Sexual health refers to the freedom from, and prevention and treatment of, infections and diseases which impact upon sexual or reproductive function – although the United Nations has offered a wider definition which includes confidence and comfort around one's sexuality (Farquhar 2001). Sexual health programmes provide services such as screening, testing, treatment, advice and education. The communication and reception of sexual health messages is complicated by the strong social taboos which inhibit the discussion of sexual practices, and the implementation by individuals of sexual health strategies such as CONDOM use can be complicated by gender and relations of power (Holland 1998; Odets 1995). Sexual violence also constitutes a serious threat to sexual health.

With the exception of HIV/AIDS campaigns focusing on gay men, public sexual health campaigns for HIV/AIDs and other STDs generally target women, not only in terms of their own sexual health, but as a public health measure to stem the spread of particular diseases (Grosz 1994). Historically, this can be seen, for example, in the 1864 Contagious Diseases Act (UK), which authorized the forcible examination and treatment of PROSTITUTES living around ports and garrisons. In the contemporary context, this can be seen in calls for routine screening of women for chlamydia to be performed alongside regular smear testing, even though the infection is also growing rapidly amongst men.

In the context of international development, sexual health becomes subsumed within programmes focusing on the control of reproduction, again concentrating primarily on women (Hartmann 1995). Population control programmes tend to promote the most reliable forms of CONTRACEPTION, such as the intra-uterine device (IUD), contraceptive implants, and sterilization, which not only involve considerable health risks for women in their own right, but which also carry risks to sexual health by moving the focus away from condom usage. (**Karen Throsby**)

Sexual orientation   A description of who and what one desires sexually, one's OBJECT CHOICE. It has achieved widespread acceptance as the most common term to refer neutrally and non-hierarchically to a range of different sexualities, for instance in anti-discrimination legislation. It is usually used to refer to whether one is heterosexual, homosexual, or bisexual; however, as Pat Califa remarks 'it is very odd that sexual orientation is defined solely in terms of the sex of one's partners' (cited in Hemmings 2002: 113). It might also refer to other fixed sexual desires such as PAEDOPHILIA, and need not refer to concrete SEXUAL PRACTICES since one may have an orientation and never act upon it. The term is sometimes, inaccurately, taken to be synonymous with SEXUAL PREFERENCE, a term with more transitory connotations, whereas 'orientation' implies a relatively fixed sexuality, and is therefore preferred in liberal activism which stresses acceptance of each individual as they are and refutes attempts to 'convert' those with socially stigmatized orientations. Orientation forms the basis for an IDENTITY, but individuals with similar orientations may form very different sexual personae. However, each of the above facets of orientation may be far from actualized if restrictions to being and expression are hindered, as is so often the case, by the institutions of PHALLOCENTRIC, patriarchal MONOGAMOUS HETERONORMATIVE conservatism and the negative internalizing influences these can have on the individual (see INTERNALIZED OPPRESSION). Ideas suggested by PSYCHO-ANALYSIS and promulgated by Kinsey and others, that sexuality is a continuum (see KINSEY SCALE and KLEIN SEXUAL ORIENTATION GRID), still wrestle with the social STIGMATIZATION of all non-heterosexual ways of being, especially homosexuality and bisexuality. All that is non-heterosexual has been seen as sexually *other*, or PERVERSIONS. The efforts of FEMINISM and LGBT politics, have increased the profile of diversity for sexualities, with commensurate calls for full citizenship rights. (**David Evans**)

Further reading

Wintemute (1995).

Sexual politics　Initially used to refer to the power relationships between men and women, in their various pairings or groupings, in the public and private spheres, FEMINISM has explored this topic in depth as it clearly displays the subordination of women. However the subject has been expanded to deal with the full range of issues where the state and other institutions impose normative standards of SEXUAL PRACTICE or IDENTITY – including bisexuality and homosexuality, INTERRACIAL relationships, SEX WORK, and SAFER SEX information – and where there are ACTIVIST or LIBERATION movements against such oppression. The concept of 'sexual politics' has gained most recognition since Kate Millet's pioneering work *Sexual Politics*, first published in 1969, and has directed scholarship in areas of literature, history, sociology and psychology. In it she identified sex as the one area in which one birth group was still dominated by another, a system of dominance and subordination operating as a patriarchy. Millet's choice of title for her work of historical and literary investigations indicated that sexuality is not just some natural experience of women and men but that 'sex is a status category with political implication' (Millet 1969: 23). The system operates on the basis of collaboration of both sexes brought about by social conditioning with regards to temperament role and status (see INTERNALIZED OPPRESSION). Millet also identified sexual politics as being established by biological, psychological, anthropological, educational, economic and sociological factors (1969: 23–58). The term recognizes the inseparability of the personal and the political (Seidler 1991: preface). This aspect has been relevant to feminists as it links the personal to the public so that a DOUBLE STANDARD should not exist which denies the rights of women for the sake of male freedom and independence. Sexual politics has moved on from its initial application to purely male–female power dynamics to encompass many facets of society's sex/gender-related issues owing to its ability to challenge any entrenched attitudes to sexual and/or political relationships, and the term 'patriarchy' has been expanded to HETEROPATRIARCHY in recognition of this. Since its inception it has been extended to include issues such as the impact of AIDS, the question of gays in the military (see DON'T ASK, DON'T TELL), and the debates surrounding teenage sex and pregnancy. Many of these campaigns are now linked together through the concept of SEXUAL CITIZENSHIP. (**Linda Kiernan**)

Sexual practice   Sexual practices refer to the kind of sexual acts people practise and as such they can provide an important basis for IDENTITIES. MASTURBATION, anal sex, ORAL SEX, SAFE(R) SEX, BAREBACKING, VANILLA SEX, TELEPHONE SEX, SM, casual sex, RECREATIONAL SEX, COTTAGING are some sexual practices from an indefinite list and while some of these sexual practices have given rise to specific sexual identities they are not necessarily confined to a specific identity. The link between sexual practice and identity is more complicated as identities are not reducible to particular types of erotic interactions or sexual practices (Weeks *et al.* 2001). Some lesbians have relationships with men or gay men have relationships with women. The category 'MEN-WHO-HAVE-SEX-WITH-MEN' was developed in the context of HIV prevention in order to capture men who hold on to their heterosexual identities but have sexual encounters with other men. Sexual practice interweaves in complex ways with sexual relationships and sexual identity in emerging debates on QUEER identities. Sexual practices are often subjected to assumptions about gender which construct female and male sexual practices in different terms, such as lesbians as ASEXUAL beings and gay men as HYPERSEXUAL beings. The nineteenth-century conception of the sexual drive as being only active in men has resulted in long-lasting constructions of male sexuality as active and female sexuality as passive. Notions of what 'sex' constitutes have also been highly influenced by heterosexual (male) understandings codifying 'real sex' as penis–vagina penetrative intercourse, thus leaving other forms of 'sex' with little language to describe it (Stevi Jackson 1995). (**Natalia Gerodetti**)

Sexual preference   Supplementary to SEXUAL ORIENTATION, 'preference' implies favoured choice. It is often used in conservative literature since while 'orientation' implies a fixed set of desires – which therefore must be accepted – 'preference' implies a casual interest, which could be corrected. A classic confusion between 'preference' and 'orientation' can be found in the UK law referred to as Section 28 of the Local Government Act 1988. This prohibited local government from 'intentionally promot[ing] homosexuality . . . [and] promot[ing] the teaching . . . of homosexuality as a pretended family relationship'. The underlying assumption is that through a form of proselytizing, it is possible to change – i.e. 'pervert' – someone. Inherent in this view is the belief that one can then 'choose' to revert back. This can also lead to INTERNALIZED OPPRESSION in the form of self-loathing if the individual imagines they should or could do something about changing the preference, and thus 'inflicts suffering by requiring some persons repress their "anti-social" urges' (Percy and Warner 1990: 1184). Those who most frequently condemn the diversity of sexual preferences traditionally hide behind a 'moral populism: the view that the majority have the right to dictate how all should live' (ibid., 1185). Conversely, sexual diversity embraces individual awareness that within orientations are choices, or preferences, for sexual fulfilment. For some, this fulfilment may be accentuated by the pleasurable involvement of certain people, positions, techniques, places, resources, FANTASY, etc. that can help achieve the satisfaction desired. The term 'sexual preference' may also embrace some of the more esoteric practices as well as those sometimes referred to or classified as the PARAPHILIAS. (**David Evans**)

Sexual space   Scholars have recently shown a great deal of interest in the impact that specific spatial environments may have, and the uses to which they might be put, in the arena of sexuality. The use of peripheral spaces of society for transgressive or taboo sex can be seen in the use of urban parks, toilets, graveyards, etc., as meeting places. Such spaces remain important to some gay and same-sex aligned men who wish to socialize without the expectations and expense that commercial gay culture requires; others enjoy the thrill of sexual encounters in hegemonically unsanctioned environments (see PUBLIC SEX); still others refuse an openly gay identity or require anonymity (see MEN-WHO-HAVE-SEX-WITH-MEN). Economic factors play a large part in the construction of sexual space: PROSTITUTION concentrates in deprived areas unlikely to be patrolled by legal forces which tend to protect property. For urban gay villages, low rents which initially permit the colonization of certain areas (see Chauncey 1995: esp. 33–45) often begin to increase as the area becomes gentrified by the influx of disposable incomes and COMMUNITY cohesion. This can lead to ill-feeling for those who feel 'pushed out'. The development of communications technologies, such as the Internet, may have removed many spatial restraints from sexual desire, undoubtedly permitting the sharing of innumerable subjects' virtual sexual encounters across the globe without regard to physical proximity. Some have argued, however, that VIRTUAL SEX has not heralded the predicted epoch-defining rupture in sexual practice. Not least, masturbation is certainly nothing new. (**Alex Evans**)

Further reading

Bell and Valentine (eds) (1995).

Sexual stratification   A term for the hierarchy that results when SEXUAL PRACTICES are subject to the approval as well as disapproval of dominant ideologies. The sexual stratifications are plural rather than singular, for there are diverse versions across history and geography. They are also contingent, under the sway of time. In one of the most influential articles on this topic, Rubin (1984), lays out 'the charmed circle', which is situated at the centre of many societies. Within this circle are validated, normative sexual practices, outside it are practices classified as DEVIANCE or PERVERSION. Every centred practice actually defines an opposed one: SM opposed to VANILLA, homosexual and bisexual opposed to STRAIGHT, MONOGAMY opposed to NON-MONOGAMY and so forth. The more accepted sexual practices are considered 'good sex' and the antagonistic ones 'bad sex', with STIGMA often imposed upon those who are engaged them. Although Rubin only mentions 12 adverse pairs, the diagram can be expended to reach ever-emerging new sexual practices. It is also noteworthy that the very same stratification functions differently for men and women – for example, men's extramarital sex is more accepted, women's is more subject to condemnation. The difference marks a DOUBLE STANDARD based on gender. Rubin also argues that although 'good sex' and 'bad sex' are fixed at the extremes in many stratifications, the battlefield for activists and conservatives is the intermediary ground. This intermediary ground accommodates quasi-acceptable practices, such as masturbation and homosexual marriage. While some practices of 'bad sex' could be abusive, many of them might be merely unconventional. Diverse opinions over types of 'bad sex' play a major role in the SEX WARS. While SEX RADICALS are fighting conservatives over the promised land of 'good sex' and the intermediary battlefield, inner debates also roar among the activists between those practices falling between the intermediary land and the social periphery of 'bad sex' – for instance, INTERGENERATIONAL SEX. (**Ta-wei Chi**)

Sexualization   The process by which certain social groups, bodily attributes, or objects, are made to seem erotic. For instance, Dworkin (1981) has argued that PORNOGRAPHY sexualizes female passivity, making women in pain or in positions of weakness, seem arousing to heterosexual men. Sexualization thus encourages a sexual response to certain situations or images which might otherwise be treated very differently. For instance, the sexualization of black people through white fantasies of INTER-RACIAL SEX leads to assumptions being made about both the supposed availability of black women and the supposed sexual threat posed by black men.

While some SOCIOBIOLOGISTS believe that certain physical attributes are naturally more desirable than others (see Ridley 1993), a historical perspective shows that social processes invest sexuality in a culturally particular manner: blonde hair, wide eyes, and high heels might be sexualized at the moment in the West, but we can be certain that this will not last forever. The fact that some things appear sexual and others not, is therefore only an effect of the particular way in which a society organizes DESIRE. Any social order defines certain subjects as supposedly inherently ASEXUAL, and reacts with shock when they are treated as having erotic potential – the sexualization of children in photography for instance.

Advertising may be said to sexualize our daily lives without our having any say in the matter – all manner of objects have been marketed as 'sexy', with their use supposedly highlighting some aspect of the sexuality of their purchasers. Once cigarettes, cars, drinks, furniture, and stereos have been sexualized, it is impossible for them not in turn to sexualize their users. In a wider sense, Foucault (1990) asks how it is that we have all come to be sexualized – to assume that sexuality is an area of particular importance in explaining who we are, rather than merely being an incidental pleasure without any necessary significance. Against this tendency, many campaigners have called for the deliberate DESEXUALIZATION of society. Foucault infamously suggested that one strategy for achieving this might be to end those laws which make RAPE a different category of crime from other acts of violence. He argued that we might be liberated from our focus on sex by ceasing to view as different many of those activities, whether pleasurable or traumatic, that happen to involve genitals rather than any other body parts (see Bell 1991). (**Jo Eadie**)

Further reading

Haug (1987).

Shame   Shame is an emotion that occurs when sexual interest or enjoyment has been initiated but is denied, REPRESSED or delayed because of SEX-NEGATIVE, personal, familial, cultural, social, and/or legal prohibitions (Tomkins 1995: 134). The effect of shame is to inhibit sexual activity or to create secrecy around sexual activity, and can lead to a denial of one's SEXUAL ORIENTATION. Although shame is often associated with non-normative sexual activity, shame pervades the discourses and practices of all forms of sexuality. Some theorists argue that there exists a contemporary 'politics of shame' in which public discussions and practices of sexuality are prohibited or severely limited. Warner, for example, argues that the United States is the 'land of sexual shame' and cites the Clinton–Lewinsky affair as evidence that public discourse around sexuality is framed by shame and discomfort (1999: 21). (See also STIGMA, FAMILY VALUES, CLOSET, and INTERNALIZED OPPRESSION.) (**Rachael Groner**)

Shaving   See PUBIC HAIR.

Situational homosexuality   Situational homosexuality is characterized by same-sex attraction and/or sexual activity in an otherwise heterosexual person (see MSM). In the 1940s and 1950s, the term was particularly viewed within the psychiatric opus of Freudian PSYCHOANALYSIS. Freudian theory led to the belief in 'pseudo homosexuals'; some people were thought to have an authentic homosexuality that lay LATENT (i.e. they will become lesbian or gay at some point) and others merely to have a homosexua potential – derived from a universal bisexuality or POLYMORPHOUS PERVERSITY – which they might express given certain circumstances. Situational homosexuality is now more appropriately set within sociological phenomena, devoid of medical pathologization, and is presumed to occur mainly in HOMOSOCIAL or same-sex institutions such as schools, religious houses, prisons and the armed forces. Men practising it may use the absence of women as their rationale for sex with men, or in other ways seek to define their same-sex activities as different in some ways from homosexuality, to which they remain HOMOPHOBICALLY opposed. Given the cultural invisibility of lesbianism in many societies, research on situational female homosexuality is minimal, but it too occurs in similar single-sex contexts such as prisons, convents, and schools. Situational homosexual acts or relationships may occur voluntarily, such as by way of 'falling in love' with a particular individual, as an experiment, under the (presumed) influence of disinhibiting substances, through loneliness, or the opportunity of the moment. They may also occur for other reasons such as in commercial SEX WORK, or through coercion. Situational homosexuality is more acceptable amongst cultures that do not rely on Westernized classifications of sexualities (Herdt 1997); however, recent research argues that the concept only makes sense within a Western framework, and should not be exported as an explanation of cultures where same-sex activity is regarded as an unexceptional feature within predominantly heterosexual lives (see Jenkins 1996). (**David Evans**)

Further reading

Klein and Wolf (1985).

Skin   The sheer range of individual and cultural practices associated with bodily surface demonstrates how 'skin becomes, rather than simply is, meaningful' (Ahmed and Stacey 2001: 1). Skins constitute the highly problematic seat of race, are the bearers of religious and spiritual inscription, and are the sites of PIERCING and tattoo, assault and mutilation. Often in the service of enhancing one's sexual attractiveness, skins are made-up, epilated, tanned, and altered through COSMETIC SURGERY. As that which is radically personal and inevitably shared, the skin can be seen as a fascinating way of thinking through both the possibilities and the limits of our embodied selves.

While Merleau-Ponty (1968) takes up questions of bodily surface and the flesh in his phenomenological investigations of perception and visibility, the majority of those who have endeavoured to make sense of the skin have been informed by PSYCHOANALYTIC theory. In Kristeva's (1982) theory of ABJECTION, the skin is figured as the primary boundary object dividing the self and its objects from the non-self and the objects that must be expelled. In Anzieu's (1989) work on the 'skin ego', the body's surface is posited as a central constituent of identity formation. Tracing the origins of the skin ego back to primitive experiences of tactility, Anzieu argues that it is the infant's experiences of maternal touch that enable the infant to acquire a spatial understanding and a narcissistic appreciation of its own body. Proper skin-to-skin contact is thus crucial to both the genesis of a coherent body image and the establishment of an outer surface invested (or 'CATHECTED') with LIBIDO. Building on Anzieu's insights, Prosser (1998) explores the notion of living without a 'skin of one's own' as it relates to transsexual embodiment. Prosser's enquiry into the transsexual 'life quest to change [the] contours' (67) of the material body shows that the self must be substantively invested in bodily surface – that the skin is, in fact, anything but 'skin deep'. Also inspired by Anzieu's work, Yang (2001) discusses how AIDS-related changes to the skin (such as Kaposi's sarcoma) both condition medical discourses of the disease itself and affect the body image of those who have contracted it. (**Marc Lafrance**)

Slash fiction   A fantastic example of fan appropriation – and a favourite cultural studies topic – slash fiction describes (usually) HOMOEROTIC depictions of relationships between characters in 'cult' TV shows and movies. Perhaps the best known in the genre are Kirk/Spock stories, comic strips and illustrations, which centre on the erotic relationship of *Star Trek*'s lead characters. But virtually every film or TV show with a same-sex pairing at its core has some slash fiction to accompany it: *Starsky and Hutch*, Bodie and Doyle from *The Professionals*, Napoleon Solo and Illya Kuryakin of *The Man From UNCLE* (Jenkins 1992). Much of this slash art and fiction is produced and consumed by STRAIGHT female fans, who playfully subvert the 'normal' codes of mainstream entertainment. Slash belongs to a larger portfolio of active fan involvement with media – fanzines, 'filk' songs and so on – that Henry Jenkins (1992) collects under the label textual poaching. Slash fiction has generated debate within the fan community, with some critics seeing its pornographic and homoerotic scripts as amounting to 'character rape'. What's more, slash fiction has generated considerable discussion within the academy, as scholars attempt to understand the motivations behind those who write and read it: why would female fans want to read about male characters in loving and sexual relationships? Some academics subject slash and its fans to PSYCHOANALYTIC analysis, uncovering layers of fantasy identification (for an overview, see Hills 2002). Fans and writers confess to a multiplicity of motivations, a knowing appropriation of styles and codes and a playful approach to identity and fantasy. (**David Bell**)

Further reading

Jenkins (1992).

SM   An abbreviation of 'sadomasochism', a word combining two terms: 'sadism', meaning an erotic love of cruelty or domination, and derived from the PORNOGRAPHIC writings of the Marquis de Sade (1740–1814); and 'masochism', meaning the erotic love of pain and submission, coined by German SEXOLOGIST Richard von Krafft-Ebing (1840–1902) in his *Psychopathia Sexualis* (see Krafft-Ebing 1965). Leopold von

Sacher-Masoch (1836–95) inspired Krafft-Ebing through his semi-autobiographical tales of subservient men admiring dominant women, *Venus in Furs* being the best known (Sacher-Masoch 2000). Although the term 'sadomasochism' is colloquially used to describe attitudes of violence and used in PSYCHOANALYTIC theory to describe innate personality traits of domination and submission, its most widespread sexual use is as the term of choice to describe communities organized around the derivation of pleasure from roleplay and the infliction of physical and/or mental pain (see Weinberg 1995). However, differences need to be acknowledged between sex which involves consensual violent roleplay, as opposed to the brutality of physical and mental cruelty often referred to as 'sadistic' behaviour. Many consensual participants therefore choose to speak of 'SM' as opposed to quasi-pathologizing 'sadomasochist', 'sadist', or 'masochist' terminology. Unfortunately, the latter terms are used in popular and legal parlance to describe those who participate in consensual practices, as well as the brutal perpetrators of acts of violence and destruction, including misogynists, rapists, homophobes, child sex abusers and those who commit atrocious war crimes.

As a sexual subculture of pleasure and freedom, SM has a distinct style in terms of dress and behaviour. Leather, latex and uniforms (e.g. military, medical), and an array of SEX TOYS, characterize SM dress. SM SCENES typically involve a TOP (sadist) and a BOTTOM (masochist), and encompass a wide range of activities that generate intense bodily and emotional arousal – including corporal punishment, INFANTILISM, BONDAGE, FISTING, mummification (the complete enclosure of the body), and PIERCING – within a context where certain limits and pleasures have been agreed by prior NEGOTIATION. CONSENT is the basis for SM practice, as is negotiation and the use of SAFEWORDS. Pro-SM theorists utilize the practice of negotiation to defend SM against the argument that it is an abuse of power, arguing that SM practice differs from so-called VANILLA sex precisely because vanilla relationships often ignore the power inequalities embedded in assumptions about what sexual partners will do (Duncan 1996). Increasingly gaining recognition in many 'open' societies, these practices have formed the basis for organized subcultures, generating their own vocabulary: variant terms including LEATHER-SEX (see Thompson 1991), SM or BDSM (Bondage and Domination/SM). The erosion of once rigid boundaries has changed the 'grammar' of this term from originally being abbreviated as 'S/M', to its current embodiment of simply 'SM' – the erasure of the slash signifying the fluidity and crossover of sadism and masochism (see SWITCH). While SM is a label of SELF-DEFINITION, there are still many other 'sexual practitioners' who do not IDENTIFY with the SM community, despite their practice of sadomasochistic acts. Indeed Beckman (2001) suggests that we have seen a recent NORMALIZATION of sadomasochism, so that it has come to be regarded as merely one more pleasurable sexual option amongst many, with handcuffs and whips being sold in relatively mainstream sex shops, and articles on sadomasochistic play featuring in *Cosmopolitan*.

As with many minority SEXUAL PREFERENCES and non-heterosexual ORIENTATIONS, SM sex and its aficionados have been the brunt of numerous psychiatric theories, criminal laws, and moral approbations (Dynes 1990b). Elements within feminism have also condemned SM practices (Hart 1998; see SEX WARS), most particularly for the linkage of heterosexist domination of male over female, and for the objectification of women (Kelly 1998). Within much feminist scholarship, there is a fear that SM enacts and mimics the kinds of violence from which feminism seeks to free women, arguing that SM asserts the inevitability of inequality, whereas FEMINISM seeks an end to inequality (Linden *et al.* 1982). Evidence shows how a key element in understanding attitudes towards the consensual use of pain as erotic pleasure is frequently founded on EROTOPHOBIA. For example, most of the world's largest religions have, at some time, praised flagellation, the use of restraints or other acts of punishment to combat the 'lusts of the flesh'. If such methods are used for the contrary purpose, of indulging in the 'lusts of the flesh', then they are deemed immoral (Scott 1996). Likewise, pain inflicted in certain sports is prized with universal trophies; if the acts were equally consensual, but for sexual gratification, they would be almost universally illegal. (**David Evans** and **Caroline J. McKenzie**)

Further reading

Thompson (1994); Weinberg (1995).

Social constructionism   A theoretical approach that proposes that sexuality is the consequence of a process of attaching particular meanings to the social objects and phenomena that constitute sexuality. This perspective argues that the context of languages, histories and institutions are crucial to understandings and experiences of sexuality and provides an explanation for the FLUID and dynamic nature of sexuality, disrupting the traditional concept of sexual orientation. Social constructionism is a response to explanations of sexuality as rooted in biological origins (e.g. SOCIOBIOLOGY), or as essential or inherent to an individual's behaviours or desires. This binary of ESSENTIALISM and social constructionism has dominated discussions of sexuality. Social constructionism is often informed by poststructuralist approaches, and uses the term 'subjectivity' to refer to the state of a person where language and culture, not biology, give meaning to our sense of self. It challenges the BINARY expectation that homosexuality or heterosexuality are fixed across time and exist as the only possibilities for sexuality. This critique extends to the idea of a predetermined and fixed DEVELOPMENTAL NARRATIVE of sexuality. The work of Michel Foucault (1990) has been influential in conceptualizing the social construction of sexuality – for instance his argument that the emergence of the category of homosexuality in the late nineteenth century reflected a shift towards understanding 'the homosexual' as a separate species, interesting to medical and psychological sciences and reliant on men who had sexual relationships with men to see *themselves* as homosexual (see MODERN SEXUALITY).

Social constructionism is not a unitary paradigm – see Nardi and Schneider (1998) for examples of early social constructionist work. The problems of a social constructionist stance are arguably a loss of politics and identity associated with LIBERATION; the realization of only a limited number of sexual categories despite its predictions of infinite possibilities; and questions about where this approach leaves considerations of the materiality of the body (see BODY POLITICS), and agency (see VOLUNTARISM). (**Sara MacBride-Stewart** and **Stefanie Rixecker**)

Further reading

Halperin (2002).

Social parent   A person who has no biological relationship to a particular child, but who nevertheless fulfils a care-giving parental role in relation to that child. Perhaps the most familiar examples of social parents are foster parents, adoptive parents and step-parents. However, reproductive technology has provided new forms of social parenthood. These include the non-biological fathers of children conceived through ARTIFICIAL INSEMINATION using donor sperm, or women who conceive using donor eggs; the non-biologically related partner in a lesbian or gay parenting context (see GAY FATHER(s) and LESBIAN MOTHER(s)); or the social parents of children conceived in surrogacy arrangements where donor gametes have been used (Pollock and Vaughan 1987; Lehmann 2001). The contemporary emphasis on the importance of genetic relationships between family members constructs social parenthood as a lesser relationship. This is apparent in the context of step-parenting, where pejorative stereotypes of the unloving stepmother and the abusive stepfather serve as an emphatic reminder of the dominant cultural belief that blood is thicker than water. Children raised by adoptive parents may choose to seek out what are constructed in the dominant discourse as their 'real' parents, thereby reinforcing the primacy of the biological over the social. The perceived primacy of the BIOLOGICAL PARENT is particularly evident when the claims of biological parents are in conflict with those of social parents. For example, where lesbian or gay couples are raising a child together that is only biologically related to one of them, the non-biologically related partner's status in relation to the child is highly precarious and ill-defined. Consequently, if a couple separates and the biological parent is hostile to further contact between the child and the social parent, it is uncertain that the social parent will be able to secure access to the child. This can also occur in the exclusion of step-parents when relationships fail. The subordinated status of social parenting marks a failure to acknowledge the raising of a child as a primarily social rather than biological activity – an exclusion which runs counter to the proliferation of non-traditional family structures evident in contemporary society. (**Karen Throsby**)

Further reading

Wright (1998).

Social purity   The Social Purity movement emerged against the background of rapid social change that accompanied industrialization in the second half of the nineteenth century (see MODERN SEXUALITY). At the centre of its concerns were sexual and moral matters such as the fight against PROSTITUTION and the regulation of young people's sexuality through the AGE OF CONSENT. The social purity movement swept across Europe emanating from England and various national and local groups emerged as well as an international federation in 1875. Jeffreys (1985) has argued that the women's social purity movement ought to be seen as part of the early FEMINIST movement. During the nineteenth century the social effects of prostitution, such as its conflict with prevailing moral norms, the exploitation of women's economic position and the spread of SEXUALLY TRANSMITTED DISEASES, were increasingly causing concern (Bland 1995). Despite existing legal and sanitary sanctions in most European countries, it was the Contagious Diseases Acts of the 1860s which prompted a wider opposition in England. In 1869 Josephine Butler founded, together with a broad coalition of social reformers, doctors and lawyers, an opposition movement to these laws, promoting the abolition of the DOUBLE STANDARD of morality and opposing the state's view that prostitution was a necessary evil. In their view, there was little difference between homosexuality and prostitution as they were both driven by male lust and male sexual selfishness. Promoting a single standard of morality for men and women, the social purity movement often directed its politics at changing men's sexual and moral conduct. While the social purity movement significantly contributed in shaping sexuality as a public and social issue there were also more contradictory positions within the movement, such as its racial politics and its aim to control particularly the working classes (Bland 1995). (**Natalia Gerodetti**)

Sociobiology   A school of thought originating from the 1970s and largely popular in the United States. A sociobiological approach theorizes human and animal societies from a genetic evolutionary perspective, making links between the two. Also referred to as 'neo-Darwinism', sociobiology focuses upon the process of genetic selection. This perspective views all social behaviour as having a biological basis and stresses the relationship between animal and human behaviour. For example, a sociobiological approach ties sexuality to reproduction, and stresses the supposed natural tendency for male promiscuity and female monogamy.

Sociologists have largely been critical of a sociobiological approach. The key source of criticism focuses upon its biological reductionist tendencies. Critics argue that sociobiology not only negates the differences between human and animal behaviour, but also that it ignores the great cultural and social diversity between human societies. Sahlins (1976) has rejected the claims that sociobiology is a distinct field of academic study by arguing that it lacks theoretical coherence, while both scientists and sociologists have questioned its use of scientific evidence. More recently, sociobiology has been associated with neo-conservatism. Rose (1984) for example has linked sociobiology to right-wing thinking in the United States, which denounces the goals of equality made by social movements such as FEMINISM and gay and lesbian groups since the

1960s. Contemporary sociologists working in the areas of gender, 'race' and sexuality are particularly critical of a sociobiological approach, which they argue is unresponsive to the distinct experiences of 'minority' social and cultural groups. Despite strong criticisms, sociobiology is now a well-established field of study. Recently an alternative strand of sociobiology has developed, which seeks to legitimize alternative sexualities by showing that they have a functional role in animal species, for example instances of mating amongst animals of the same sex. (**Sally Hines**)

Further reading

Rose *et al.* (1984).

Sodomy　Sodomy and BUGGERY: frequently interchangeable terms of separate etymologies. Like 'buggery', in its earliest uses the term had connotations of heresy and blasphemy. Sodomy has traditionally been an offence punishable by death, but has also been a highly political term, deployed with motives beyond the punishment of sexual DEVIANCE – Henry VIII used it as a weapon in his war on the Catholic Church, directing it against the clergy, as a result of which English law of the MEDIEVAL and EARLY MODERN periods fluctuated in its treatment of sodomy as for many years the crime was taken on and off the statute books, while English monarchs vied over whether England should become a Protestant or Catholic nation (Smith 1994: 41–9). But contemporary scholars revisiting the Biblical origin of the 'Sin of Sodom' have suggested that it should more properly be seen as 'inhospitality' (Boswell 1981), a position gaining credence in those who forgo centuries of intransigent interpretation of later, alternative, readings that exalt procreative patriarchal hegemonies. Earliest traditions of the myth (Genesis 19) mention visiting male dignitaries or (depending upon translation) angels, who are threatened with violence and rape by the citizens of Sodom for not following tribal procedures. Rather than contravene his obligations as host, Lot offers to placate the aggressors by offering up his own daughters in their place. The only reference to Sodom by Christianity's cornerstone, Jesus of Nazareth, is in the context of inhospitality (Matthew 10:15), a point glossed over by followers for most of 2,000 years since. Importantly, he makes no reference to same-sex sex. Superimposing nineteenth-century psychopathological nomenclature – 'homosexuality' – backwards through the ages, and re-identifying it with this Old Testament incident of MALE RAPE perpetuates internalized HOMOPHOBIA for many lesbian and gay religious people, as well as justifying states and individuals with crimes of hatred all in the name of a religion that once (arguably mistakenly) associated modern sexual identities with Sodom, 'the city of sin'. This tradition of recurring negative sodomitical motifs include the sterility of sex-for-pleasure and infection. Infection is taken as a sign of corrupting and 'violating the social order' (Goldberg 1994:5), as well as a personal punishment, images which have played a shaping role in those social representations of AIDS which link sewerage, plague, pollution and the 'wrath of God' (Watney 1994). Within this context, sodomy is *the* act of sexual rebellion, challenging patriarchy by fucking society up the bum, in a communion between the phallus of generation and the site of the most ABJECT, pleasurable non-procreation. (**David Evans**)

Further reading

Goldberg (1994).

Soft core   See EROTICA; PORNOGRAPHY.

Sperm donor   A sperm donor provides sperm to be used in ARTIFICIAL INSEMINATION procedures which enable women for whom conception through vaginal intercourse with a man is not possible or desired, including lesbian (Saffron 1994) and single women, and heterosexual women whose male partners are infertile or unable to have penetrative intercourse (Mason 1993). The majority of sperm donors donate to sperm banks, where donors are screened for genetic disorders, and samples are tested for infections. Samples are frozen and stored for six months and then re-tested for infection before use. Although it is illegal in the United Kingdom to pay egg or sperm donors, a small sum can be offered to cover expenses. Donors are required by law to give their name and birth date, which will be held confidentially by the Human Fertilization and Embryology Authority (HFEA). Donors are also asked to provide non-identifying additional information such as eye or hair colour, or occupation, and this additional information may be provided on request to any subsequent children born as a result of that donation. Currently, there is no legal relationship between a sperm donor and a child born as a result of that donation, although children have the legal right to know whether they were born using donor eggs or sperm. Except for those cases where the right to anonymity is waived by the sperm donor – for example, where lesbian couples recruit donors privately and establish co-parenting relationships with them (Hogben and Coupland 2000) – no identifying information can be given to those children about the donor. This restriction is currently under debate within the United Kingdom, and while many argue that it is necessary for children born using AI to know about their biological parents, it is speculated that the number of donors in the future will be severely reduced if the right to anonymity is removed. (**Karen Throsby**)

STD   Acronym for sexually transmitted disease, a term for any one of a host of infections acquired mainly but not exclusively through sexual contact. STDs are classified on the basis of aetiology or clinical manifestation into five categories: bacteria, ectoparasites, fungi, protozoa or viruses. Timeworn STDs include lymphogranuloma venereum (LGV) a viral infection caused by chlamydia involving the genital lymph glands; a bacterial infection of the genital region known as granuloma inguinale (donovanosis), chancroid, gonorrhea and syphilis. Other common STDs are hepatitis viruses (HBV, HCV, etc.), herpes, human immunodeficiency virus (HIV), human papillomavirus (HPV), molluscum contagiosum, non-gonococcal urethritis (NGU), pelvic inflammatory disease (PID), and vaginitis. With the exception of HIV (identified in 1985) these diseases are among 20 that in the 1960s were grouped together and labelled sexually transmitted diseases, replacing the previous fifteenth-century term venereal disease (from the Latin *venereus* as in Venus, goddess of love and sexual desire). Today, sexually transmitted infection (STI) is the term most often preferred for its accuracy as most STDs can be asymptomatic and undetected. Although frequently stigmatized, STDs occur in all plants and animals that reproduce sexually (Baskin 1999). STDs are generally more serious in women than men because women are physiologically more susceptible to these infections and their effects. In addition, diagnosis and treatment of women is often more difficult than for men. Morally, women have been labelled vectors of infection, particularly prostitutes even though most sexually transmitted infections are more easily transmitted from a man to a woman or from a man to a man than from a woman to a man or woman (Eng and Butler 1997). Screening for STDs and other measures such as CONDOM use are considered preventive, but EROTOPHOBIC public health campaigns often urge abstinence and have consequently been seen to be using fears about STDs to attempt to control sexual behaviour (Mort 1987). (**Dan Allman**)

Sterilization   See CONTRACEPTION; MODERN SEXUALITY; SEXUAL HEALTH.

Stigma   A stigma is a mark or sign that identifies someone as being different from, and often inferior to, 'the norm'. The problem lies with the presupposition that a 'norm' exists and that it is justifiably exalted above the stigmatized person (hence: abnormal, PERVERTED, unnatural, bent and other such pejorative discriminators). Goffman (1990) categorized stigmas according to physical, mental, moral character, or socio-cultural origin. Certain stigmas may be 'passed off', or hidden, from others, a phenomenon which Jones *et al.* (1984) refer to as the stigma's 'concealability'. The stigma's 'course' describes the handling of the stigma by the marked individual and others, both when the stigma is (apparently) concealed, and when revealed. Many sexual stigmas are historically and culturally specific, and tend to discriminate against all those who are seen to deviate from an arbitrary 'norm'. In effect, the privileged forms of sexuality in a society are: heterosexuality, MONOGAMY, reproductive sex, the (post-pubescent) young, able-bodied, 'beautiful' people (see BODY FASCISM). Individuals with characteristics that deviate from these, and many similar preferential identifiers, are often treated as sick, perverted, and even evil. Sexual stigmas may predispose the marked person to verbal or physical abuse from others, including invisibility of sexual needs, RAPE and QUEERBASHING. The history of most cultures abounds with EROTOPHOBIC stigma-orientated myths and negative stereotypes frequently perpetuated through ancient religious and superstitious beliefs (Evans 2000: 1162) and now include HIV and

AIDS stigmas (Evans 2001: 104). Stigmas are also routinely affiliated with forms of social exclusion. The internalized effects of stigma on the individual can predispose to negative beliefs and destructive behaviours, such as low self-esteem, unsafe sex, substance abuse and suicide (see INTERNALIZED OPPRESSION). (**David Evans**)

Further reading

Goffman (1990).

Stone butch   In Anglo-American lesbian communities, a BUTCH who does not allow her partners to touch her in sexual interaction. The stone butch is altruistic in the attention accorded to lovers' pleasure, and yet impenetrable to their sexual touch. The triumphs and trials of stone butch experience in mid-twentieth century United States have been powerfully recounted by Feinberg (1993). More recently, stone butch has come to occupy a prominent place in QUEER THEORY debates. Halberstam (1998: 123) notes that stone butch is a peculiar IDENTITY, in that it is articulated in the negative: what sexual practices the subject does *not* engage in and what physical boundaries are *not* to be breached in sexual activity. She further argues that the stone butch profoundly unsettles a number of assumptions: the combination of masculinity and sexual untouchability of the stone butch challenges supposed commonalities of SEXUAL PRACTICE among lesbians, sexual desire among women and grounds of masculine identification among butches (ibid., 21). A key marker of butch variability, the stone butch is in Halberstam's analysis located within a spectrum of FEMALE MASCULINITY. In the context of an analysis of transsexual autobiographies, Prosser (1998) disputes this point and argues instead for an understanding of the stone butch in terms of a subjectivity that is specifically TRANSGENDER. Despite QUEER THEORY's anti-ESSENTIALIST theoretical propensities, Prosser considers the claims to embodiment made by the protagonist of Feinberg's novel, and makes a case for the acknowledgement of the place of ESSENTIALISM in transsexual and transgender narratives. According to Hale (1998) the stone butch, thus positioned to mark a liminal space between BUTCH and FTM, becomes a 'border zone' and the site of 'border wars', struggles over territory and legitimacy which are partly the products of residual BINARY thinking. Such violent appropriations should be resisted in favour of alliances grounded on respect of specificities. (**Silvia Posocco**)

Straight   In sexuality studies, straight is conventionally used to mean HETEROSEXUAL as opposed to gay/lesbian/bisexual, queer or perverse. British feminist Lynne Segal (1992, 1994, 1997) has long attributed a certain perversity to heterosexual desire and pleasure. Discarding what she views as the consensus of 'feminism as anti-heterosexual pleasure and heterosexual pleasure as anti-woman' (1997: 77), she outlines the continuing need to rethink heterosexuality in terms of what it means materially and psychosexually for women, in tandem with shifting definitions of MASCULINITY for straight men. Segal urges us to attack the hegemonic images of PHALLIC prowess, and to sexualize those of female activity. The archaic gender polarity of male activity and female passivity supposedly at the centre of heterosexual relations masks the more complex reality of male desire for vulnerability and passivity in sex. In other words, straight sex in practice is far more diverse than its enemies care to admit. Whereas the sexual moralizing line would see sex as confirming gender oppression, Segal turns the argument around, positing sex (and subversive fantasy) as that which potentially troubles the status quo of gender polarity. Segal attempts to undermine the naturalized link between manhood and heterosexuality by re-signifying 'straight' as in actual fact 'perverse'. Much heterosexual discontent is projected onto PORNOGRAPHY; what she describes as 'the pains and pleasures of heterosexual desire' (1992: 65) are worked out on the slag heap of sexual representation – the revulsion and appeal of pornography are intricately bound up in fraught negotiations around the intimate questions of sex: how can heterosexual women conceive of an enjoyable, active, egalitarian sexuality with men; how do they become *subjects* of desire? (For a counter-argument, see SEPARATISM and WOMAN-IDENTIFIED WOMAN.) (**Nicholas Rees-Roberts**)

Straight acting   A term within gay male culture used to refer to men who adopt a conventionally – or even stereotypically – masculine persona modelled on hegemonic heterosexual MASCULINITY: no piercings, no flamboyant clothes, and no public same-sex affection. This is very different from a CLONE identity, which mimics conventional masculinity but is deliberately visibly identifiable as gay. In essence, straight acting is appealing to HETERONORMATIVE social structures (Fee 2000) that associate gayness with EFFEMINACY and CAMP. Petersen (1998) says the male 'homosexual', in particular, came to signify the antithesis of the 'normal' male 'heterosexual', and was seen to possess an effeminate body having its own distinct desires and pathologies. 'Straight acting' gay, bisexual or other MEN-WHO-HAVE-SEX-WITH-MEN may thus dislike the perceptions of men like themselves in their culture, and therefore wish to appear different. It is thus simplistic in its conceptualization of male heterosexuality, which it wrongly presumes never to be effeminate or camp. Where hyper-masculine cultures exist, such as in certain professions or other 'testosterone-charged' environments, 'straight acting' may be *de rigueur*, and not an option. For example, straight acting can be a way of concealing non-heterosexual orientations especially in times, cultures or places where COMING OUT is unsafe. Straight acting may also be the result of INTERNALIZED OPPRESSIONS, such as internalized HOMO- and BIPHOBIA. Straight acting may also be a way of protecting oneself from the violence and abuse characteristically meted out by homophobes and biphobes in HETEROSEXIST cultures (see PASSING). Finally, straight acting men may constitute a SEXUAL PREFERENCE, in that the *persona sexualis* of so-called 'real men' is a typically prized asset for those who are attracted to such an image. (**David Evans**)

Straight mind   According to Wittig, 'the discourses which particularly oppress all of us, lesbians, women, and homosexual men, are those which take for granted that what founds society, any society, is heterosexuality'. These apolitical discourses which naturalize heterosexuality rely on a foundational notion of SEXUAL DIFFERENCE: 'this necessity of the different/other is an ontological one for the whole conglomerate of sciences and disciplines that I call the straight mind' (Wittig 1992: 24–5). Under attack is the systematic interdisciplinarity of heterosexual myths, principally Lacanian psychoanalysis and structuralist anthropology, hence Wittig's parody of the title of Lévi-Strauss's *Savage Mind*. The difficulty with tackling heterosexuality politically is its apparent invisibility. Wittig defines heterosexuality as 'a nonexistent object, a fetish, an ideological form which cannot be grasped in reality, except through its effects' (ibid., 41). Thus, Wittig concludes, the overthrowing of straight concepts (woman, man, sex, difference) engenders panic, for those who are severing the heterosexual contract create a paradigm shift. Going beyond heterosexual difference, the lesbian, according to Wittig's axiom, is not a woman. In Butler's (1990) reading, Wittig's political theory is said to reject dominant terms, thereby refusing reformist or subversive positions. Butler's argument goes on to describe heterosexuality as a comedy, containing elements that allow it to subvert itself, thus denying Wittig's full-scale refusal; 'even that refusal', Butler maintains, 'constitutes an engagement and, ultimately, a radical dependence on the very terms that lesbianism purports to transcend' (ibid., 124). Thus for Butler, a radical split between homo- and heterosexuality is not politically viable or psychically possible. Bersani echoes this point, arguing that Wittig fails to differentiate between the heterosexual and the HETEROSEXIST (Bersani, 1995: 38). (**Nicholas Rees-Roberts**)

Strap-on   A strap-on is a DILDO (an artificial phallus) worn against the body by means of straps or ties. Dildos may have straps affixed or may be used with a harness, a leather or cloth garment designed to secure a dildo in place. Various types of harness are available, including thong and jock-strap models. Strap-ons are most often worn against the pubic bone, but newer models allow a dildo to be worn on the thigh. Unlike hand-held dildos, strap-ons allow 'hands free' sex (Newman 1999: 138–40; Winks and Semans 2002: 196–9). In addition to their sexual use, strap-on dildos may also be worn under the clothing, a practice known as PACKING. Strap-ons may be used by people of all sexes and genders (including men with erectile difficulties), but they are employed most often by women who wish to take on a penetrative role – ORAL, ANAL or VAGINAL – in sexual intercourse. During the SEX WARS of the late 1970s and early 1980s, some lesbian feminists condemned the use of strap-ons and dildos as a patriarchal practice (Lotney 2000: xi). Strap-ons are favoured by many BUTCH women and TRANSGENDER men who wish to take on what traditionally has been defined as a masculine role in sex. In 2000 Karlyn Lotney, a San Francisco sex educator, wrote the first book dedicated solely to strap-on sex. At the turn of the twenty-first century the practice of women penetrating their male partners with strap-ons (dubbed 'pegging' by syndicated sex advice columnist Dan Savage 2001) gained public popularity, advanced by media representations such as SIR Video's sex-positive educational video *Bend Over Boyfriend* (1998). (**Liz Highleyman**)

Stripping   See RED LIGHT DISTRICT; SEX INDUSTRY; SEX WORK; VOYEURISM.

Swinging   Experiments in sex and relationships have taken many forms at different times, and some are afforded more coverage than others. So, while sociologists such as Giddens (1992a) can discuss excitedly concepts such as the PURE RELATIONSHIP or PLASTIC SEXUALITY, he shies away – as do most other commentators – from discussing swinging. Nevertheless, swinging as a sociological phenomenon remains of some significance, even if its inner workings as a 'scene' have yet to be fully mapped. Synonymous with what used to be known as wife swapping and with 'key parties', associated with orgies and a certain level of BICURIOSITY (at the least), the swinging scene remains tainted with the sexual excesses of the 1960s and 1970s – hence, perhaps, its academic sidelining: it sounds clichéd and embarrassing, conjuring images of British sexploitation movies with titles like *Suburban Wives* (see Hunt 1998). It is definitively a scene for couples, the kind that describe themselves as 'open minded' or 'straight but not narrow' in personal ads or on the Internet, yet it has never been cited as a place for SEX RADICALISM. It's too cosy and domestic for that, and conceived as staunchly apolitical and hedonistic – there's no 'swingers pride'. However, the sizeable scene includes private SEX PARTIES, members' clubs, and a vibrant set of web-based resources. But it remains outside both the sexual mainstream and sex radicalism, only ever the subject of tabloid titillation and PORNOGRAPHY. Under the general heading of swinging, we can also include other 'fringe' sexual practices, such as the curious mixed ecology of VOYEURISM and EXHIBITIONISM, and 'dogging', in which couples have sex in cars while others watch. (**David Bell**)

Switch   A term from SM culture, referring to someone who takes on multiple sexual ROLES. Although they may have a primary role they occupy, typically a switch alternates between TOP and BOTTOM, or dominant and submissive roles, being a top in one SCENE, but a bottom in another, either trying different roles with different partners, or in different scenes with a regular partner. Switch is a newer term, arising from the exploration of less clear-cut roles than in the past, where people were assumed to be either top or bottom, and there was no foreseeable or acceptable alternative where one could move from one role to another. A person in several SM relationships may maintain a dominant status with their slave or submissive, but may also maintain a submissive status to their top. Likewise, some tops in the SM community believe in experiencing everything their bottoms/submissives do, so they take on a bottom/submissive role for this purpose. For some in the SM community, there are negative connotations to the term; switches may be seen as less serious than those who identify strictly as tops or bottoms. Their preferences may seem less intense, which is similar to the STIGMA attached to BISEXUALITY (Tan 1995) and other HYBRID identities, where those who do not fit into BINARY classifications are often labelled as misfits or failures. However, as Highleyman (1996) suggests, the very foregrounding of the constructedness of roles within SM play leads to a heightened awareness of their artificiality and hence changeability. Switching may therefore be seen by some as the full realization of the promise of sexual liberation into a world free from limits (Tan, 1995), while others feel that sex is more intense if rigid limits are set upon it. (**Caroline J. McKenzie**)

T

Tea-room   See COTTAGING.

Teledildonics   With the coming of new technologies come new SEXUAL PRACTICES and products. The printing press brought the dirty book; the movie camera the porn film. The arrival of cyberspace and the Internet has similarly seen a flourishing of sexual activity, mostly new outlets for PORNOGRAPHY, new ways to meet sexual partners, and new modes of computer-mediated eroticism. However, by and large the actual embodied sexual practices materialize offline rather than online; as Kaloski (1999) writes, much 'online sex' equates to one-handed typing. However, virtual reality (VR) – an offshoot of cyberspace in which participants experience a full computer-generated environment – seemed for a time to offer new and unique sexual possibilities. Beginning with a special visor to give 360-degree visibility, and soon developing to include first a sensory data-glove and then a full data-suit, VR was heralded as signalling a new phase in human–computer (and human–computer–human) interaction: remote human actors could now engage with each other via the Internet, but could experience 'co-presence': they could be 'virtually' in the same place (Rheingold 1992). Data-gloves and data-suits provided sensory connection beyond the visual, making cyberspace a tactile environment, too. It should come as no surprise that these developments were soon woven into scenarios about the future of sex. In the era of AIDS panic, moreover, VIRTUAL SEX or teledildonics offered the ultimate in SAFE(R) SEX. It also offered endless fantasy possibilities, given that cyberspace and VR also provide opportunities to use alternate personae, to play with identity. However, these fantasies might hold their own dangers, and the bridge between the real and virtual worlds can be breached (as in, for example, debates about 'virtual rape'; see Dibbell 1999). The heat generated by teledildonics – and indeed by VR more broadly – has subsided somewhat in recent years, mainly due to the technology's inability to deliver the fantasy of immersive, embodied experience online. (**David Bell**)

Telephone sex   No history book records Alexander Graham Bell and Mr Watson engaging in telephone sex. Nevertheless, during history's first telephone call in the spring of 1876, the former is reported to have asked the latter to 'come here'. Before 'Hello' or 'What are you wearing?' or 'I'm going to cum', Western wankers have had the ability to 'reach out and touch' a voice, that Weatherford suggests is little more than a VIRTUAL SEX prop utilized to help a caller 'pretend they are doing something other than manipulating themselves to ORGASM' (1986: 37). In the course of a century and a quarter, the telephone has become the quintessential POSTMODERN SEX TOY, first as a potentially potent hub of iniquity, devoid of the dangers of physical if not emotional INTIMACY, and second, as a DESEXUALIZED and PUBLIC SEX tool where diallers can bunker down with as many personas or FANTASIES as their erotic virtuosity will allow (Gordon 1980). As the years progress, the telephone has become a FLUID mainstay of a seemingly inevitable erotic climate, itself a by-product of this technosexual innovation at work. From Woody Allen's *Sleeper* (1973) to the history of modern presidents and principalities, the telephone has the potential to be every household's medium of communication, consumption, convenience, entertainment and service. Imagine a plastic launching pad to a world where the size and shape of an operator's privates are decidedly less revealing than the dimensions of their vocabulary, then – 'let your fingers do the walking'. Whether enjoyed commercially or between sweethearts, as bridge or a barrier; be it headset or hands-free, 'only in telephone sex, robot sex, computer sex, is there escape from ugliness and cruelty. Machine sex is the only kind left that is uncontaminated, antiseptic, clean, even a little mysterious' (Andy Warhol quoted in Ultra Violet, 1988: 14). (**Dan Allman**)

Testicles   The male reproductive organs which produce sperm, as well as male sex hormones (especially testosterone). In humans, the testicles are external, situated in the scrotum. This is because the optimum temperature for the production of viable sperm is two degrees lower than the 37 degrees Celsius of the human body, so the scrotum has the function of cooling the testicles. Because the testicles are of great genetic significance, they are also extremely sensitive, which has in turn allowed for their treatment as a sexual part, especially through licking and fondling, or through more aggressive torture in SM scenes. Testicles have a symbolic function as well as a biological one. Apart from allowing men to produce children and to hormonally make the physical transition from boyhood to adulthood, testicles represent male wholeness and power – hence the language of 'having the balls' to do something. Women's self-defence classes have sought to challenge this mythology by emphasizing the vulnerability of the testicles, and the relative success of deterring male assailants by a forceful kick to the groin (Marcus 1992). The current belief that testicles confer MASCULINITY runs counter to the earlier Western medical tradition in which the ovaries were also called testicles, and it was assumed that women possessed similar, but internal, organs with similar functions (Laqueur 1990). But so fundamental is the testicles–masculinity link that even commercial DILDOS are often manufactured with sculpted balls, as an alternative to which lesbian designers and consumers have manufactured their own testicle-free options. FTM transsexuals would also argue that testicles are not essential for maleness, and that an equally authentic masculine identity can be constructed without them. (**Ivan Crozier** and **Jo Eadie**)

Third sex   The term 'third sex' has its roots in SEXOLOGY of the nineteenth century, and generally refers to individuals who are attracted to members of their own sex. In the 1860s, a German lawyer, Karl Ulrichs, developed a scientific theory to account for men who engaged in same-sex erotic acts. He named these individuals 'Urnings', as love between two men is ascribed to the god Uranus in Plato's *Symposium*. Influenced by early medical writings about HERMAPHRODITES, Ulrichs believed that men who were attracted to men have some inborn 'female' sexual tendencies. He believed such individuals (himself included) constituted a third sex, and considered this a natural and healthy phenomenon (Wikholm 1999). Richard von Krafft-Ebing and Havelock Ellis further developed the theory that an individual might have an inborn sex identity different from their anatomical sex. These sexologists constructed a theory of sexual INVERSION, which not only encompassed same-sex erotic behaviour, but 'connoted a total reversal of one's sex role' (Chauncey 1983: 119), conflating sex, gender, and sexual OBJECT CHOICE. In addition, sexologists began increasingly to view inverts as suffering from mental disease and hereditary degeneration. In the early twentieth century, Magnus Hirschfeld, a German sex researcher, took Ulrichs's theory of a third sex and further expanded on it, positing an 'intermediate sexual type' that existed as a third sex somewhere between male and female. Like Ulrichs, Hirschfeld was unapologetic about his homosexuality. Hirschfeld became unpopular during the Nazis' rise to power, not only because of his leftist politics and Jewish heritage, but also because of his 'work on behalf of homosexual rights . . . and his ceaseless campaign for repeal of Paragraph 175, the German sodomy law' (Haeberle 1989: 367). The notion that homosexuals constitute a third sex fell out of favour as more complex psychological theories that separated biological sex, gender role identity, and sexual object choice such as PSYCHOANALYSIS, took its place. Nevertheless, the ubiquitous idea that female homosexuals are somehow male and male homosexuals are somehow female shows the depth to which the belief in a third sex has permeated Western culture, even up to the present time. (**Linnea Stenson**)

Tomboy   See FEMALE MASCULINITY; FTM; IDENTIFICATION.

Top   This term is primarily used as a noun in relation to anal sex amongst gay men and SADO-MASOCHISTIC roles with both heterosexual and same-sex partners. Amongst gay men 'top' refers to the partner who takes the insertive role in penetrative anal sex. For some men this relates to a stable preference and may form an integral part of sexual identity whilst other men may enjoy performing both top and BOTTOM roles across or within sexual encounters (Underwood 2003). Whilst it should be noted that many gay men eschew the term because of its association with unequal power relations and HETEROSEXIST stereotypes that gay relationships mimic traditional gender roles (see Wegesin, Elwood and Bowen 2000), the term remains in widespread usage in many gay communities as evidenced by Bartholome, Tewksbury and Bruzzone (2000) in their study of gay personal ads. It is likely that the expression has greater currency in navigating casual sexual encounters than in long-term gay male relationships. The term is also widespread amongst individuals of all genders and sexualities who practise sado-masochism and other non-VANILLA sexual activities including FISTING and BONDAGE. Top refers to the partner who is symbolically seen as holding the powerful or dominant role. This generally involves the more active and penetrative role (where appropriate). Many participants are versatile enjoying both dominant and submissive roles within and across sexual SCRIPTS (see SWITCH). Contrary to popular stereotypes 'tops' do not reliably demonstrate certain personality traits, childhood experiences or underlying pathology (Weinberg 1995). (**Iain Williamson**)

Trans   Describing persons whose gender does not conform to norms, e.g. a transman, the transcommunity. This is taken from the prefix used with several words used to describe gender variance, i.e. transvestite, transsexual, transgender. It is sometimes used as a less controversial synonym of 'transgender', in that 'trans' references, but does not specify, transvestite, transsexual and transgender people, as well as other gender variances. This makes it a fluid descriptor which is a broad, yet specific reference depending on context, which avoids the problems of the term transgender. 'Transgender' is problematic on several grounds. While the term 'transgenderist' was originally created to contrast with the terms transvestite and transsexual, referring to those who live in a sex role different from their anatomical sex, but who do not desire sex reassignment surgery (Holly 1991: 31), 'transgender' has been extended by some to refer to all gender-variant people – including, for instance, DRAG QUEENS, DRAG KINGS, and others practising GENDERFUCK. Some criticize this extension on the grounds that it creates a problematic category which unites persons of differing, and perhaps conflicting political interests. Moreover, the understanding of 'transgender' as implying that gender is a social or psychological construct can ironically result in a solidification of the binary nature of 'biological' sex (Valentine 2000: 2). Further complicating the picture, 'transgender' is a 'discourse in motion', a term controversial even among those whom it purports to describe, and is primarily a white middle-class US and UK identifier, thus reproducing social hierarchies of race, class and gender (ibid., 7–8). For these reasons, many people prefer to use the term 'trans'. The dispute surrounding the term transgender, leading to a preference for trans, has been described as follows:

> Who knows what to call transpeople these days? The dominant discourse in the transcommunity is at best a moving target. . . . Transgender began as an

umbrella term, one defined by its inclusions rather than its boundaries, coined to embrace anyone who was (in Kate Bornstein's felicitous phrase) 'transgressively gendered'... Increasingly, the term has hardened to become an identity rather than a descriptor... But at some point such efforts simply extend the linguistic fiction that real identities (however inclusive) actually exist prior to the political systems that create and require them. (Wilchins 1997: 15–17) (**Jill Weiss**)

Trans studies An academic field of study focusing on the experience of TRANS people. This is a relatively new field of study which 'promises to offer important new insights into such fundamental questions as how bodies mean or what constitutes human personhood' (Stryker 1998: 155). While it is often subsumed under LESBIAN AND GAY STUDIES or QUEER THEORY, it is at the same time disruptive of structured sexualities such as 'gay' and 'lesbian' (Stone 1991: 296). It encompasses many disciplines, such as sociology (Devor 1997), anthropology (Valentine 2000), psychology (Brown and Rounsley 1996), philosophy (Butler 1990), law (Whittle 2002), and history (Meyerowitz 2002). Some of the main tensions of the field include debates over why trans people are not accepted by society, whether transgender is properly a part of the 'LGBT' community, whether there is a spectrum of genders between or beyond male and female, whether those who do not 'change sex' are transgender, and whether those who are trans are properly classified as men, women, both or neither for social, legal and other purposes. (**Jill Weiss**)

Trans theory 'Trans' refers to a movement through or beyond. Thus, trans theory concerns itself with theorizing phenomena that demonstrate a process or movement through or beyond current conceptualizations. Within gender and sexuality studies, trans theory most often turns its attention to TRANSGENDERISM. Kessler and McKenna (2000) detail three meanings of 'trans' within transgender theory. In a first sense, 'trans' means change, as in the transformation of individuals to the gender they feel they always were (the definition of transsexual). In a second sense, 'trans' means to move across genders without necessarily any physical changes taking place. Although purporting FLUIDITY between genders, this meaning of 'trans' accepts that there are two genders (women and men) that certain individuals move between. The third meaning of 'trans' is to move beyond or through gender. This is the most radical of meanings, as it suggests that gender has become an anachronism within MODERN SEXUALITY. Trans theory tends to emphasize this third meaning in contemplations of the erasure or elimination of gender (Hird 2002).

Within the fields of sexuality and SEXUAL DIFFERENCE, trans theory has most recently turned to the interaction of culture and nature. Donna Haraway (1997) theorizes transspecies, transfusions, transgene and transgenics that disturb the hierarchy of taxonomic categories (genus, family, class, order, kingdom) derived from 'nature'. For Haraway, trans 'cross a culturally salient line between nature and artifice, and they greatly increase the density of all kinds of other traffic on the bridge between what counts as nature and culture' (1997: 56). Here again we see the third meaning of trans theory, as it signifies movement both between and within matter that confounds traditional notions of the constitution of 'culture' and 'nature'. (**Myra Hird**)

Further reading

Bornstein (1994).

Transgender   A term describing a range of states in which an individual, through dress, behaviour or body modification, displays attributes which are different from the social and cultural expectations of their gender. Male and female transgender practices have a long history in the West. It is believed that prior to the dominance of Christian thought, gender categories were seen to be more fluid and transgender identities were accepted (see PREMODERN SEXUALITY). The influence of Christianity in the West led to transgender practices being seen as 'unnatural'. The development of SEXOLOGY in the nineteenth century pathologized transgender identities and attempted to 'cure' or 'treat' transgender people. In many non-Western cultures, transgender people have lived as integrated members of their communities, for example the indigenous BERDACHE and TWO-SPIRIT. In the 1970s a transgender person or *transgenderist* was seen to be someone whose gender IDENTIFICATION was that of the opposite sex to which they were born, but who did not have surgery to change their body. Transgender people have also been described as non-operative TRANSSEXUALS (Whittle 2000: 65). However, since the 1990s transgender has come to be used as a much broader umbrella term to include a range of people who do not identify with the orthodox gender BINARIES of male and female. The term includes people who self-identify as transsexual, TRANSVESTITE, INTERSEX, ANDROGYNOUS, third gendered, bi-gendered, transgender DYKE, BUTCH LESBIAN, DRAG KING and DRAG QUEEN. It is inclusive of people who take cross-sex hormones and have gender reassignment surgery to change their bodies, and of those who change their gender in less permanent ways. The term includes FTM and MTF practices and can encompass a range of sexualities. For some transgender people PASSING is important, while others seek to visibly disrupt the BINARIES of male and female (see GENDER CAPITAL).

The issue of transgender continues to be controversial within FEMINIST and gay and lesbian theory and politics. Radical feminists for example argue that gender is linked to biological sex and cannot be altered. Many feminists have been hostile to transgender people and have refused to accept their SELF-DEFINITION as male or female. This has had particular implications for MtF people who identify as feminists and/or lesbians, who have been rejected from feminist and/or lesbian circles. Other feminist and/or lesbian critics however, dismiss this perspective and argue for a more diverse analysis of gender, which is inclusive of transgender individuals. Since the 1990s transgender communities have organized politically for equal civil rights and opportunities. However, transgender people continue to face a wide range of discriminatory practices and personal attacks. Comparable to HOMOPHOBIA, the term TRANSPHOBIA has been developed to describe all forms of discrimination against transgender people.

There are many debates concerning the aetiology of a transgender identity. Some follow the idea of the *wrong body*, which suggests that a person's genetic make-up and anatomical sex is dissimilar to their 'true' gender. Others dispute a biological approach by arguing that transgender practices illustrate the fallibility of a two-gender model which, rather than being 'natural', is socially and culturally constructed (see SEXUAL DIMORPHISM). From this perspective it can be argued that we are all transgendered. Gender is thus seen as a category that can be disrupted, as suggested by the concept of gender PERFORMATIVITY. Some transgender writers explore a future of embodiment in which male and female body parts can be chosen because they *suit*, rather than because they are *given*. (**Sally Hines**)

Further reading

Califia (1997b).

Transman   A man of transsexual experience, referring to one who was assigned female sex at birth, but who lives as a male, with or without medical or surgical intervention (cf. TRANSWOMAN). Cromwell describes its meaning as follows:

> In its original coinage, transman was intended to be an encompassing term
> that included anyone assigned female at birth but who identifies somewhere
> on the so-called continuum between male/female and man/woman. They may
> or may not take testosterone and may or may not have body-altering surgeries
> but live either some or all of the time as men. Some transmen still use 'FTM' as a
> way to reinforce the fact that they have a female socialization and history.
> Others use 'transman' instead to distance themselves from anything that
> connotes female or feminine. Still others use the term to distance themselves
> from their transsexual status. (Cromwell 1999: 28) (**Jill Weiss**)

Transphobia   Prejudice and/or discrimination towards anyone transsexual, transgendered or perceived to transgress prescribed societal gender roles and rules, or those who may exhibit ambiguity in gender cues. Transphobia stems from a belief in an absolute and natural gender polarity and is therefore closely connected to HETEROSEXISM, COMPULSORY HETEROSEXUALITY and HOMOPHOBIA. Transphobic acts can range from overt harassment and violence to restricting access to resources, such as medical and legal assistance. Asking a trans-identified person about the appearance of their genitals is transphobic. One of the best-known cases of transphobia involved the death of female-to-male transsexual Brandon Teena (1972–93), who was murdered on 31 December 1993 in Humboldt, Nebraska. Teena's life has been depicted in a documentary, *The Brandon Teena Story* (1998) and the film *Boys Don't Cry* (1999). Subtle forms of transphobia include mistaking a person's sex(ual)/gender IDENTITY, refusing to acknowledge a person's declaration of their trans status, as well as thinking an MTF is not a 'real' woman or that an FTM is not a 'real' man (see Hale 1996). The Michigan Womyn's Music Festival, the 'mother' of WOMYN's music festivals, is often criticized for its 'womyn-born-womyn' policy which discriminates against MTF transsexuals and TRANSWOMEN.

Califia (1997b) provides a history and critique of transphobia, emanating from certain quarters of feminism, the lesbian community and the psychological field, specifically the *Diagnostic and Statistical Manual* (*DSM-IV*) which assesses issues surrounding sex-reassignment surgery (SRS) and gender identity disorder (GID). Within academia, charges of transphobia have been made against feminists like Janice G. Raymond, author of *The Transsexual Empire* (1979), who characterizes male–to–female transsexuals as 'male-to-*constructed*-females'. Califia rejects Raymond's argument that transwomen are the 'dupes of the patriarchy' (103) and characterizes Raymond as a 'gender supremacist' (106). Furthermore, trans activists have been quick to point out the lesbian appropriation of transpeople in the fight for lesbian visibility (Feinberg 1997). Some have argued that transsexuals are more readily accepted than gay men and lesbians since there is a medical procedure (sex-reassignment surgery) which can rectify their 'problem', while homosexuals, on the other hand, are often seen as hopelessly deviant. However, the pressure to put the oppression of transpeople and homosexuals into a hierarchy is symptomatic of the BINARY thinking perpetuated by Western thought. These divide and conquer tactics exaggerate the differences between trans and LGB communities, making coalition efforts difficult. In December of 1990, JoAnn Roberts published a Bill of Gender Rights (http://www.tgf-mall.com/pw/bgr.html) fighting for the right to assume and express gender roles, which has been adopted by many queer activist groups and formed the basis for the 1995 International Bill of Gender Rights (http://www.altsex.org/transgender/ibgr.html). (**Caroline J. McKenzie**)

Further reading

Bornstein (1994).

Transsexual   A term used to describe people who experience an incompatibility between their anatomical and psychological sex. The term refers to both FTMS and MTFS. Most transsexual people seek to alter their bodies through hormone therapy and/or what is medically known as gender reassignment surgery, though many transsexual people prefer to use the term 'gender realignment surgery', as a more adequate reflection of the conflict between their sex and gender. The incongruity of sex and gender is medically referred to as GENDER DYSPHORIA.

Although the history of TRANSGENDER people in the West reaches back to Ancient Greece, the term 'transsexual' was developed within twentieth-century medical discourse and was first used in medical literature in 1954 by Harry Benjamin, a doctor who specialized in hormone therapy (Whittle 2000: 11). In this way it can be argued that medical discourse *created* transsexualism as a distinct identity, which was later to be pathologized and seen as 'unnatural' (Hausman 1995). As such, many reject the label of transsexual and prefer the term TRANSMAN or TRANSWOMAN, or simply male or female. Within medical discourse and the growing field of SEXOLOGY, transsexualism was viewed as a pathological 'condition' and various forms of curative 'treatment' followed diagnosis.

There are conflicting accounts of the aetiology of transsexualism. While some transsexuals support the medical position that transsexualism is an inborn 'condition' rooted in the brain, others reject a biological determinist position and offer more fluid discussions of the changing meanings of sex and gender. The extent to which transsexuality represents the fluidity of gender categories however, is a central area of debate within TRANS THEORY. While Stone (1991) for example views transsexuality as representative of a POSTMODERN gender flux, Prosser (1998) argues that transsexuality is an ESSENTIAL embodied identity. Radical feminists have viewed transsexualism as a process whereby a patriarchal medical system created sex role stereotypes, and have refused to accept the self-articulated gender of trans people. Other critics have dismissed this perspective as representative of TRANSPHOBIA, however there continues to be much division over the extent to which feminism should be inclusive of trans people. The key issues of debate within the transgender community concern the desirability of legislative changes, such as the rights to marry and to change birth certificates following transition. While some transsexual activists see these issues as instrumental to social inclusion, others oppose them as conservative demands. (**Sally Hines**)

Further reading

Moore and Whittle (eds) (1999).

Transvestite   A term used to describe CROSS-DRESSING practitioners. The term may be used to incorporate DRAG QUEENS and DRAG KINGS who dress and/or perform as their opposite gender, as well as individuals who cross-dress less publicly. Sex researcher and reformer of anti-homosexual legislation Magnus Hirschfeld originally coined the term in 1910. From a contemporary perspective Hirschfeld's work can be criticized for conflating transvestism and homosexuality; and similarly, sex researchers and psychiatrists have frequently associated transvestism with transsexuality. For example Harry Benjamin who pioneered research into transsexuality and was the first medical authority to advocate sex reassignment, theorized transvestites, transsexuals and homosexuals as 'sex-split personalities' (quoted in Califia 1997b: 57). Critics now argue strongly against an association between SEXUAL ORIENTATION and cross-dressing practices. Likewise, there is a distinction between transvestism and transsexuality. Although some transsexuals may have identified as transvestite at an early point during their transition, most transvestites do not identify as transsexual. Thus, transvestites generally do not identify as the opposite gender, but rather choose to dress as women or men for particular occasions. Unlike transsexualism then, transvestite practices are largely based around bodily appearance, rather than embodied feelings of cross-gender identification. While some transsexuals strongly disassociate themselves from transvestites, others welcome transvestites into the TRANSGENDER community and argue that it is important to build a plural transgender – or GENDERQUEER – politics, which works on behalf of all sections of the community. (**Sally Hines**)

Further reading

Whittle (2000).

Transwoman   Referring to one who was assigned male sex at birth, but who lives as a female, with or without medical or surgical intervention. This has a different connotation from MTF (Male to Female), a term which emphasizes the male origins of the subject. It is also contrasted with the term 'woman of transsexual/transgender experience', which emphasizes femaleness (as opposed to FEMININITY) by placing 'woman' first and gender variance second (Valentine 2001: 186 n2). 'She-male' is a term associated by some with the sex industry, but adopted by some transwomen as a marker of both their HYPERSEXUALITY and their non-operative status. While it might seem to some that 'transwoman' is a simple opposite to 'TRANSMAN', politically, transwomen are distinguishable from transmen because of (1) the different histories of transmen and transwomen, (2) different social locations, including transwomen's male privilege and FTM social invisibility, and (3) superior MtF surgical technology (the reasons for which may lie in the prior two distinctions). (**Jill Weiss**)

Triad   A triad is a group of three persons who love each other sexually and otherwise. As opposed to a threesome, which is often referred to as a sexual act involving three persons, a triad is more stable. The word describes both the relationship and its members. The concept has been developed in the context of POLYAMORY, a sexual culture that rejects MONOGAMY and opts for inclusive relationships. The members of a triad relate both sexually and as part of an expanded family. They can all be sexually involved with one another, or one can be sexually involved with the other two, while they are not. This formation is referred to as a V. Polyamorous triads are often formed by one person of one gender, and two of the other. Members of a triad can be bisexual, or not. If the two members who are not sexual with each other are of the same gender, the triad is not bisexual. If all three members relate sexually to each other, it obviously is, unless the members have the same gender. Members of a triad can all live together, or not. If two members live together, the third can be a more external member who lives somewhere else and is still part of the triadic committed relationship. If all members live separately, they can all function interdependently. Some triads include two members who are officially married and some do not. A basic tenet of triadic relationships is that 'compersion' replaces jealousy. Compersion is the ability to enjoy the sexual and affectional joy of one's partners without participating in them directly (see also MÉNAGE À TROIS). (**Serena Anderlini-D'Onofrio**)

Tribadism   A term that today describes the erotic practice of one woman rubbing her CLITORIS on the pubic bone, genitals, thigh, hip, or other area of her female partner (Sisley and Harris 1977). The word itself comes from the Greek 'tribas', meaning 'to rub'. Historically, it was believed that a woman with an enlarged clitoris was able to penetrate another woman, and so in late antiquity the term became associated with female same-sex erotic activity (Traub 1995). A woman who engaged in these activities was called a 'tribade'. Halberstam (1998: 61–2) notes that in contemporary lesbian SEXUAL PRACTICES, tribadism involves 'various modes of sexual gendering at play, and many of them turn on which partner is on top' and that the practice is 'often accompanied by penetration of a partner with fingers or a DILDO, and so mutuality and reciprocation tend not to be the main objective, although satisfaction for both partners through different means most definitely is its aim'. A contemporary slang term for this practice is 'dyking'. (**Linnea Stenson**)

Two-spirit   As a term to describe NON-HETEROSEXUAL components of Native American and First Nations populations, two-spirit has been recently and rapidly adopted to replace the more Eurocentric term BERDACHE. Historically, there has been debate as to the variance of gender IDENTITY within Native North American communities, and the construction of community members as either one or several of three or four gender categories. In its broadest sense two-spirit refers to gay and lesbian people, traditions of gender diversity, transvestite, transgender and transsexual people – in short an entire LGBT community (Jacobs *et al.* 1997). Two-spirit is most frequently defined as either a male who fills an established social status other than man or woman, a male or female who behaves and dresses as a member of the opposite sex, or a male or female who occupy established third or fourth genders. In much the same way as the creation of self-chosen terminology has been part of the history of African-American, feminist, and lesbian and gay movements, so too do we find its use in contemporary Aboriginal discourse (Roscoe, 1988). Jacobs *et al.* (1997) trace the use of the term two-spirit (or two-spirited) to the third Native American/First Nations Gay and Lesbian conference held in Winnipeg, Manitoba in 1990. There, the term was consistently used to deliberately distance Aboriginal non-heterosexuals from non-native gays and lesbians. By replacing an older terminology (berdache) with two-spirit, Native peoples essentially reject a colonialist study of sexuality which conceives sex and gender as having two components: something natural and something social. In contrast, Native North American communities and First Nations have recognized a FLUIDITY to sexual expression and sexual orientation that many Western cultures have not. For these peoples, the concepts of gender and sex are viewed as something social (gender) and something that is also social – i.e. the manner in which a society or culture envisions, and indeed limits biological sex (Goulet 1996). (**Dan Allman**)

Universalizing   See MINORITIZING.

Urolagnia   See WATERSPORTS.

Vagina   The term used to anatomically define the tunnel before the cervix has come to stand in for the whole of the female genitalia, including the labia majora and minora, the CLITORIS, and the vagina proper. The vagina attracted much attention during the twentieth century in terms of the so-called 'vaginal' ORGASM, or orgasm by penetration, promulgated by Sigmund Freud and others, and later with the much-discussed discovery of the g-spot, by Ernest Grafenberg (1950), the sensitive area on the front wall of the vagina that has been linked to vaginal orgasm. Within much early SEXOLOGY, its primary purpose was constructed as being to facilitate male pleasure and male orgasm, with women's pleasure supposedly being deferred onto the childbirth that would eventually follow. However, although it had previously been argued that the vagina had no sexual sensation, Freud stressed the importance of vaginal pleasure because such a biology appears to underwrite heterosexual intercourse (Laqueur 1990). At the same time, with the vagina imaged merely as an absence of the penis, it is read as signifying a lack of sexual desire itself. The converse of this, is that any expression of desire on the part of women is read as aberrant, diseased or threatening; indeed, much masculinist discourse evinces a fear of the hungry (i.e. desiring) vagina

– encapsulated in the image of the VAGINA DENTATA. Creed (1993: 105–21) argues that this imagery of the vagina as lack or wound is in fact a displacement of the more fearful possibility, that men cannot fulfil female sexual appetite, or a fear of SEXUAL DIFFERENCE itself. This fear is often translated into a punitive hatred, expressed in terms of physical revulsion at its sight or smell (colloquially called 'chopped liver syndrome' amongst some gay men).

Against these hostilities, feminism has articulated a language that valorizes the vagina – most recently in the popular success of *The Vagina Monologues* (Ensler 2001) – celebrating it as a source of PRIDE and pleasure for women – whether for MASTURBATION, egalitarian intercourse, or ORAL SEX – and reclaiming terms like 'cunt' and 'pussy' as playful signifiers of female desire. Alongside this, lesbian culture has sought to articulate an alternative vaginal imagery, in which it exists as a source of pleasure in its own right and breaks from the heterosexual male fantasy that its purpose is to complement the PENIS (Chisholm 1995). (**Ivan Crozier** and **Jo Eadie**)

Further reading

Muscio (1998).

Vagina dentata   The *toothed vagina* appears in mythology – including that of ancient India, southern Africa and the Americas – in Freudian PSYCHOANALYSIS, and consequently, in sections of feminism (Creed 1993: 105–21). As Paglia (1990) says, the myth of the toothed vagina is a gruesomely direct transcription of female power and male fear (see CASTRATION COMPLEX). It symbolizes a male fear of the female body, and at the same time attributes power to women. Therefore it has been an ambivalent image within feminist discourse, since it is misogynistic but might be reclaimed as an image of female sexual autonomy, and resistance to male sexual attention. The toothed vagina is a potent symbol of the gate-keeping accoutrements for the regulation of sex and procreation, accentuating mystery surrounding female sexuality, especially genital anatomy and its power. The *vagina dentata* is also the epitome of a sexualized Eve image. As the mythological Eve was subjugated to 'man' on account of her sexual appetite, consequently she (woman) is described as suffering in the physicality of womanhood, including her unquenched desire for union with man, and in the pain of childbirth. Thus, where Eve is viewed as the primordial mother through sexual desire, and her antithesis is the Virgin Mary, so the ultimate dynamism of sexualized women is found in an image that portrays not only complete control of sexual regulation but its domination, too. The *vagina dentata* turns the myth of Eve around allowing woman to keep her sexual desires for man, as well as control of regulating his entry into her, rather than vice versa. The ultimate representation of this phenomenon is the black widow spider; she permits mating for the sake of reproduction, and then kills her mate. The *vagina dentata* too can permit penetration, only to emasculate after the event. (**David Evans**)

Vanilla   'Vanilla' refers to those SEXUAL PRACTICES that are supposedly the most ordinary. The term is borrowed from the menu of ice cream flavours, from which vanilla is the most commonly accepted – and blandest – flavour. At first, the term was adopted by SM aficionados, who considered the sexually unadventurous to be as plain as vanilla. SM is the opposite of vanilla: with its spectacular paraphernalia and verbal performance, SM appears weird and outlandish to outsiders, while vanilla represents the acceptable familial norm. It is no wonder that, in popular literature and film, the 'good' characters often perform vanilla sex whereas their predators are SM practitioners. From the viewpoint of the SM community, the vanilla people are tasteless – while, in wider society the vanilla people are normative while the SM aficionados are marginalized. In a heterosexual MARRIAGE, vanilla can refer to the convention that the husband is active while the wife is responsive. Within the lesbian and gay community, vanilla stands for the milder sexual practices, such as those without SEX TOYS or role-play. Vanilla becomes a moralistic measure in the scheme of SEXUAL STRATIFICATION: in the scheme, vanilla sex is assumed to be 'the original', while other sexual practices are derivatives, DEVIANCES or PERVERSIONS. Vanilla is established as the norm, and as a result other practices are 'abnormal'. While other practices are sometimes thought to be adventurous and tantalizing, they might also be condemned as dangerous or illegal or both, and in some religious communities, any sex other than vanilla deserves punishment. The symbolic function of the supremacy of vanilla sex is therefore to hand down social regulations, according to which other sexual behaviours are rumoured to corrupt the society. By naming it comically, SM practitioners have aimed to dethrone it from this position. (**Ta-wei Chi**)

Viagra   Viagra is the tradename for sildenafil citrate, the first oral drug approved for the medical treatment of 'erectile dysfunction' (IMPOTENCE). The arrival of Viagra heralded a significant change in the conceptualization and treatment of sexual difficulties affecting men; the previous association of impotence with psychological factors was replaced by a focus on the bio-mechanics of erections. While much is known about the physical effects of Viagra for men (including the side effects of the drug), and research is continuing on the possibilities of similar drugs for the treatment of sexual difficulties affecting women, there has been less interest by the scientific and medical communities in the broader socio-cultural implications of the development and use of sexuopharmaceuticals. Such issues are being investigated by feminist and critical social theorists, who argue that the recent proliferation and popularity of drugs like Viagra is indicative of the cultural trend to medicalize male (and female) sexuality. Criticism has been directed at the medical construction of 'normal' and 'healthy' male sexuality, which stresses the ability to produce an ERECTION and experience male ORGASM via heterosexual penetration (Tiefer 1995), thereby reinforcing the COITAL IMPERATIVE and disregarding other modes of sexual pleasure (Potts 2002). Mamo and Fishman (2002) propose that Viagra is a contemporary 'sexual technology' that predominantly reinstalls conventional (hetero)sexual scripts and ideas about gender and sexuality (in particular, notions of 'natural' masculine sexuality as active and penetrating), but that may also be used by those wishing to resist or transgress normative sex. They also argue that drugs like Viagra, which are readily purchased via the Internet, represent the contemporary COMMODIFICATION of sex; Fishman and Mamo (2002: 181) claim such 'prescription drugs are fast becoming popular consumer products; a capitalist fetish where one is encouraged to think of such drugs as a means through which to improve one's life'. (**Annie Potts**)

Vibrator   A general term used to describe a battery-operated or electric device, used for sexual stimulation. Unlike the DILDO, the vibrator has a history of medical use evolving at the end of the nineteenth century from previous massage therapies used to treat 'women's complaints' such as HYSTERIA. Since MASTURBATION was seen as unhealthy for women and androcentric models of sexuality routinely fell short of effecting orgasm in most women, it fell to doctors to cure women suffering from these ail ments. These purported 'diseases' were treated by bringing women to ORGASM through genital massage. The emergence of an electromechanical instrument provided doctor with a more efficient manner to administer this treatment, increasing their success, as well as their income (Maines 1999). In the early twentieth century, the vibrator was marketed in periodicals to women as a home appliance. Vibrator attachments could be found for 'a home motor that also drove attachments for churning, mixing, . . . and operating a fan' (Maines 1999: 20). As understandings of women's sexuality increased the vibrator's visibility as a health device decreased. In the 1960s, the vibrator re emerged as a sex aid, widely available and clearly marketed with the intent of produc ing sexual pleasure in women. Rubin notes that the use of 'manufactured objects' for sexual pleasure places individuals outside the 'charmed circle' of 'good, normal, nat ural, blessed sexuality' (1984: 281). While vibrators are primarily seen as devices for women, today they come in a variety of models for use by men as well. Vibrators are largely seen as one of a variety of SEX TOYS that an individual may use for AUTOEROTICISM or that couples and groups may utilize for sex play. (**Linnea Stenson**)

Virginity   The term virgin generally refers to those people that have never engaged in sexual intercourse. Though often regarded as a female trait, strictly speaking anyone male or female, who has not engaged in sexual intercourse can be referred to as a virgin. While male virginity may not be easily determined physically, with women the breaking of the hymen during first sexual intercourse is often regarded as the loss of virginity. That said, the hymen may be 'ruptured by tampon use or exercise' (Brooke 1998: 548). In both the CLASSICAL and MEDIEVAL tradition, virginity was regarded as a female trait and valued in a bride. Indeed, women were classified in Medieval Europe as virgins, wives, or widows. Christian writers, such as St Ambrose, stressed the integrity, both bodily and spiritual, in virginity. While the idea that women should be virgins upon marriage passed after the mid-twentieth century, a recent study argues for three periods of distinct sexual attitudes and behaviour in Europe: the generations of sexual restraint, of sexual revolution, and of gender equalization (Haavio-Mannila *et al.* 2002: xiv). With the generation of gender equalization, this study has indicated that virginity can be regarded as a burden and some women attempt to lose their virginity before marriage (ibid., 76). With the 1980s and the growing concern over AIDS, however, the generation of gender equalization has become more cautious in sexual activity (ibid., 7). Protection from sexually transmitted diseases (STDS) such as AIDS is not as simple as remaining a virgin. As Gorna has pointed out, while women may remain sexually inactive by choice, male sexual violence (RAPE) can place women at risk (1996: 62). Interestingly, modern commentators do not treat virginity as a lifestyle choice; rather virginity is viewed as a temporary stage of life corresponding to childhood. (**Andrew Cranmer**)

Virility   See CLASSICAL SEXUALITY; ERECTION; FEMALE MASCULINITY; IMPOTENCE; LESBIAN MOTHER(S); VIAGRA.

Virtual sex   Virtual or cyber sex refers to sexual interactions that take place in a computer-mediated simulated environment. These can include 'tiny sex' (Turkle 1995), that is on-screen encounters between characters (known as avatars) in simulated environments such as Multi-User Dungeons (MUDs). These interactions are purely textual – for instance 'Mandy runs her hand down Darren's thigh' – but, given the long-term investment that many people put into developing their avatars and participating in these communities, these interactions can be very emotive, as shown by the outrage evoked in these communities at attempts of 'virtual rape' (when a user hijacks an avatar and forces the character to interact sexually against its owner's wishes). Other online sexual interactions may take place in chat rooms, jokingly referred to as 'one-handed typing'. Virtual sex has the potential for a great deal of gender PERFORMATIVITY, with the online gender expressed by an avatar often differing from an individual's gender in real life. Some MUDs allow avatars to change gender at will or offer more choices than the usual male/female binary – allowing for online experimentation that would be impossible to achieve in 'real life'. However, some users express anxiety at the thought that their online partners may not 'really' be of the gender they claim, which can lead to flaming when a user's online identity is believed to be fake. Recent technological advances have enabled virtual sex to move beyond text exchange with the development of TELEDILDONICS (Haraway 1997) – interactive devices that can be strapped to the pelvic region. (**Mark Mclelland**)

Further reading

Rheingold (1992).

Visibility   Sexual activities and identities have arguably become more visible and public throughout the twentieth and twenty-first centuries. One's sexual identity, for example, may be a matter of public record through marriage licences, through the reporting of HIV test results to government offices and/or employers, or through the act of COMING OUT of the CLOSET to friends, family, or strangers. These forms of visibility tend to be IDENTIFICATORY, and serve to codify sexual acts and identities either publicly or privately. At the same time, gay, lesbian, bisexual, transgender, and queer activists argue that the entirety of sexuality, particularly non-normative sexual acts and identities, are becoming less visible in the public sphere. In New York City, for example, the elimination of gay bars, sex shops, pornographic theatres, and prostitutes from Times Square has been an erasure of so-called 'DEVIANT' sex, so that Times Square is now populated by family- and tourist-friendly stores and theatres. Warner (1999) argues that the re-zoning of businesses based around sex in New York City has rendered sexuality less visible, and has reduced the amount of public space in the city overall, not just for sexual practices but for any and all public activities. In addition, gay, lesbian, bisexual, transgender, and queer activists are divided about how to make the non-normative sexualities visible. In the late 1980s and early 1990s, for example, OUTING was a practice that made individuals visible without their consent, but this practice drew criticism from other activists for placing an unfair burden on individuals, rather than groups or movements. (See also PUBLIC/PRIVATE.) (**Rachael Groner**)

Voluntarism   Voluntarism refers to the notion that individuals create and act in their own worlds independently of the wider social contexts in which they are embedded. When applied to sexuality, a purely voluntaristic argument would suggest that one 'chooses' one's own sexual IDENTITY and SEXUAL PRACTICES in isolation from the influence of prevailing cultural meanings and relations of power. One example is the idea that sexual orientation is purely a matter of individual 'choice'. Voluntarism is thus strongly associated with liberal individualism. Its direct opposite is determinism, according to which individual will plays no part in the creation of one's sexual actions, feelings and identities. Examples include the biological determinist argument that the characteristics of individuals' sexualities are purely the outcome of biological processes, such as the GAY GENE, or the suggestion that sexual identities are determined by economic relationships.

Many theorists in fact suggest that a middle path between voluntarism and determinism offers the most promise for the study of sexuality. For example, Jackson and Scott (1996: 6) suggest the importance of recognizing that we do actively construct our own understandings of sexuality within the constraints imposed by cultural and historical contexts as well as social structures (such as HETERONORMATIVITY, COMPULSORY HETEROSEXUALITY and male domination). We are therefore neither wholly determined by our environment nor expressive of a sexuality which arises entirely within ourselves. One specific approach is offered by Gagnon and Simon's (1973) theory of sexual

SCRIPTS in which individuals fashion sexual selves as they negotiate the social meanings and conventions provided by the surrounding culture. Such middle-ground approaches are reflexive in suggesting that individuals' own actions and meaning-making processes both influence and are influenced by wider social contexts. (**Chris Brickell**)

Voyeurism   To look at others for pleasure – particularly to watch others while masturbating. Within PSYCHOANALYSIS voyeurism is seen as a central component of human sexuality, and derives from a more basic impulse to accumulate knowledge about the adult world. Since sexual knowledge is routinely hidden from children within contemporary culture, we all to some extent grow up as voyeurs, easily aroused by catching a glimpse of what has been forbidden us (Kaplan 1993: 30). Feminism has argued that this desire to look is particularly central to male heterosexuality, hence the prevalence of peep-shows, pornography, lap-dancing, striptease, and the female NUDE as the preferred subject of male art (Neade 1992). In these situations, men are able to have a distance which allows them to keep control of the sexual situation, since the privilege of looking implies that the woman has been tamed (Kaplan 1983: 311–12). However, Cowie (1992) notes that the psychoanalytic model also complicates this simplistic account: the voyeur may want to be caught out and punished; may be watching because they feel inadequate and unsure that they can fully please the one they watch; may be watching adoringly from a position of powerlessness; may feel pleasure because of experiencing an IDENTIFICATION with the one who is on display. While voyeurism has traditionally been defined as a feature of male heterosexuality, more recent theorization points out the importance of voyeurism to female sexuality (Gamman and Marshment 1988). Jeffreys (1993:175) argues that this merely repeats the heterosexual male dynamics of objectification. But others suggest that the lesbian gaze, when cast on another lesbian, necessarily assumes that the other woman may look back, and hence takes part in a more playful and mutually voyeuristic relationship, where power relations are not fixed and always open to change (Kaplan 1983: 324–5). (**Jo Eadie**)

Watersports   A general term for sex involving urine, also called golden showers, yellow sex, or within SEXOLOGY, urophilia and urolagnia (drinking urine). Practices may include pissing oneself, sharing one's piss with another/others, competitions to see who can 'pee' the furthest, urinating onto another (naked or clothed), drinking piss, controlling urination (e.g. by the use of urinary catheters), role-playing INFANTILIST scenes of wetting nappies/diapers, or pissing inside a partner during unprotected vaginal or anal intercourse. Motives for practising watersports can be as broad as the need to achieve any sexual satisfaction in life, from the liberation of breaking cultural taboos, feeling the warmth of a womb-like experience, showing closeness to another, to domination and humiliation (see SM). Some people attend 'piss parties' or clubs where 'piss slaves' are available for golden showers and urolagnia. The use of urinary catheters in sex might be employed to control the urination of a 'slave', or to add liquids, such as the urine from the dominant partner, directly into the bladder.

Fresh urine is generally sterile; when going onto unbroken skin it causes no health problems. A person with infectious pathogens, such as hepatitis B, cytomegalovirus, gonorrhoea or chlamydia, could pass these on if the contaminated urine enters the blood stream or body of another. Catheterization, even when performed under strict aseptic (surgically clean) conditions, is never totally risk free. Inserting an object and germs into the urethra can cause trauma. Trauma and local infection can lead to scarring in the narrow urethra; ascending infections can ultimately lead to potentially life-damaging conditions such as serious kidney infections. Thus, under the umbrella term of watersports, a broad spectrum of safe and pleasurable through to potentially dangerous practices can be experienced. (**David Evans**)

Further reading

www.sexuality.org (2002).

Whore   The term whore has currently the same meaning as the term PROSTITUTE. Although it is usually used as a deprecatory term or an insult, against SEX WORKERS or sexually active women, there is a trend within the sex workers' rights movement to reclaim this term as a positive one, and many prostitutes refer to themselves as whores (Nagle 1997). For example, the sex workers' organization CORP have publicly politicized the positive identity of whore by producing and distributing pamphlets and banners reading 'whore-power', 'whores are safe sex pros', and 'proud to be a whore'. Sex work ACTIVISTS have identified and defined the 'whore stigma':

> The whore label is attached to anyone who works or has worked in the sex
> industry as . . . a provider of sexual service or entertainment . . . But not only
> prostitutes are labelled whores. Any woman may be designated 'whore' within
> a particular cultural setting, especially if she is a migrant, target of racist
> discrimination, independent worker or victim of abuse. (Pheterson 1989: 4)
> (**Ana Lopes**)

Wimmin   See WOMYN.

Woman-identified woman   A coinage that first appeared in print in the classic manifesto, 'The Woman-Identified Woman' (Radicalesbians 1970). The term, referring to 'the primacy of women relating to women' (ibid., 4), was used euphemistically in place of the more charged term, 'LESBIAN'. As one of the authors of the collaboratively generated manifesto, put it, 'we . . . called ourselves "women-identified women" – that is, those who chose to work with and for others of our gender. It was a term even heterosexuals could feel comfortable claiming' (Jay 1999: 141). As such, while 'woman-identified woman' was and is still often interpreted within and beyond FEMINIST circles as 'lesbian-ness', the term is not an exclusively lesbian marker. It is, instead, a feminist marker. For, as Lorde explains, 'there are lesbians, God knows . . . who [are] not feminist and would not call themselves feminists. But the true feminist deals out of a lesbian consciousness whether or not she ever sleeps with women' (as cited by Hammond 1980: 18). (**Tamarah Cohen**)

Womyn   'Womyn' (pl. 'wimmin') is a non-generic radical FEMINIST coinage, derived from the generic term 'woman' and designed to circumvent the 'man' perceived in 'woman'. It is inextricably linked to lesbian feminist women, but not necessarily to the exclusion of non-lesbian feminists. A female-specific expression of solidarity, 'womyn' conveys a range of nuances, depending on the speech community employing it. In its genesis, the neologism and its many variants (including 'womin', 'wimyn', 'womon', 'wo/man', 'womn', 'wom'n', and 'womnn') self-referred to a political subset of the whole class of women, i.e. radical feminists and those non-lesbian feminists with shared radical politics. It originated as a word that categorized biological females on the basis of political consciousness and activism rather than allowing sexuality to be the defining feature, and as such, signified the radical feminist conviction that women who identified sexually as heterosexual could have a radical feminist consciousness. Thus, 'womyn' originally reflected WOMAN-IDENTIFIED-ness, a concept that is often interpreted within and beyond women-identified feminist circles as 'lesbian-ness'. By the 1980s, however, many non-lesbian feminists as well as mainstream lexicographers began to define 'womyn' in such a way as to rid it of lesbian associations, avoiding reference to its lesbian-specific semantic antecedents. For example, ' "wimmin" (1983) A semi-phonetic spelling of women, recently adopted by some feminists' (Oxford English Dictionary 1989).

'Womyn' is currently an ambiguous referent in that it has several synonyms that are not themselves synonyms of each other, including: 'adult female', 'black feminist', 'black lesbian feminist', 'heterosexual feminist', 'lesbian feminist', 'lesbian'. Many (primarily lesbian) women assert that 'womyn' might best be restricted to its lesbian-positive application – a synonym for 'woman' minus the HET mark – and its pseudo-generic (heterosexual) activation avoided in the service of conceptual clarity.

When applied to non-lesbians, 'womyn' inadvertently perpetuates lesbian invisibility. If, the argument continues, 'womyn' and its orthographic variants are to be used now to reference political values, they might at least, in deference to its radical feminist origin, be used inclusively, that is, to include lesbians by inference, not mere implication. Others simply see 'womyn' as dated, a word on its way out of usage. (**Tamarah Cohen**)

Z

Zami   Originally a word from the Caribbean island Carriacou for women working together as both lovers and friends, the term is most closely associated with Audre Lorde (1934–92), an American black lesbian feminist writer and political activist. In *Zami: A New Spelling of My Name*, Lorde (1984) charts her passionate relationship with her mother, and her experience of growing up as a 'gaygirl' in New York in the 1950s. *Zami* is a tale of surviving racism, misogyny and homophobia against the odds. In its form and content *Zami* challenges the linearity of white, HETEROSEXIST narratives of the world, valuing black, working-class and lesbian perspectives on the world as critical knowledge to be treasured in a hostile world. The term Zami has thus been extended to mean a particular location (black, working class, lesbian) and the particular knowledges that such a position produces. It also signifies the persistent racial and class exclusions of the term LESBIAN. In this sense the term is similar to Walker's 'womanist' (1984), that she develops as more appropriate than 'feminist' to the specific experiences of black women. (**Clare Hemmings**)

Further reading

Hill Collins (2000).

Bibliography

Abelove, Henry, Barale, Michèle Aina and Halperin, David M. (eds) (1993) *The Lesbian and Gay Studies Reader*, New York and London: Routledge.

Acevedo, Cynthia (1990) Too much denial, in The ACT UP/NY Women and AIDS Book Group (eds) *Women AIDS and Activism*, Boston: South End Press, 119–22

Adam, Barry D. (1998) Theorizing homophobia. *Sexualities* 1 (4): 387–404.

Adams, Parveen (1996) *The Emptiness of the Image*, London: Routledge.

Ahmed, Sara (1999) She'll wake up one of these days and find she's turned into a nigger. *Theory, Culture and Society* 16(2): 87–106.

Ahmed, Sara and Stacey, Jackie (2001) *Thinking Through the Skin*, London: Routledge.

Aidsmap (2001) http://www.aidsmap.com/web/pb3/eng/31A92CCD-AB30-4A1E-A58C-73B6A88ECD0A.htm

Allram, R.D. (2000) Autoerotic asphyxiation syndrome, http://www.studioja.com/ryan.htm

Allyn, David (2000) *Make Love Not War. The Sexual Revolution: An Unfettered History*, Boston, New York and London: Little, Brown and Company.

Altman, Dennis (1982) *The Homosexualization of America, the Americanization of the Homosexual*, New York: St Martin's Press.

Altman, Dennis (1986) *Aids and the New Puritanism*, London: Pluto Press.

Altman, Dennis, and Wecks, Jeffrey, (1993) *Homosexual Oppression and Liberation*, New York: New York University Press.

Anapol, Deborah (1997) *Polyamory: The New Love Without Limits*, San Rafael, CA: Internet Resource Center.

Andermahr, Sonya, Lovell, Terry and Wolkowitz, Carol (2000) *A Glossary of Feminist Theory*, London: Arnold.

Anderson, D. and Berman, M. (2002) *Sex Tips for Straight Women from a Gay Man*, London: Thorsons.

Andrews L.B. (1999) *The Clone Age: Adventures in the New World of Reproductive Technology*, New York: Henry Holt and Company.

Angelides, Steven (2001) *A History of Bisexuality*, Chicago: University of Chicago Press.

Angier, Natalie (1999) *Woman: An Intimate Geography*, Boston: Houghton-Mifflin.

Anonymous (1999) Mistresses could have it all. *The Times*, May 29, 1999: 36.

Anzieu, Didier (1989) *The Skin Ego: A Psychoanalytic Approach to the Self*, New Haven: Yale University Press.

Archard, David (1998) *Sexual Consent,* Oxford: Westview.

Arguelles, J.R. (1991) A history of Filipino sexuality, *Maganda Magazine* Vol. 3, http://www.magandamagazine.org/03/content.html

Ariès, Philippe and Béjin, André (eds) (1985) *Western Sexuality: Practice and Precept in Past and Present Times,* Oxford: Blackwell.

Ashley, Kathleen M. and Plesch, Véronique (2002) The cultural processes of 'appropriation'. *Journal of Medieval and Early Modern Studies* 32(1): 1–15.

Ault, Amber (1999 [1996]) Ambiguous identity in an unambiguous sex/gender structure: the case of bisexual women, in Merl Storr (ed.) *Bisexuality: A Critical Reader,* London: Routledge, 167–85.

Austin, J. L (1962) *How to Do Things with Words,* Cambridge, MA: Harvard University Press.

Ayto, John (1990) *Dictionary of Word Origins,* New York: Arcade.

Baker, Paul (2002) *Polari: The Lost Language of Gay Men,* London: Routledge.

Baker, Roger (1994) *Drag,* London: Cassell.

Barker, Isabelle (2000) Editing pornography, in Drucilla Cornell, (ed.) *Feminism and Pornography*, Oxford: Oxford University Press, 643–52.

Barry, K. (1979) *Female Sexual Slavery,* New York: Avon Books.

Bartholome, A., Tewksbury, R. and Bruzzone, A. (2000) 'I want a man': patterns of attraction in all-male personal ads. *Journal Of Men's Studies* 8(3): 309–21.

Baskin, Y. (1999) Birds, bees, and STDs, *Natural History* 108(1): 52–5.

Bayrd, Bayle (2002) Debunking bed death: forget what you've heard about the curse of long-term lesbian couplehood. *Curve,* April: 30–4.

Beauvoir, Simone de. (1953) *The Second Sex,* tr. H. M. Parskley, New York: Knopf.

Bech, Henning (1997) *When Men Meet: Homosexuality and Modernity*, Cambridge: Polity Press.

Beck, Ulrich and Beck-Gernsheim, Elisabeth (1995) *The Normal Chaos of Love.* Cambridge: Polity Press.

Beckman, Andrea (2001) Deconstructing myths: the social construction of 'sado-masochism' versus the 'subjugated knowledges' of practitioners of consensual 'SM'. *Journal of Criminal Justice and Popular Culture* 8(2): 66–95. http://www.albany.edu/scj/jcjpc/vol8is2/beckmann.pdf

Beemyn, Brett and Eliason, Mickey (eds) (1996) *Queer Studies: A Lesbian, Gay, Bisexual, and Transgender Anthology,* New York and London: New York University Press.

Beemyn, Brett and Steinman, Erich (2001) (eds) *Bisexuality in the Lives of Men: Facts and Fictions,* Binghampton, NY: Harrington Park Press.

Beemyn, Brett and Steinman, Erich (2002)(eds) *Bisexual Men in Culture and Society.* Binghampton, NY: Harrington Park Press.

Bell, David (1997) One-handed geographies: an archaeology of public sex, in Gordon Brent Ingram, Anne-Marie Bouthillette and Yolanda Reiter (eds) *Queers in Space*, Seattle: Bay Press, 81–7.

Bell, David (2000) Eroticizing the rural, in Richard Phillips, Diane Watt and David Shuttleton (eds) *De-Centring Sexualities: Politics and Representation Beyond the Metropolis*, London: Routledge, 83–101.

Bell, David and Binnie, Jon (2000) *The Sexual Citizen: Queer Politics and Beyond*, Cambridge: Polity Press.

Bell, David and Holliday, Ruth (2000) Naked as nature intended. *Body and Society* 6(3–4): 127–40.

Bell, David and Valentine, Jill (eds) (1995) *Mapping Desire: Geographies of Sexualities*, London: Routledge.

Bell, V. (1991) Beyond the thorny question: feminism, Foucault, and the desexualization of rape. *International Journal of the Sociology of Law* 19: 83–100.

Benjamin, Jessica (1983) Master and slave: the fantasy of erotic domination, in Ann Snitow, Christiane Stansell and Sharon Thompson (eds) *Powers of Desire*, New York: Monthly Review Press, 280–99.

Benjamin, Jessica (1988) *The Bonds of Love: Psychoanalysis, Feminism and Domination*, New York: Pantheon.

Berer, M. (1993) *Women and HIV/AIDS: an International Resource Book: Information, Action and Resources on Women and HIV/AIDS, Reproductive Health and Sexual Relationships*, London: Pandora.

Berry, Sarah. (2000) *Screen Style: Fashion and Femininity in 1930s Hollywood*, Minneapolis, MN: University of Minnesota Press.

Bersani, Leo (1988) Is the rectum a grave?, in D. Crimp (ed.), *AIDS: Cultural Analysis, Cultural Activism*, London: The MIT Press, 197–222.

Bersani, Leo (1995) *Homos*, London: Harvard University Press.

Bhavnani, Kum-Kum (ed.) (2000) *Feminism and Race: a Reader*, Oxford: Oxford University Press.

Bi Academic Intervention (eds)(1997) *The Bisexual Imaginary*, London: Cassell.

Bindman, J. (1997) Rethinking prostitution as sex work on the international agenda, http://www.walnet.org/csis/papers/redefining.html

Bland, Lucy (1995) *Banishing the Beast: English Feminism and Sexual Morality 1885–1914*, London: Penguin.

Bland, Lucy and Doan, Laura (1998) *Sexology in Culture. Labelling Bodies and Desires*, Chicago and London: University of Chicago Press.

Blasius, Mark (ed.) (2001) *Sexual Identities, Queer Politics*, New Jersey: Princeton University Press.

Blasius, Mark and Phelan, Shane (eds) (1997) *We Are Everywhere: A Historical Sourcebook of Gay and Lesbian Politics*, New York and London: Routledge.

Bleys, Rudi C (1996) *The Geography of Perversion*, London: Cassell.

Bloomquist, Eric (2000) Responsible non-monogamy: a brief introduction to polyamory, http://www.biresource.org/pamphlets/nonmonogamy.html

Bloor, M. (1995) *The Sociology of HIV Transmission*, London: Sage Publications.

Blumenfeld, Warren and Hemmings, Clare (1996) Reading 'monosexual'. *Journal of Gay, Lesbian, and Bisexual Identity* 1 (4): 311–21.

Bogus, SDiane A. (1990) The 'queen B' figure in black literature, in Karla Jay and Joanna Glasgow (eds) *Lesbian Texts and Contexts: Radical Revisions*, New York: New York University Press, 1990, 275–90.

Bordo, Susan (1993) *Unbearable Weight: Feminism, Western Culture, and the Body*, Berkeley: University of California Press.

Bornstein, K. (1994) *Gender Outlaw: On Men, Women and the Rest of Us*, New York and London: Routledge.

Boston Women's Health Book Collective (1998) *Our Bodies, Ourselves For the New Century*, New York: Touchstone Books.

Boswell, John (1981) *Christianity, Social Tolerance and Homosexuality*, Chicago and London: The University of Chicago Press.

Boswell, John (1995) *The Marriage of Likeness: Same-Sex Unions in Pre-modern Europe*, London: HarperCollins.

Bourdieu, Pierre (1984) *Distinction: A Social Critique of Judgements of Taste*, London: Routledge and Kegan Paul.

Braidotti, Rosi (1991) *Patterns of Dissonance*, New York: Routledge.

Bright, Susie (1990) *Susie Sexpert's Lesbian Sex World*, Pittsburgh and San Francisco: Cleis Press.

Bristow, Joseph (1989) Homophobia/misogyny: sexual fears, sexual definitions, in Simon Shepherd and Mick Wallis (eds) *Coming On Strong: Gay Politics and Culture*, London: Unwin Hyman, 54–75.

Brooker, Christine (1998) *Human Structure and Function: Nursing Applications in Clinical Practice*, London: Mosby.

Brown, Mildred L. and Rounsley, Chloe Ann (1996) *True Selves: Understanding Transsexualism*, San Francisco: Jossey-Bass Publishers.

Brown, Peter (1988) *The Body and Society: Men, Women and Sexual Renunciation in Early Christianity*, New York: Columbia University Press.

Brownmiller, Susan (1975) *Against Our Will: Men, Women and Rape*, New York: Fawcett Columbine.

Brownmiller, Susan (1986) *Femininity*, London: Paladin.

Brundage, James A. (1987) *Law, Sex, and Christian Society in Medieval Europe*, Chicago: University of Chicago Press.

Bulcroft, K. (1999) *Romancing the Honeymoon: Consummating Marriage in Modern Society*, Thousand Oaks, CA: Sage.

Bullough, Vern L. (1976) *Sexual Variance in Society and History*, London: University of Chicago Press.

Bullough, Vern L. and Brundage, James A. (eds) (1996) *Handbook of Medieval Sexuality*, London: Garland Publishing.

Bullough, Vern L. and Bullough, Bonnie (1987) *Women and Prostitution*, New York: Buffalo.

Bullough, Vern L., and Bullough, Bonnie (1993) *Crossdressing, Sex, and Gender*, Philadelphia: University of Pennsylvania Press.

Bunch, Charlotte (1972) Lesbians in revolt, http://scriptorium.lib.duke.edu/wlm/furies

Burana, Lily Roxxie and Due, Linnea (eds) (1994) *Dagger: On Butch Women*, San Francisco: Cleis Press.

Burgess, Jacquelin (1998) But is it worth taking the risk: how women negotiate access to urban woodland, in Rosa Ainley (ed.) *New Frontiers Of Space, Bodies And Gender*, London: Routledge, 115–28.

Burton, Peter (1985) *Parallel Lives*, London: Gay Men's Press.

Butler, Judith (1990) *Gender Trouble: Feminism and the Subversion of Identity*, New York: Routledge.

Butler, Judith (1993) *Bodies That Matter: On the Discursive Limits of 'Sex'*, New York: Routledge.

Butler, Judith (1997) Melancholy gender/refused identification, in *The Psychic Life of Power: Theories in Subjection*, Stanford, CA: Stanford University Press, 132–50.

Butler Judith (1998) Merely cultural. *New Left Review* 227: 33–44.

Butler, Judith (1999) From interiority to gender performatives, in Fabio Cleto (ed.) *Camp: Queer Aesthetics and the Performing Subject: A Reader*, Ann Arbor: University of Michigan Press, 361–8.

Cabello-Santamaria, Francisco (1997) Female ejaculation: myths and reality. Paper presented at the 13th World Congress of Sexology, Barcelona, Spain.

Cadden, Joan (1996) Western medicine and natural philosophy, in J. A. Brundage and V.L. Bullough (eds) *Handbook of Medieval Sexuality*, London: Garland Publishing, 1996, 51–80.

Califia, Pat (1994) *Public Sex: The Culture of Radical Sex*, San Francisco: Cleis Press.

Califia, Pat (ed.)(1995) *Doing It for Daddy: Short Sexy Fiction about a Very Forbidden Fantasy*, Boston: Alyson.

Califia, Pat (1997a) San Francisco: revisiting 'the city of desire', in Gordon Brent Ingram, Anne-Marie Bouthillette and Yolanda Retter (eds) *Queers in Space: Communities/ Public Places/Sites of Resistance*, Seattle: Bay Press, 177–96.

Califia, Pat (1997b) *Sex Changes: The Politics of Transgenderism*, San Francisco: Cleis Press.

Callery, P. (1998) Sex and children in the past and present, in T Harrison (ed.), *Children and Sexuality: Perspectives in Health Care*, London: Bailliere Tindall / RCN, 1–18.

Cantarella, Eva (1992) *Bisexuality in the Ancient World*, New Haven: Yale University Press.

Carlisle, C. (2001) HIV and AIDS, in T. Mason, C. Carlisle, C. Watkins and E. Whitehead (eds) *Stigma and Social Exclusion in Health Care*, London and New York: Routledge, 117–26.

Carlson, Margaret (1993) Then there was Nunn. *Time* 26 July: 40–1.

Carol, Avedon (1993) Porn, perversion and sexual ethics, in Victoria Harwood, David Oswell, Kay Parkinson and Anna Ward (eds) *Pleasure Principles: Politics, Sexuality and Ethics*, London: Lawrence and Wishart, 149–56.

Carrera, M. (1992) *The Language of Sex: An A to Z Guide*, New York and Oxford: Facts On File.

Case, Sue-Ellen (1989) Towards a butch-femme aesthetic, *Discourse* 11 (Winter 1988–9): 55–73.

Case, Sue-Ellen, Brett, Philip, and Foster, Susan Leigh (eds) (1995) *Cruising the Performative: Interventions into the Representation of Ethnicity, Nationality, and Sexuality*, Bloomington: Indiana University Press.

Cauldwell, D. (2001 [1950]) Questions and answers on the sex life and sexual problems of trans-sexuals. *International Journal of Transgenderism*, 5(3): 1–37. http://www.symposion.com/ijt/cauldwell/alt/cauldwell_04.htm

Cawson, P., Wattam, C., Brooker, S., and Kelly, G. (2000) *Child Maltreatment in the UK: A Study of the Prevalence of Child Abuse and Neglect*, London: NSPCC.

Chalker, Rebecca (1987) *The Complete Cervical Cap Guide*, New York: Harper and Row.

Chalker, Rebecca (2000), *The Clitoral Truth*, New York: Seven Stories Press.

Chase, C. (1998) Hermaphrodites with attitude: mapping the emergence of intersex political activism. *GLQ* 4(2): 189–212.

Chapkis, Wendy (1997) *Live Sex Acts*, New York: Routledge.

Chasin, Alexandra (2000) *Selling Out: The Gay and Lesbian Liberation Movement Goes to Market*, New York: Palgrave.

Chauncey, George (1983) From sexual inversion to homosexuality: medicine and the changing conceptualization of female deviance. *Salmagundi: A Quarterly of the Humanities and Social Sciences* 58–9: 114–46.

Chauncey, George (1995) *Gay New York: The Making of the Gay Male World, 1890–1940*, London: Flamingo.

Chisholm, Dianne (1995) The 'cunning lingua' of desire: bodies-language and perverse performativity, in Elizabeth Grosz and Elspeth Probyn (eds) *Sexy Bodies: The Strange Carnalities of Feminism*, London: Routledge, 19–41.

Chvany, Peter (1999) Burden of proof. *The Slant* (October): 20.

Cixous, Hélène (1973) L'Essort de Plusje, *L'Arc* 54: 46–52.

Cixous, Hélène (1976) The laugh of the Medusa, tr. Keith Cohen and Paula Cohen, *Signs* 1(4): 875–93.

Cixous, Hélène (1986) *The Newly Born Woman*, tr. Betsy Wing. Manchester: Manchester University Press.

CJPOA (1994) Criminal Justice and Public Order Act 1994, http://www.hmso.gov.uk/acts/acts1994/Ukpga_19940033_en_15.htm

Clark, Elizabeth (ed.) (1996) *St Augustine on Marriage and Sexuality*, Washington: The Catholic University of America.

Clarke, A. E. (2000) Maverick reproductive scientists and the production of contraceptive, 1915–2000+, in A. R. Saetnan, N. Oudshoorn and M. Kirejczyk (eds) *Bodies of Technology: Women's Involvement in Reproductive Medicine*, Columbus: Ohio State University Press, 37–89.

Cleland, John. (1994 [1748–1749]) *Fanny Hill Or Memoirs Of A Woman Of Pleasure*, London: Penguin.

Cleto, Fabio (ed.) (1999a) *Camp: A Reader*, Edinburgh: Edinburgh University Press.

Cleto, Fabio (1999b) Introduction: queering the camp, pp 1– 42 in Fabio Cleto (ed.) *Camp: A Reader*, Edinburgh: Edinburgh University Press

Cockburn, Cynthia. (1990) Men's power in organizations: 'equal opportunities' intervenes, in Jeff Hearn and David Morgan (eds) *Men, Masculinities and Social Theory*, London: Unwin Hyman, 72–89.

Cohen, David (1991) *Law, Sexuality And Society: The Enforcement Of Morals In Classical Athens*, Cambridge: Cambridge University Press.

Cohen, Tamarah (2002) 'Gay' and the disappearing [+female]. *The Gay and Lesbian Review, Worldwide* 9(6): 22–4.

Coleman, J. and Roker, D. (eds) (1998) *Teenage Sexuality: Health, Risk and Education*, Amsterdam: Harwood Academic Press.

The Combahee River Collective (1983 [1977]) A black feminist statement, in Cherrie Moraga and Gloria Anzaldua (eds) *This Bridge Called My Back: Writings by Radical Women of Color*, New York: Kitchen Table Women of Color Press, 210–18.

Connell, R.W. (1987) *Gender and Power*, Stanford: Stanford University Press.

Connell, R. and G. Dowsett (1999) 'The unclean motion of the generative parts': frameworks in Western thought on sexuality, in R. Parker and P. Aggleton (eds) *Culture, Society and Sexuality*, London: UCL Press, 79–196.

Cook, M. and Howells, K (1981) *Adult Sexual Interest In Children*, London. Academic Press.

Cooper, Davina (1993) The citizen's charter and radical democracy: empowerment and exclusion within citizenship discourse. *Social and Legal Studies* 2(2): 149–71.

Core, Philip (1984) From 'Camp: the lie that tells the truth', in Fabio Cleto (ed.) *Camp: A Reader*, Edinburgh: Edinburgh University Press, 80–6.

Cornell, Drucilla (2000a) Introduction, in *Feminism and Pornography*, Oxford: Oxford University Press, 1–15.

Cornell, Drucilla (2000b) (ed.) *Feminism and Pornography*, Oxford: Oxford University Press.

Corrigan, Annette and Meredyth, Denise (2001) The body politic, in Kate Pritchard Hughes (ed.) *Contemporary Australian Feminism 2: 2nd edition*, South Melbourne: Longman, 52–75.

Cott, Nancy F. (1987) *The Grounding of Modern Feminism*, New Haven, CT: Yale University Press.

Cowie, Elizabeth (1992) Pornography and fantasy: psychoanalytic perspectives, in Lynn Segal and Mary McIntosh (eds) *Sex Exposed: Sexuality and the Pornography Debate*, London: Virago, 132–52.

Cowie, Elizabeth (1997) Fantasia, in *Representing the Woman: Cinema and Psychoanalysis*, London: Macmillan, 123–65.

Cowling, Mark (1998) *Date Rape and Consent*, Aldershot: Ashgate

Coxell, A., King, M., Mezey, G. and Gordon, D. (1999) Lifetime prevalence, characteristics, and associated problems of non-consensual sex in men: cross-sectional survey. *British Medical Journal* 318: 846–50, http://bmj.com/cgi/reprint/318/7187/846.pdf

Creed, Barbara (1993) *The Monstrous Feminine: Film, Feminism, Psychoanalysis*, London and New York: Routledge.

Crimp, Douglas (ed.) (1988) *AIDS: Cultural Analysis, Cultural Activism*, Boston: Cambridge, MA: MIT Press

Cromwell, Jason (1999) *Transmen & FTMs: Identities, Bodies, Genders and Sexualities*, Urbana and Chicago: University of Illinois Press.

Dajenya (1995) Bisexual lesbian, in Naomi Tucker (ed.) *Bisexual Politics: Theories, Queries and Visions*, New York: Harrington Park Press, 195–7.

Daly, M (1978) *Gyn/ecology: the Metaethics of Radical Feminism*, London: Women's Press

Dangerous Bedfellows (eds) (1996) *Policing Public Sex: Queer Politics and the Future of AIDS Activism*, Boston: South End Press.

D'Augelli, A. R. and Patterson, C. J. (eds) (2001) *Lesbian, Gay And Bisexual Identities And Youth: Psychological Perspectives*, New York: Oxford University Press.

Davenport-Hines, Richard (1990) *Sex, Death and Punishment*, London: Fontana.

Davis, Angela (1982) *Women, Race and Class*, London: Women's Press.

Davis, Kathy (1995) *Reshaping the Female Body: The Dilemma of Cosmetic Surgery*, New York and London: Routledge.

Davis, Lennard J. (ed.) (1997) *The Disability Studies Reader*, London: Routledge.

Davy, Kate (1994) Fe/male impersonation – the discourse of camp, in Moe Meyer (ed.) *The Politics and Poetics of Camp*, London: Routledge, 130–48.

Dean, Tim (2000) *Beyond Sexuality*, Chicago: The University of Chicago Press.

Dekkers, Midas (1994) *Dearest Pet: On Bestiality*, London: Verso.

De Lauretis, Teresa (1990) The practice of sexual difference and feminist thought in Italy an introductory essay, in The Milan Women's Bookstore Collective, *Sexual Difference A Theory of Social-Symbolic Practice*, Bloomington: Indiana University Press, 1–21.

De Lauretis, Teresa (1993) Sexual indifference and lesbian representation, in H. Abelove M.A. Barale and D.M. Halperin (eds) *The Lesbian and Gay Studies Reader*, New York: Routledge, 141–58.

De Lauretis, Teresa (1994) *The Practice of Love: Lesbian Sexuality and Perverse Desire* Bloomington: Indiana University Press.

Delacoste, Frédérique and Alexander, Priscilla (1987) *Sex Work*, San Francisco: Cleis Press.

Delany, Samuel R. (1997) Coming/out, in Patrick Merla (ed.) *Boys Like Us: Gay Writers Tell Their Coming Out Stories*, London: Fourth Estate, 1–26.

Delphy, Christine (1993) Rethinking sex and gender. *Women's Studies International Forum* 16(1): 1–9.

D'Emilio, John (1986) Making and unmaking minorities: the tensions between gay politics and history, in Wayne R. Dynes and Stephen Donaldson (eds) *Studies in Homosexuality: Homosexuality and Government, Politics, and Prisons*, New York and London: Garland Publishing, 1992, 109–16.

D'Emilio, John (1992) Gay and lesbian studies: new kid on the block?, in *Making Trouble: Essays on Gay History, Politics, and the University*, New York and London: Routledge, 160–75.

Densmore, Dana (1968) On celibacy, http://scriptorium.lib.duke.edu/wlm/fun-games1/#celibacy

Derrida, Jacques (1978) [1967] *Writing and Difference*, tr. Alan Bass. London: Routledge and Kegan Paul.

Devor, Holly (1989) *Gender Blending: Confronting the Limits of Duality*, Bloomington: Indiana University Press.

Devor, Holly (1997) *FTM: Female-to-Male Transsexuals in Society*, Bloomington and Indianapolis: Indiana University Press.

Dibbell, Julian (1999) A rape in cyberspace; or how an evil clown, a Haitian trickster spirit, two wizards, and a cast of dozens turned a database into a society, in Peter Ludlow (ed.) *High Noon on the Electronic Frontier: Conceptual Issues in Cyberspace*, Cambridge, MA: MIT Press, 375–96.

Doan, Laura (2000) *Fashioning Sapphism: The Origins of a Modern English Lesbian Culture*, New York: Columbia University Press.

Dollimore, Jonathan (1991) *Sexual Dissidence: Augustine to Wilde, Freud to Foucault*, Oxford: Clarendon Press.

Donaldson, S. and W. Dynes (1990) Typology of homosexuality, in W. Dynes, W. Johansson and W. Percy (eds) *Encyclopedia of Homosexuality*, Chicago and London: St James Press, 1332–7.

Dorkenoo, Efua (1994) *Cutting the Rose: Female Genital Mutilation: The Practice and its Prevention*, London: Minority Rights Publications.

Dover, K. J. (1979) *Greek Homosexuality*, London: Gerald Duckworth and Co.

Dowling, Linda (1994) *Hellenism and Homosexuality in Victorian Oxford*, Ithaca and London: Cornell University Press.

Doyle, Laura (1994) *Bordering on the Body*, Oxford: Oxford University Press.

Dreger, A. (1998) *Hermaphrodites and the Medical Invention of Sex*, Cambridge, MA, and London: Harvard University Press.

Dressler, Joshua (1995) When 'heterosexual' men kill 'homosexual' men: reflections on provocation law, sexual advances, and the 'reasonable man'. *Journal of Criminal Law and Criminology* 85(3): 726–63.

Dryden C. (1999) *Being Married, Doing Gender: A Critical Analysis of Gender Relationships in Marriage,* London: Routledge.

Duggan, Lisa and Hunter, Nan (1995) *Sex Wars: Sexual Dissent and American Political Culture,* London: Routledge.

Durkheim, Émile (1982 [1893]) *The Rules of Sociological Method,* London: Macmillan.

Duesburg, P. (2001) *Duesburg on AIDS,* http://www.duesberg.com/

Duncan, Patricia (1996) Identity, power and difference: negotiating conflict in an S/M dyke community, in Brett Beemyn and Mickey Eliason (eds) *Queer Studies: A Lesbian, Gay, Bisexual and Transgender Anthology,* New York: New York University Press, 87–114.

Dundes, Alan (1985) The American game of 'smear the queer' and the homosexual component of male competitive sport and warfare. *The Journal of Psychoanalytic Anthropology* 8(3): 115–29.

Dutton, Kenneth R. (1995) *The Perfectible Body,* London: Cassell.

Dworkin, Andrea (1981) *Pornography: Men Possessing Women,* London: The Women's Press.

Dworkin, Andrea (1987) *Intercourse,* New York: Free Press.

Dyer, Richard (1985) Gay male porn: coming to terms. *Jump Cut* 30: 27–9.

Dyer, Richard (1999 [1976]) It's being so camp as keeps us going, in Fabio Cleto (ed.) *Camp: Queer Aesthetics and the Performing Subject: A Reader,* Ann Arbor: University of Michigan Press, 110–16.

Dynes, W. (1990a) Buggery, in W. Dynes, W. Johansson and W. Percy (eds) *Encyclopedia of Homosexuality,* Chicago and London: St James Press, 171–3.

Dynes, W. (1990b) Sadomasochism (S/M), in W. Dynes, W. Johansson and W. Percy, *Encyclopedia of Homosexuality,* Chicago and London: St James Press, 1143–6.

Dynes, W., Johansson, W. and Percy, W. (eds)(1990) *Encyclopedia of Homosexuality.* Chicago and London: St James Press.

Eadie, Jo (1993) Activating bisexuality: towards a bi/sexual politics, in J. Bristow and A. Wilson (eds) *Activating Theory. Lesbian, Gay and Bisexual Politics,* London: Lawrence and Wishart, 139–70.

Eadie, Jo (1994) The motley crew: what's at stake in the production of bisexual identity. *Paragraph* 17(1): 17–26.

Eadie, Jo (1996) Indigestion: diagnosing the gay malady, in Mark Simpson, (ed.) *Anti-Gay,* London: Cassell, 66–83.

Edwards, Tim (1994) *Erotics and Politics: Gay Male Sexuality, Masculinity and Feminism.* London: Routledge.

Ekins, Richard. (1997) *Male Femaling: A Grounded Theory Approach to Cross-dressing and Sex-changing,* London and New York: Routledge.

Ekins, Richard and King, Dave (1997) Blending gender: contributions to the emerging field of gender studies. *International Journal of Transgender* 1(1), http://www.symposion.com/ijt/ijtc0101.htm

Elias, James E., Bullough, Vern L., Elias, Veronica and Brewer, Gwen (eds) (1998) *Prostitution: On Whores, Hustlers, and Johns,* Amherst, NY: Prometheus Books.

Ellis, Havelock (1931 [1903]) *Analysis of the Sexual Impulse: Studies in the Psychology of Sex, Vol.III.* Philadelphia: F.A. Davis.

Ellis, Havelock (1898) Autoerotism: a psychological study. *Alienist and Neurologist* 19: 260–99.

Ellis, Havelock and Symonds, John A. (1897) *Sexual Inversion,* London: Wilson and Macmillan.

Ember, Carol, Ember, Melvin and Peregrine, Peter (1992) *Anthropology,* Upper Saddle River, NJ: Prentice Hall.

Eng, T. and Butler, W. (eds) (1997) *The Hidden Epidemic: Confronting Sexually Transmitted Diseases,* Washington, DC: National Academy Press.

Ensler, Eve (2001) *The Vagina Monologues,* New York: Villard.

Epstein, Steven (1998) Gay politics, ethnic identity: the limits of social constructionism, in Peter M. Nardi and Beth Schneider (eds) *Social Perspectives in Lesbian and Gay Studies,* London and New York: Routledge, 134–59.

Ericsson, J. (2000) Male rape: a personal story. *Axiom* (39): 25–7.

Evans, David (1993) *Sexual Citizenship: The Material Construction of Sexualities,* London: Routledge.

Evans, D.T. (2000) Speaking of sex: the need to dispel myths and overcome fears. *British Journal of Nursing* 9(10): 1162–9.

Evans, D.T. (2001) The stigma of sexuality: concealability and course, in T. Mason, C. Carlisle, C. Watkins and E. Whitehead (eds), *Stigma and Social Exclusion in Health Care,* London: Routledge, 104–16.

Evans, Dylan (1998) From Kantian ethics to mystical experience: an exploration of jouissance, in Danny Nobus (ed.) *Key Concepts in Lacanian Psychoanalysis,* London: Rebus Press, 1–28.

Faderman, Lilian (1981) *Surpassing the Love of Men: Romantic Friendship And Love Between Women from the Renaissance to the Present,* London: The Women's Press.

Faderman, Lilian (1991) *Odd Girls and Twilight Lovers: A History of Lesbian Life in Twentieth-Century America,* London: Penguin.

Faderman, Lilian (1992) The return of butch and femme: a phenomenon in lesbian sexuality of the 1980s and 1990s. *Journal of the History of Sexuality* 2(4): 578–96.

Faludi, Susan (1992) *Backlash,* London: Vintage.

Farquhar, Clare, Bailey, Julia and Whittaker, Dawn (2002) Are lesbians sexually healthy?, *South Bank University Papers,* http://www.lsbu.ac.uk/fhss/sexuality/reports

Fausto-Sterling, Anne (1993) The five sexes: why male and female are not enough. *The Sciences* (March–April): 20–4.

Fausto-Sterling, Anne (2000) *Sexing the Body: Gender Politics and the Construction of Sexuality*, New York: Basic Books.

Featherstone, Mike (2000) *Body Modification*, London: Sage.

Federation of Feminist Women's Health Centers (1991) *A New View of a Woman's Body*, Los Angeles: Feminist Health Press.

Fee, D. (2000) 'One of the guys': instrumentality and intimacy in gay men's friendships with straight men, in P. Nardi (ed.) *Gay Masculinities*, London: Sage, 44–65.

Feinberg, Leslie (1993) *Stone Butch Blues*, Milford, CT: Firebrand Books.

Feinberg, Leslie (1996) *Transgender Warriors: Making History from Joan of Arc to RuPaul*, Boston: Beacon Press.

Fell, Christine (1984) *Women in Anglo-Saxon England*, Oxford: Blackwell.

Feminists Against Censorship (2001) Submission to the BBFC, http://www.fiawol.demon.co.uk/FAC/femejac.htm

Field, Nicola (1995) *Over the Rainbow: Money, Class and Homophobia*, London: Pluto Press.

Finger, Anne (1997) Forbidden fruit, in Estelle Disch (ed.) *Reconstructing Gender: A Multicultural Anthology*, London and Toronto: Mayfield Publishing Company, 244–7.

Finkler, Lilith and Chater, Nancy (1995) 'Traversing wide territories': a journey from lesbianism to bisexuality, in The Bisexual Anthology Collective (eds), *Plural Desires. Writing Bisexual Women's Realities*, Toronto: SisterVision, 14–36.

Firestone, S. (1971) *The Dialectic of Sex*, London: Cape.

Fisher, H.E. (1992) *Anatomy of Love: The Natural History of Monogamy, Adultery, and Divorce*, London: Simon and Schuster.

Fishman, Jennifer and Mamo, Laura (2001) What's in a disorder: a cultural analysis of medical and pharmaceutical constructions of male and female sexual dysfunctions, in Ellyn Kaschak and Leonore Tiefer (eds) *A New View Of Women's Sexual Problems*, New York: Haworth Press, 179–93.

Foucault, Michel (1977) *Discipline and Punish*, tr. Robert Hurley. London: Tavistock.

Foucault, Michel (1990[1976]) *The History of Sexuality: An Introduction*, tr. Robert Hurley, Harmondsworth: Penguin.

Foucault, Michel (1985 [1984]) *The History of Sexuality, Volume 2: The Use of Pleasure*, tr. Robert Hurley, Harmondsworth: Random House.

Foucault, Michel (1997 [1982]) Sex, power, and the politics of identity, in Paul Rabinow (ed.) *Ethics, Subjectivity and Truth. The Essential Works of Foucault, Volume I 1954–1984*, New York: New Press, 163–74.

Fout, John C. (1992) *Forbidden History: The State, Society, And The Regulation Of Sexuality In Modern Europe*, Chicago and London: University of Chicago Press.

Fox, Ronald C. (1996) Bisexuality in perspective: a review of theory and research, in Beth A. Firestein (ed.) *Bisexuality: The Psychology and Politics of an Invisible Minority*, Thousand Oaks, CA: Sage, 3–50.

Foyster, E.A. (1999) *Manhood In Early Modern England: Honour, Sex And Marriage*, London: Longman.

Frankel, D. (1994) US surgeon general forced to resign. *The Lancet* 34: 1695.

Franklin, Adrian (1999) *Animals and Modern Cultures: A Sociology of Human–Animal Relations in Modernity*, London: Sage.

Franklin, S. (1997) *Embodied Progress. A Cultural Account of Assisted Conception*, London: Routledge.

Fraser, Mariam (1999) *Identity Without Selfhood: Simone de Beauvoir and Bisexuality*, Cambridge: Cambridge University Press.

Fraser, Nancy (1998) Heterosexism, misrecognition and capitalism: a response to Judith Butler. *New Left Review* 228: 140–9.

Freeman, M.D.A. (1996) *Divorce: Where Next?* Aldershot, Hants: Dartmouth Publishing Company.

Freud, Sigmund (1905a) Fragment of an analysis of a case of hysteria, in *The Standard Edition of the Complete Psychological Works of Sigmund Freud*, (ed.) James Strachey (tr.), Vol. 7, London: The Hogarth Press, 1–122.

Freud, Sigmund (1905b) Three essays on the theory of sexuality, in *The Standard Edition of the Complete Psychological Works of Sigmund Freud*, (ed.) James Strachey (tr.), Vol. 7, London: The Hogarth Press, 123–245.

Freud, Sigmund (1908) On the sexual theories of children, in *The Standard Edition of the Complete Psychological Works of Sigmund Freud*, (ed.) James Strachey (tr.), Vol. 9, London: The Hogarth Press, 205–26.

Freud, Sigmund (1909) Analysis of a phobia in a five-year-old boy, in *The Standard Edition of the Complete Psychological Works of Sigmund Freud*, (ed.) James Strachey (tr.), Vol. 10, London: The Hogarth Press, 3–150.

Freud, Sigmund (1912) On the universal tendency to debasement in the sphere of love, in *The Standard Edition of the Complete Psychological Works of Sigmund Freud*, (ed.) James Strachey (tr.), Vol. 11, London: The Hogarth Press, 177–90.

Freud, Sigmund (1914a) On narcissism: an introduction, in *The Standard Edition of the Complete Psychological Works of Sigmund Freud*, (ed.) James Strachey, Vol. 14, London: The Hogarth Press, 67–104.

Freud, Sigmund (1914b) Repression, in *The Standard Edition of the Complete Psychological Works of Sigmund Freud*, (ed.) James Strachey (tr.), Vol. 14, London: The Hogarth Press, 141–58.

Freud, Sigmund (1921) Group psychology and the analysis of the ego, in *The Standard Edition of the Complete Psychological Works of Sigmund Freud*, (ed.) James Strachey (tr.), Vol. 18, London: The Hogarth Press, 67–143.

Freud, Sigmund (1924) The dissolution of the oedipus complex, in *The Standard Edition of the Complete Psychological Works of Sigmund Freud*, (ed.) James Strachey (tr.), Vol. 19, London: The Hogarth Press, 173–9.

Freud, Sigmund (1925) Negation, in *The Standard Edition of the Complete Psychologica* *Works of Sigmund Freud*, (ed.) James Strachey (tr.), Vol. 19, London: The Hogarth Press, 235–9.

Freud, Sigmund (1933) On femininity, in *The Standard Edition of the Complete Psychological works of Sigmund Freud*, (ed.) James Strachey (tr.), Vol. 22, London: The Hogarth Press, 136–57.

Freud, Sigmund (1991a [1927]) Fetishism, in *On Sexuality* (Penguin Freud Library, Vol. 7), Harmondsworth: Penguin.

Freud, Sigmund (1991b[1920]) The psychogenesis of a case of homosexuality in a woman, in *Case Histories II* (Penguin Freud Library Vol. 9) Harmondsworth: Penguin, 367–400.

Friedan, Betty (1963) *The Feminine Mystique*, New York: W.W. Norton.

Friedman, David (2001) *A Mind of Its Own: A Cultural History of the Penis*, New York: Free Press.

Frye, M. (1983) *The Politics of Reality*, Trumansburg: Crossing Press.

Furman, C. Sue (1995) *Turning Point: The Myths and Realities of Menopause*, Oxford: Oxford University Press.

Fuss, Diana (1990) *Essentially Speaking*, London: Routledge.

Fuss, Diana (1995) *Identification Papers*, New York: Routledge.

Gage, Carolyn (1997) *Like There's No Tomorrow: Meditations for Women Leaving Patriarchy*, Monroe, ME: Common Courage Press.

Gagnon, John and Simon, William (1973) *Sexual Conduct: The Social Sources of Human Sexuality*, Chicago: Aldine.

Gamman, L. and Makinen, M. (1994) *Female Fetishism: A New Look*, London: Lawrence and Wishart.

Gamman, Lorraine and Marshment, Margaret (1988) *The Female Gaze: Women a. Viewers of Popular Culture*, London: The Women's Press.

Gamson, Joshua (1998) Must identity movements self-destruct: a queer dilemma, in Peter M. Nardi and Beth E. Schneider (eds), *Social Perspectives in Lesbian and Gay Studies*, New York: Routledge, 589–604.

Garber, Eric (1988) Gladys Bentley: the bulldagger who sang the blues. *Out/Look* 1 52–61.

Garber, Marjorie (1992) *Vested Interests: Cross-Dressing and Cultural Anxiety*, New York Routledge.

Garber, Marjorie (1995) *Vice Versa: Bisexuality and the Eroticism of Everyday Life* London: Hamish Hamilton.

Garland, Rodney [Adam de Hegedus] (1995 [1953]) *The Heart in Exile*, Brighton Millivres.

Garlinger, Patrick Paul (1999) 'Homo-ness' and the fear of femininity. *Diacritics* 29 (1) 57–71.

Gates, Henry Louis Jr. (1987) *Figures in Black: Words, Signs and the 'Racial' Self*, New York and London: Oxford University Press.

Gates, Henry Louis Jr (1995) *Colored People*, Harmondsworth: Penguin.

Gayle, P. (1994) *The Hand Book: A Practical Guide to Your Arse, Douching, Dildoes and Fisting for Gay Men*, London: BottomLiners.

George, Susan (1993) *Women and Bisexuality*, London: Scarlet Press.

George, Susan (2001) Making sense of bisexual personal ads, *Journal of Bisexuality* 1(4), 33–58. http://www.haworthpressinc.com/store/SampleText/J159.pdf

Giddens, Anthony (1992a) *The Transformation of Intimacy: Sexuality, Love and Eroticism in Modern Societies*, Cambridge: Polity Press.

Giddens, Anthony (1992b) *Sociology*, Oxford: Polity Press.

Gill, Linda (2001) Women beware! The appropriation of women in Hollywood's revisioning of Mary Shelley's 'Frankenstein'. *Journal of American and Comparative Cultures* 24(3–4): 93–8.

Gilman, Sander (1993) *Disease and Representation: Images of Illness from Madness to AIDS*, New York: Cornell University Press.

Gilmartin, Brian (1987) *Shyness and Love: Causes, Consequences, and Treatment*, New York: University Press of America, Inc.

Ginzberg, R. (1994) audre lorde's (nonessentialist) lesbian eros, in C. Card (ed.) *Adventures in Lesbian Philosophy*, Bloomington: Indiana University Press.

Gittins, D. (1993) *The Family in Question: Changing Households and Familiar Ideologies*, London: Macmillan Press, 81–97.

Goergen, D. (1976) *The Sexual Celibate*, London: SPCK.

Goffman, E. (1990 [1963]) *Stigma: Notes on the Management of Spoiled Identity*, London: Penguin.

Goldberg, J., (ed.) (1994) *Reclaiming Sodom*, London: Routledge.

Gollaher, David (2000) *Circumcision: A History of the World's Most Controversial Surgery*, New York: Basic Books.

Goodwin, L. (2002) Pansexuality and separatism, http://www.lauragoodwin.org/pansexual.htm

Gordon, G.N. (1980) *Erotic Communications: Studies in Sex, Sin, and Censorship*, New York: Hastings House.

Gorna, Robin (1996) *Vamps, Virgins, and Victims: How Can Women Fight AIDS?* London: Cassell.

Goulet, Jean-Guy A. (1996) The 'berdache'/'two-spirit': a comparison of anthropological and native constructions of gendered identities among the northern Athapaskans. *Journal of the Royal Anthropological Institute* 2(4): 683–701.

Grafenberg, E. (1950) The role of the urethra in female orgasm. *International Journal of Sexology* 3: 145–8.

Grahn, Judy (1984) *Another Mother Tongue*, Boston: Beacon Press.

Green, Victoria (1999) *The Point Behind the Needle: An Investigation into Body Piercing in Western Society*, Keele: Keele University Working Papers in Social Relations.

Greer, Germaine (1999) *The Whole Woman*, London: Doubleday.

Grey, A. (1993) *Speaking of Sex: The Limits of Language*, London: Cassell.

Groocock, Veronica (1994) Lesbian journalism: mainstream and alternative press, in Liz Gibbs (ed.) *Daring to Dissent*, London: Cassell, 91–119.

Grosz, Elizabeth (1994) *Volatile Bodies*, Indianapolis and Bloomington: University of Indiana Press.

Gupta, Sunil (1989) Black, *brown* and white, in Simon Shepherd and Mick Wallis (eds) *Coming On Strong: Gay Politics and Culture*, London: Unwin Hyman, 163–79.

Gutterman, David (2001) Postmodernism and the interrogation of masculinity, in Stephen Whitehead and Frank Barrett (eds) *The Masculinities Reader*, Cambridge: Polity, 56–72.

Haavio-Mannila, Elina, Kontula, Osmo, Rotkirch, Anna and Campling, Jo (2002) *Sexual Lifestyles in the Twentieth Century: A Research Study*, Basingstoke: Palgrave.

Hadley, D.M. (ed.) (1999) *Masculinity in Medieval Europe*, London: Longman.

Hadley, J. (1997) *Abortion: Between Freedom and Necessity*, London: Virago Press.

Haeberle, Edwin J. (1989) Swastika, pink triangle, and yellow star: the destruction of sexology and the persecution of homosexuals in Nazi Germany, in Martin Duberman, Martha Vicinus, and George Chauncey (eds) *Hidden from History: Reclaiming the Gay and Lesbian Past*, New York: Penguin/New American Library, 365–79.

Hagland, Paul EeNam Park (1998) Undressing the oriental boy: the gay Asian male in the social imaginary of the gay white male, in Dawn Atkins (ed.) *Looking Queer: Body Image and Identity in Lesbian, Bisexual, Gay and Transgender Communities*, New York, London: Harrington Park Press, 277–93.

Halberstam, Judith (1998) *Female Masculinity*, Durham and London: Duke University Press.

Hale, Jacob (1996) Writing rules: suggested rules for non-transsexuals writing about transsexuals, transsexuality, transsexualism, or transsexual, http://www.twenty-club.org/news/july96.html

Hale, C. Jacob (1998) Consuming the living, dis(re)membering the dead in the butch/ftm borderlands. *GLQ* 4(2): 311–48.

Hall, Lesley A. (2000) *Sex, Gender and Social Change in Britain Since 1880*, New York: St Martin's Press.

Hall, Donald E. and Pramaggiore, Maria (eds) (1996) *RePresenting Bisexualities: Subjects and Cultures of Fluid Desire*, New York: New York University Press.

Hall, Radclyffe (1950 [1928]) *The Well of Loneliness*, New York: Pocket Books.

Halperin, David M. (2002) *How To Do the History of Homosexuality*, Chicago: University of Chicago Press.

Hammond, Karla (1980) An interview with Audre Lorde. *American Poetry Review* March/April: 18–21.

Hancock, Ian (1984) Shelta and Polari, in Peter Trudgill (ed.) *The Language of the British Isles*, Cambridge: Cambridge University Press, 384–403.

Hanley, Susan B. (1997) *Everyday Things in Premodern Japan: The Hidden Legacy of Material Culture*, London: University of California Press.

Haraway, Donna (1990) Investment strategies for the evolving portfolio of primate females, in Mary Jacobus, Evelyn Fox Keller, and Sally Shuttleworth (eds), *Body/Politics: Women and the Discourses of Science*, London: Routledge, 139–62.

Haraway, Donna (1997) *Modest-Witness@Second-Millennium. FemaleMan-Meets-OncoMouse: Feminism and Technoscience*, New York: Routledge.

Harding, Jennifer (1997) Bodies at risk: sex, surveillance and hormone replacement therapy, in Alan Peterson and Robin Burton (eds) *Foucault, Health and Medicine*, London and New York: Routledge, 134–50.

Harper, Phillip Brian (1994) Private affairs: race, sex, property and persons. *GLQ* 1(2): 111–33.

Hart, Lynda (1998) *Between the Body and the Flesh: Performing Sadomasochism*, New York: Columbia University Press.

Hartmann, B. (1995) *Reproductive Rights and Wrongs: The Global Politics of Population Control (Revised)*, Boston: South End Press.

Hartouni, V (1997) *Cultural Conceptions: On Reproductive Technologies and the Remaking of Life*, London: University of Minnesota Press.

Haug, Frigga (1987) *Female Sexualization*, tr. Erica Carter. London: Verso.

Hausman, Bernice (1995) *Changing Sex: Transsexualism, Technology and the Idea of Gender*, Durham, NC: Duke University Press.

Healey, Emma (1996) *Lesbian Sex Wars*, London: Virago.

Healy, Murray (1996) *Gay Skins: Class, Masculinity and Queer Appropriation*, London: Cassell.

Heine, Ken (2002) To pack or not to pack. *Womonspace Newsletter*, May 2002, http://www.gaycanada.com/womonspace/nl2002/may02/nl0502_a10.html

Heins, Marjorie (2001) *Not in Front of the Children: 'Indecency', Censorship, and the Innocence of Youth*, New York: Hill and Wang.

Hemmings, Clare (1998) Waiting for no man: bisexual femme subjectivity and cultural repudiation, in Sally Munt (ed.) *Butch/Femme: Inside Lesbian Gender*, London: Cassell, 90–100.

Hemmings, Clare (2002) *Bisexual Spaces: A Geography of Sexuality and Gender*, London: Routledge.

Henkin, William A. (1989) Tales from the crib: a review of *Psychosexual infantilism in adults: the eroticization of regression*, by Thomas John Speaker, http://www.sexuality.org/l/wh/whinfant.html

Henkin, William A (1998) Scat: ask the therapist, http://www.sexuality.org/l/wh/att80.html

Herdt, Gilbert (1984) Ritualized homosexual behavior in the male cults of Melanesia: an introduction, in Gilbert Herdt (ed.) *Ritualized Homosexuality in Melanesia*, Berkeley: University of California Press, 1–81.

Herdt, Gilbert (ed.) (1994) *Third Sex, Third Gender: Beyond Sexual Dimorphism in Culture and History*, New York: Zone.

Herdt, G. (1997) *Same Sex, Different Cultures*, Boulder: Westview Press.

Herek, G.M. (ed.) (1998) *Stigma and Sexual Orientation: Understanding Prejudice Against Lesbians, Gay Men and Bisexuals*, London: Sage Publications.

Herek, G.M., and Berrill, K.T. (1992) *Hate Crimes: Confronting Violence Against Lesbians and Gay Men*, London: Sage.

Herek, G.M., Cogan, J.C. and Gillis, J.R. (2002) Victim experiences in hate crimes based on sexual orientation, http://psychology.ucdavis.edu/rainbow/html/jsi_2002.pdf

Highleyman, Liz A. (1992) Identity and ideas: strategies for bisexuals, in Naomi Tucker (ed.) *Closer to Home: Bisexuality and Feminism*, Seattle: Seal Press, 73–92.

Highleyman, Liz (1996) Kinky bisexuals: ultimate switches or ultimate outcasts?, http://www.sexuality.org/l/cu/bism_24.html

Hill Collins, Patricia (2000) Black feminist epistemology, in *Black Feminist Thought: Knowledge, Consciousness and the Politics of Empowerment*, New York: Routledge, 251–71.

Hills, Matt (2002) *Fan Cultures*, London: Routledge.

Hird, M.J. (2000) Gender's nature: intersexuals, transsexuals and the 'sex'/ 'gender' binary. *Feminist Theory* 1(3): 347–64.

Hird, M.J. (2002) For a sociology of transsexualism. *Sociology* 36(3): 573–91.

Hird, M.J. and Germon, J. (2001) The intersexual body and the medical regulation of gender, in K. Backett-Milburn and L. McKie. (eds) *Constructing Gendered Bodies*, London: Palgrave, 162–78.

Hirschfeld, Magnus (1991 [1910]) *Transvestites: The Erotic Drive to Cross-Dress*, tr. Vern Bullough, Amherst, NY: Prometheus Books.

Hitchcock, Tim (2002) Redefining sex in eighteenth-century England, in Kim M. Phillips and Barry Reay (eds) *Sexualities in History*, London: Routledge, 185–221.

Hoad, Neville (1998) Neoliberalism, homosexuality, Africa, the Anglican Church: The World Conference of Anglican Bishops at Lambeth, July 18–August 9, 1998. http://www.umanitoba.ca/faculties/arts/english/media/workshop/papers

Hoagland, Sarah Lucia and Penelope, Julia (eds) (1988) *For Lesbians Only: A Separatist Anthology*, London: Onlywomen.

Hodes, Martha (1997) *White Women, Black Men: Illicit Sex in the Nineteenth Century South*, New Haven, CT: Yale University Press.

Hogben, S. and Coupland, J (2000) 'Egg seeks sperm: end of story. . .?': articulating gay parenting in small ads for reproductive partners. *Discourse and Society* 11(4): 459–85.

Holland, J. (1998) *The Male in the Head: Young People, Heterosexuality and Power*, London: Tufnell.

Holland, Janet, Ramazanoglu, Caroline and Sharpe, Sue (1993) *Wimp or Gladiator: Contradictions in Acquiring Masculine Sexuality*, London: The Tufnell Press.

Holloway, Wendy and Jefferson, Tony (1998) 'A kiss is just a kiss': date rape, gender and subjectivity. *Sexualities* 1(4): 405–23.

Holly (1991) The transgender alternative. *TV/TS Tapestry Journal* 59:31–3.

hooks, bell (1986) *Ain't I a Woman: Black Women and Feminism*, London: Pluto Press.

Hopper, Jim (2003) *Child Abuse: Statistics, Research, and Resources,* http://www.jimhopper.com/abstats

Hosken, Fran (1982) *The Hosken Report: Genital and Sexual Mutilation of Females*, Lexington, MA: International Network News.

Houppert, Karen (1999) *The Curse: Confronting the Last Unmentionable Taboo – Menstruation*, New York: Farrar, Straus and Giroux.

Housk, Randall (2002) *Piercing: A Modern Anthology*, London: Salamander Books.

Humphreys, Laud (1970) *Tearoom Trade*, London: Duckworth.

Hunt, Leon (1998) *British Low Culture: From Safari Suits to Sexploitation*, London: Routledge.

Hunter, Nan D. (1995) Sexual dissent and the family: the Sharon Kowalski case, in Lisa Duggan and Nan D. Hunter (eds) *Sex Wars: Sexual Dissent and Political Culture*, New York: Routledge, 101–6.

Huntley, Rebecca (2000) Sexing the belly: an exploration of sex and the pregnant body. *Sexualities* 3(3): 347–62.

Hutchins, Lorraine and Ka'ahumanu, Lani (1990) 'Glossary', in Lorraine Hutchins and Lani Ka'ahumanu (eds) *Bi Any Other Name: Bisexual People Speak Out,* Boston: Alyson Publications, 369–71.

Hutchins, Lorraine, and Ka'ahumanu, Lani (eds)(1990) *Bi Any Other Name: Bisexual People Speak Out,* Boston: Alyson Publications.

Hyde, Janet Shibley and DeLamater, John D. (1997) *Understanding Human Sexuality,* Boston: McGraw-Hill Press.

Ingraham, Chrys (1999) *White Weddings*, New York: Routledge.

Innes, Sherrie A. and Lloyd, Michele E (1996) G.I. Joes in barbie land: recontextualizing butch in twentieth-century lesbian culture, in Brett Beemyn and Mickey Eliason (eds) *Queer Studies: A Lesbian, Gay, Bisexual, and Transgender Anthology*, New York and London: New York University Press, 9–34.

Irigaray, Luce (1985a) [1974] *Speculum of the Other Woman*, tr. Gillan C. Gill, Ithaca: Cornell University Press.

Irigaray, Luce (1985b) [1977] *This Sex Which Is Not One*, tr. Catherine Porter, Ithaca: Cornell University Press.

ISNA (2003a) On the word 'hermaphrodite', http://www.isna.org/faq/language.html.

ISNA (2003b) What is an intersex condition? What do these diagnoses mean? http://www.isna.org/faq/faq-medical.html

Jackson, Earl Jr. (1995) *Strategies of Deviance: Studies in Gay Male Representation*, Bloomington: Indiana University Press.

Jackson, Stevi (1995) Gender and heterosexuality: a materialist feminist analysis, in Mary Maynard and June Purvis (eds) *(Hetero)sexual Politics*, London: Taylor and Francis, 11–25.

Jackson, Stevi (1999) *Heterosexuality in Question*, London: Sage.

Jackson, Stevi and Scott, Sue (eds) (1996) *Feminism and Sexuality: A Reader*, New York: Columbia University Press.

Jacobs, Sue-Ellen, Thomas, Wesley, and Lang, Sabine (eds) (1997) *Two-Spirit People: Native American Gender Identity, Sexuality, and Spirituality*, Urbana and Chicago: University of Illinois Press.

Jagose, Annamarie (1996) *Queer Theory: An Introduction*, New York: New York University Press.

Jakobsen, Janet (1998) *Working Alliances and the Politics of Difference*, Bloomington and Indianapolis: Indiana University Press.

James, Wendy and Kedgley, Susan Jane (1973) *The Mistress*, London: Abelard and Schuman.

Jamieson, Lynn (1998) *Intimacy: Personal Relationships in Modern Societies*, Cambridge: Polity Press.

Jamieson, Lynn (1999) Intimacy transformed? A critical look at the 'pure relationship'. *Sociology* 33(3): 477–94.

Jansen, H., Kesler, B. and Poldervaart, S. (eds) (2002) *Contemporary Utopian Struggles*, Somerset, NJ: Transaction Publishers.

Jay, Karla (1999) *Tales of the Lavender Menace: A Memoir of Liberation*, New York: Basic Books.

Jeffreys, Sheila (1985) *The Spinster and Her Enemies: Feminism and Sexuality, 1880–1930*, London: Pandora.

Jeffreys, Sheila, (1989) Butch and femme: now and then, in The Lesbian History Group (eds) *Not a Passing Phase: Reclaiming Lesbians in History 1840–1985*, London: The Women's Press, 158–87.

Jeffreys, Sheila (1993) *The Lesbian Heresy*, London: The Women's Press.

Jeffreys, Sheila (2003) *Unpacking Queer Politics: A Lesbian Feminist Perspective*, Cambridge: Polity Press.

Jenkins, Carol L. (1996) The homosexual context of heterosexual practice in Papua New Guinea, in Peter Aggleton (ed.) *Bisexualities and AIDS*, London: Taylor and Francis, 191–206.

Jenkins, Henry (1992) *Textual Poachers: Television Fans and Participatory Culture*, London: Routledge.

Jenness, Valerie, and Broad, Kendal (1997) *Hate Crimes: New Social Movements and the Politics of Violence*, Hawthorne, NY: Aldine de Gruyter.

Jochens, Jenny (1996) Old Norse sexuality: men, women, and beasts, in Vern L. Bullough and James A. Brundage (eds) *Handbook of Medieval Sexuality*, London: Garland Publishing, 369–400.

Johansson, Warren and Percy, William A. (1996) Homosexuality, in Vern L. Bullough and James A. Brundage (eds) *Handbook of Medieval Sexuality*, London: Garland Publishing, 155–89.

Johnson, Lee (1994) Lesbian bed death: a radical interpretation. *Hera* 31: 5.

Johnson, S. (2002) *The Gay Baby Boom: The Psychology of Gay Parenthood*, New York: New York University Press.

Jones, Constance (1996) *Sexual Harassment*, New York: Facts on File.

Jones, E.E., Farina, A., Hastorf, A.H., Markus, H., Miller, D.T., Scott, R.A. and de French, S. (eds) (1984) *Social Stigma: The Psychology of Marked Relationships*, New York: W H Freeman.

Jones, Kevin (2000) (ed.) *Safety at Work 7: Special Issue on Safety in the Workplace and the Sex Industry*. http://www.walnet.org/csis/safety/safetyatwork.html

Jose, Jim and Bacchi, Carol (1994) Dealing with sexual harassment: persuade, discipline or punish? *Australian Journal of Law and Society*, 10: 1–13. http://www.learnline.ntu.edu.au/studyskills/nm/nmDocs/JJCB-AJLS.pdf

Kaloski, Ann (1999) Bisexuals making out with cyborgs: politics, pleasure, con/fusion, in Merl Storr (ed.) *Bisexuality: a Critical Reader*, London: Routledge, 201–10.

Kaplan, E Ann (1983) Is the gaze male?, in Ann Snitow, Christiane Stansell and Sharon Thompson (eds) *Powers of Desire*, New York: Monthly Review Press 309–27.

Kaplan, Louise J (1993) *Female Perversions*, Harmondsworth: Penguin.

Karras, Ruth Mazo (1996) Prostitution in medieval Europe, in Vern L. Bullough and James A. Brundage (eds) *Handbook of Medieval Sexuality*, London: Garland Publishing, 243–60.

Kelly, L. (1998) 'It's everywhere': sexual violence as a continuum, in S. Jackson and S. Scott (eds) *Feminism and Sexuality: A Reader*, Edinburgh, Edinburgh University Press, 191–207.

Kempadoo, K. and Doezema, J. (eds) (1998) *Global Sex Workers: Rights, Resistance and Redefinition*, New York and London: Routledge.

Kennedy, Elisabeth Lapovski and Davis, Madeline D. (1993) *Boots of Leather, Slippers of Gold: The History of a Lesbian Community*, New York and London: Routledge.

Kessler, Suzanne (1998) *Lessons from the Intersexed*, New Brunswick: Rutgers University Press.

Kessler, Suzanne, and McKenna, Wendy (2000) Who put the 'trans' in transgender? Gender theory and everyday life. *International Journal of Transgenderism*, 4(3): 1–5, http://www.symposion.com/ijt/gilbert/kessler.htm

Kimmel, Michael (1990) After fifteen years: the impact of the sociology of masculinity on the masculinity of sociology, in Jeff Hearn and David Morgan (eds) *Men, Masculinities and Social Theory*, London: Unwin Hyman, 93–109.

Kincaid, J. R. (1993) *Child-Loving: The Erotic Child and Victorian Culture*, London: Routledge, 93–109.

Kincaid, James R. (1998) *Erotic Innocence: The Culture of Child Molesting*, Durham, NC: Duke University Press.

King, Edward (1993) *Safety in Numbers: Safer Sex and Gay Men*, London: Cassell

King, Heather and Hayes, Jordan. (1999) *A Guide to Surviving Life as a Mistress*, London: Robert Hale.

Kinsey, Alfred, Pomeroy, W.B. and Martin, C.E. . (1948) *Sexual Behavior in the Human Male*, Philadelphia and London: W.B. Saunders Company.

Kirsch, Max (2000) *Queer Theory and Social Change*, London: Routledge.

Kitzinger, Celia (1989) *The Social Construction of Lesbianism*, London: Sage.

Klein, Fritz (1978) *The Bisexual Option: A Concept of One Hundred Percent Intimacy*, New York: Priam Books.

Klein, Fritz and Wolf, Timothy J. (eds)(1985) *Two Lives to Lead: Bisexuality in Men and Women*, New York: Harrington Park Press.

Klein, Fritz, Sepekoff, Barry and Wolf, Timothy, J. (1985) Sexual orientation: a multi-variable dynamic process. *Journal of Homosexuality* 11(1–2): 35–49.

Klein, R.D. (ed.) (1989) *Infertiliy: Women Speak Out About Their Experiences of Reproductive Medicine*, London: Pandora Press.

Kolodny, Deborah (2000) *Blessed Bi Spirit: Bisexual People of Faith*, New York: Continuum International Publishing.

Komesaroff, Paul, Rothfield, Philippa and Daly, Jeanne (eds) (1997) *Reinterpreting the Menopause: Cultural and Philosophical Issues*, London and New York: Routledge.

Koss, Mary and Cook, Sarah (1993) Facing the facts: date and acquaintance rape are significant problems for women, in Richard Gelles and Domileen Loseke (eds), *Current Controversies on Family Violence*, Thousand Oaks, CA: Sage, 104–19.

Krafft-Ebbing, Richard von (1965 [1886–1903]) *Psychopathia Sexualis*, tr. Franklin S. Klaf, London: Staples Press.

Kramarae, Cheris and Spender, Dale (gen. eds.) (2000) *Routledge International Encyclopedia of Women: Global Women's Issues and Knowledge*, New York and London: Routledge.

Kramarae, Cheris, and. Treichler, Paula A (1992) *Amazons, Bluestockings and Crones: A Feminist Dictionary*, London: Pandora Press.

Kramer, Larry (1995) *Reports from the Holocaust: The Story of an AIDS Activist* London: Cassell.

Krishnaswamy, R. (2002) The economy of colonial desire, in R. Adams and D. Savran. *The Masculinity Studies Reader*, Oxford: Blackwell, 292–317.

Kristeva, Julia (1980) *Desire in Language*, tr. Leon Roudiez. New York: Columbia University Press.

Kristeva, Julia (1982) *Powers of Horror: An Essay on Abjection*, tr. Leon Roudiez, New York: Columbia University Press.

Kroker, Arthur and Kroker, Marilouise (eds) (1987) *Body Invaders: Panic Sex in America*, Montreal: New World Perspectives.

Kuefler, Mathew (2001) *The Manly Eunuch: Masculinity, Gender Ambiguity, and Christian Ideology in Late Antiquity*, London: The University of Chicago Press.

Lacan, Jacques (1933) Motives of paranoiac crime: the crime of the Papin sisters, http://www.lacan.com/papin.htm

Lacan, Jacques (1977a) *Écrits: A Selection*, tr. Alan Sheridan, New York: Norton.

Lacan, Jacques (1977b [1958]) The signification of the phallus, tr. Alan Sheridan, in *Ecrits: A Selection*, London: Routledge, 281–91.

Lacan, Jacques (1977c [1960]) Subversion of the subject and dialectic of desire, tr. Alan Sheridan, in *Ecrits: A Selection*, London: Routledge, 293–325.

La Fontaine J (1990) *Child Sexual Abuse*, Cambridge: Polity Press.

Laird, J. (ed.) (1999) *Lesbians and Lesbian Families: Reflections on Theory and Practice*, New York: Columbia University Press.

Lano, Kevin and Parry, Claire (eds) (1995) *Breaking the Barriers to Desire: New Approaches to Multiple Relationships*, Nottingham: Five Leaves Press.

Laplanche, Jean and Pontalis, J.B. (1974) *The Language of Psychoanalysis*, New York: W.W. Norton and Company.

Laplanche, Jean and Pontalis, J.B. (1986) Fantasy and the origins of sexuality, in V. Burgin, J. Donald and C. Kaplan (eds) *Formations Of Fantasy*, London: Methuen, 5–27.

Laqueur, Thomas (1990) *Making Sex: Body and Gender from the Greeks to Freud*, Cambridge, MA: Harvard University Press.

Laqueur, Thomas (2003) *Solitary Sex: A Cultural History of Masturbation*, New York: Zone Books.

Latteier, Carolyn (1998) *Breasts: The Women's Perspective on an American Obsession*, Haworth Press.

Leap, William (ed.) (1999) *Public Sex, Gay Space*, New York: Columbia University Press.

Lees, Sue (1997) *Ruling Passions: Sexual Violence, Reputation and the Law*, Milton Keynes: Open University Press.

Lehmann, J.M. (ed.) (2001) *The Gay and Lesbian Marriage Reader: Analyses of Problems and Prospects for the 21st Century*, New York: Gordian Knot Books.

Leigh, Carol (2003) *Unrepentant Whore*, San Francisco: Last Gasp.

Lesko, N. (1996) Past, present and future conceptions of adolescence. *Educational Theory*, 46 (4): 453–72.

Lestrade, Didier (2000) *Act Up: Une Histoire*, Paris: Denoël.

Leupp, Gary (1995) *Male Colors: The Construction of Homosexuality in Modern Japan*, Berkeley: University of California Press.

LeVay, Simon (1996) *Queer Science: The Use and Abuse of Research into Homosexuality*, Cambridge, MA: MIT Press.

Lévi-Strauss, Claude (1969) *The Elementary Structures of Kinship*, tr. J. H. Belle and J. R. von Sturmer, London: Eyre and Spottiswoode.

Levine, Martin P. (1998) *Gay Macho: The Life and Death of the Homosexual Clone*, New York: New York University Press.

Lewes, K. (1989) *The Psychoanalytic Theory of Male Homosexuality*, London and New York: Quartet Books.

Lieshout, Maurice (1997) Leather nights in the woods: locating male homosexuality in a Dutch highway rest area, in Gordon Brent Ingram, Anne-Marie Bouthillette and Yolanda Retter (eds) *Queers in Space: Communities/Public Places/Sites of Resistance*, Seattle: Bay Press, 339–56.

Linden, Robin Ruth, Pagano, Darlene R., Russell, Diana E.H. and Star, Susan Leigh (eds) (1982) *Against Sadomasochism*, East Palo Alto, CA: Frog in the Well Press.

Longhurst, Robyn (1998) (Re)presenting shopping centres and bodies: questions of pregnancy, in Rosa Ainley (ed.) *New Frontiers of Space, Bodies and Gender*, London: Routledge, 20–34.

Lorde, Audre (1984) *Zami: A New Spelling of My Name*, London: Sheba Feminist Publishers.

Lotney, Karlyn (2000) *The Ultimate Guide to Strap-on Sex*, San Francisco: Cleis Press.

Love, B. (2002) *Encyclopedia of Unusual Sex Practices*, London: Greenwich.

Love, Susan and Lindsey, Karen (2000 [1991]) *Dr. Susan Love's Breast Book*, New York: Perseus Publishing.

Loving More (2002a) About polyamory, http://www.lovemore.com/aboutpoly.html

Loving More (2002b) Links and References, http://www.lovemore.com/polysites.html

Loving More (2002c) Terms and definitions, http://www.lovemore.com/terms.html

Lucas, Ian (1994) *Impertinent Decorum: Gay Theatrical Manoeuvres*, London: Cassell.

Lucas, Ian (1997) The color of his eyes: polari and the sisters of perpetual indulgence, in Anna Livia and Kira Hall (eds) *Queerly Phrased*, Oxford: Oxford Studies in Sociolinguistics, 1997, 85–94.

Lupton, Deborah (1995) *The Imperative of Health: Public Health and the Regulated Body*, London: Sage.

Lydia (1995) Sibling love. *Bifrost: The Rainbow Bridge* 39: 12–13.

Lyotard, Jean-François (1993 [1974]) *Libidinal Economy*, tr. Iain Hamilton Grant. Bloomington and Indianapolis: Indiana University Press.

Macaluso, Maurizio, Kelaghan, Joseph, Artz, Lynn, Austin, Harland, Fleenor, Michael, Hook, Edward W. and Valappil, Thamban (1999) Mechanical failure of the latex condom in a cohort of women at high STD risk. *Sexually Transmitted Diseases* 26(8): 450–8.

MacKinnon, Catherine (1979) *Sexual Harassment of Working Women*, New Haven, CT: Yale University Press.

MacKinnon, Catherine (1994) *Only Words*, London: Harper Collins.

Maines, Rachel P. (1999) *The Technology of Orgasm: 'Hysteria', the Vibrator, and Women's Sexual Satisfaction*, Baltimore: Johns Hopkins University Press.

Mamo, Laura and Fishman, Jennifer (2002) Potency in all the right places: viagra as a technology of the gendered body. *Body and Society* 7(4): 13–35.

Marcus, Sharon (1992) Fighting bodies, fighting words: a theory and politics of rape prevention, in Judith Butler and Joan Scott (eds) *Feminists Theorize the Political*, New York: Routledge, 385–403.

markc63 (1996) The autoerotic asphyxiation syndrome in adolescent and young adult males, http://members.aol.com/bj022038/AEA.htm

Marks, Lara M. (2001) *Sexual Chemistry: A History of the Contraceptive Pill*, New Haven And London: Yale University Press.

Martin, Biddy. (1996) *Femininity Played Straight: The Significance of Being Lesbian*, London: Routledge.

Martin, Del and Lyon, Phyllis (1972) *Lesbian/Woman*, New York: Bantam Books.

Martin, Emily (1987) *The Woman in the Body*, Boston: Beacon Press.

Mason, M. (1993) *Male Infertility: Men Talking*, London: Routledge.

Mason, T., Carlisle, C., Watkins, C. and Whitehead, E. (eds) (2001) *Stigma and Social Exclusion in Health Care*, London: Routledge.

Masters, William H. and Johnson, Virginia E. (1966) *Human Sexual Response*, Boston: Little, Brown and Company.

McClintock, Anne (1993) Maid to order: commercial fetishism and gender power. *Social Text* 37: 87–116.

McClure, Laura K. (ed.) (2002) *Sexuality and Gender in the Classical World*, Oxford: Blackwell.

McColgan, Aileen (1996) *The Case for Taking the Date Out of Rape*, London: Rivers Oram Press.

McLaren, Angus (1999) *Twentieth Century Sexuality: A History*, Oxford: Blackwell.

McLelland, Mark (2000) *Male Homosexuality in Modern Japan: Cultural Myths and Social Realities*, London: Routledge.

McFarlane, L. (1998) *Diagnosis: Homophobic. The Experiences of Lesbians, Gay Men and Bisexuals in Mental Health Services*, London: P.A.C.E.

Melody, Edward and. Peterson, Linda M. (1999) *Teaching America about Sex: Marriage Guides and Sex Manuals from the Late Victorians to Dr. Ruth*, New York: New York University Press.

Mercer, Kobena (1993) Reading racial fetishism: the photographs of Robert Mapplethorpe, in Emily Apter and William Pietz (eds), *Fetishism as Cultural Discourse*, New York: Cornell University Press, 307–30.

Merleau-Ponty, Maurice (1968) *The Visible and the Invisible*, tr. Alphonso Lingis, Evanston, IL: Northwestern University Press.

Meyer, Moe (1994) Introduction: reclaiming the discourse of camp, in Moe Meyer (ed.) *The Politics and Poetics of Camp*, London: Routledge, 1–22.

Meyer, Richard (1993) Robert Mapplethorpe and the discipline of photography, in Henry Abelove, Michele Aina Barale and David M. Halperin (eds). *The Lesbian and Gay Studies Reader*, London: Routledge, 360–80.

Meyerowitz, Joanne (2002) *How Sex Changed: A History of Transsexuality in the United States*, London and Cambridge, MA: Harvard University Press.

Mezey, Gilian C. and King, Michael B. (eds) (2000) *Male Victims of Sexual Assault*, New York: Oxford University Press.

Milk, Harvey (1997[1978]) The hope speech, in Mark Blasius and Shane Phelan (eds) *We Are Everywhere: A Historical Sourcebook of Gay and Lesbian Politics*, New York: Routledge, 450–3.

Miller, Neil (1995) *Out of the Past: Gay and Lesbian History from 1869 to the Present*, London: Vintage.

Millett, Kate (1969) *Sexual Politics*, New York: Doubleday.

Mills, Charles (1997) *The Racial Contract*, Ithaca, NY: Cornell University Press.

Mindel, Adrian (2000) *Condoms*, London: BMJ Books.

Mitchell, Juliet (1974) *Psychoanalysis and Feminism*, London: Allen.

Moench, T. Chipato, T., and Padian, N. (2001) Preventing disease by protecting the cervix: the unexplored promise of internal vaginal barrier devices. *AIDS: The Official Journal Of The International AIDS Society*, 15(1): 1–8.

Moghissi, Heideh (1999) Oriental Sexuality: Real and Imagined, *Feminism and Islamic Fundamentalism: the Limits of Postmodern Analysis*, London: Zed Books, 13–32.

Moll, Albert (1933 [1897]), *Libido Sexualis: Studies in the Psychosexual Laws of Love Verified by Clinical Sexual Case Histories*, New York: American Ethnological Press.

Money, John (1999) *The Lovemap Guidebook*, London: Continuum.

Moon, D. (1995) Insult and inclusion: the term 'fag hag' and gay male 'community'. *Social Forces* 74: 487–510.

Moore, Kate and Whittle, Stephen (eds) (1999) *Reclaiming Genders: Transsexual Grammars at the Fin de Siècle*, London: Cassell.

Moore, O. (1996) *PWA: Looking AIDS in the Face*, London: Picador.

Moraga, Cherrie and Anzaldua, Gloria (eds) (1983) *This Bridge Called My Back: Writings by Radical Women of Color*, New York: Kitchen Table Women of Color Press.

Morgan, Kathryn P. (1991) Women and the knife: cosmetic surgery and the colonization of women's bodies. *Hypatia* 6: 25–53.

Morris, Gary (1997) When is a kiss not a kiss? When it's a queer kiss. *Bright Lights* 20. http://www.brightlightsfilm.com/20/20_queerkiss.html

Mort, Frank (1987) *Dangerous Sexualities: Medico-moral Politics in England Since 1830*, London: Routledge and Kegan Paul.

Mort, Frank (1996) *Cultures of Consumption*, London: Routledge.

Muñoz, José (1999) *Disidentifications: Queers of Color and the Performance of Politics*, Minneapolis, MN: University of Minnesota Press.

Munt, Sally (1998a) *Heroic Desire: Lesbian Identity and Cultural Space*, London: Cassell.

Munt, Sally R. (ed.) (1998b) *Butch/Femme: Inside Lesbian Gender*, London and Washington: Cassell.

Murray, Jacqueline (1996) Introduction, in Jacqueline Murray and Konrad Eisenbichler (eds) *Desire and Discipline: Sex and Sexuality in the Premodern West*, London: University of Toronto Press, ix–xxviii.

Murray, Stephen O. (2000) *Homosexualities*, Chicago: University of Otago Press.

Murray, Suellen (1998) Keeping their secret safe: menstrual etiquette in Australia, 1900–1960. *Hecate* 24(1): 63–81.

Muscio, I (1998) *Cunt: A Declaration of Independence*, Toronto, Seal Press.

Nagel, Joane (2003) *Race, Ethnicity, and Sexuality: Intimate Intersections, Forbidden Frontiers*, Oxford: Oxford University Press.

Nagle, Jill (ed.) (1997) *Whores and Other Feminists*, New York and London: Routledge.

NAIAD (1999) Evidence HIV causes AIDS: definitions and arguments, National Institute of Allergy and Infectious Diseases, http://www.avert.org/evidence.htm.

Nardi, Peter M. and Schneider, Beth E. (1998) (eds) *Social Perspectives in Lesbian and Gay Studies: A Reader*, London: Routledge

Neade, Lynda (1992) The female nude: pornography, art and sexuality, in Lynne Segal and Mary McIntosh (eds) *Sex Exposed*, London: Virago, 280–94.

Nestle, Joan (1987) *A Restricted Country*, Ithaca, NY: Firebrand Books.

Nestle, Joan (ed.) (1992) *The Persistent Desire: A Femme-Butch Reader*, Boston, MA: Alyson Publications.

Nestle, Joan (2002) Genders on my mind, in Joan Nestle, Clare Howell and Riki Wilchins (eds) *Genderqueer: Voices from Beyond the Sexual Binary*. Los Angeles: Alyson Publications, 3–10.

Newman, Felice (1999) *The Whole Lesbian Sex Book*, San Francisco: Cleis Press.

Newman, Jenny (ed.) (1988) *The Faber Book of Seductions*, London: Faber

Newton, Esther (1972) *Mother Camp: Female Impersonators in America*, Chicago: University of Chicago Press.

Newton, Esther (1984) The mythic mannish lesbian: Radclyffe Hall and the new woman. *Signs* 9(4): 557–75.

Newton, Esther (1999 [1972]) From 'Mother camp: female impersonators in America', in Fabio Cleto (ed.) *Camp: A Reader*, Edinburgh: Edinburgh University Press, 96–109.

Nordhoff, Charles (1875) *The Communistic Societies of the United States: From Personal Visit and Observation*, New York: Harper and Brothers.

Norton, Rictor (1992) *Mother Clap's Molly House: The Gay Subculture in England 1700–1830*, London: GMP.

Noyes, George Wallingford (comp.), and Foster, Lawrence (ed.) (2001) *Free Love in Utopia: John Humphrey Noyes and the Origin of the Oneida Community*, Champaign, IL: University of Illinois Press.

Nye, Robert A. (ed.) (1999) *Sexuality*, Oxford: Oxford University Press.

Odets, Walt (1995) *In the Shadow of the Epidemic: Being HIV-Negative in the Age of AIDS*, London: Cassell.

Offer, D. and Schonert-Reichl, K.A. (1992) Debunking the myths of adolescence: findings from recent research. *Journal of the American Academy of child and Adolescent Psychiatry* 31: 1003–14.

Omolade, Barbara (1983) Heart of darkness, in Ann Snitow, Christine Stansell, and Sharon Thompson (eds) *Powers of Desire: The Politics of Sexuality*, New York: Monthly Review Press, 350–67.

Oosterhuis, Harry (2000) *Stepchildren of Nature: Krafft-Ebing, Psychiatry, and the Making of Sexual Identity*, Chicago and London: University of Chicago Press.

Osbourne, Peter (1996) (ed.) *A Critical Sense: Interviews with Intellectuals*, London: Routledge.

Oudshoorn, N. (2000) Imagined men: representations of masculinities in discourses on male contraceptive technology, in A.R. Saetnan, N. Oudshoorn and M. Kirejczyk (eds) *Bodies of Technology: Women's Involvement in Reproductive Medicine*, Columbus: Ohio State University Press, 123–45.

Overs, C. (1997) Red lights: a brief history of sex work activism in the age of AIDS, in J. Oppenheimer and H. Reckitt (eds) *Acting on AIDS: Sex, Drugs and Politics*, London: Serpent's Tail, 328–38.

Owen, L. (1993) *Her Blood is Gold: Reclaiming the Power of Menstruation*, London: Aquarian / Thorsons.

Paglia, C. (1990) *Sexual Personae: Art and Decadence from Nefertiti to Emily Dickinson*, London and New Haven: Yale University Press.

Panati, Charles (1998) *Sexy Origins and Intimate Things*, New York: Penguin.

Parisot, Jeannette (1987) *Johnny Come Lately: A Short History of the Condom*, Translated and enlarged by Bill McCann, London: Journeyman.

Parker, Andrew, and Sedgwick, Eve Kosofsky (eds) (1995) *Performativity and Performance*, New York: Routledge.

Parlee, Mary Brown (1994) The social construction of premenstrual syndrome: a case study of scientific discourse as cultural construction, in Mary G. Winkler and Letha B. Cole (eds) *The Good Body: Asceticism in Contemporary Culture*, New Haven and London: Yale University Press, 91–107.

Pateman, Carole (1988) *The Sexual Contract*, Cambridge: Polity Press.

Patten, Fionna (1997) The economy of pleasure and the laws of desire, in J.J. Mathews (ed.) *Sex in Public*, Sydney: Allen and Unwin, 31–49.

Patton, Cindy (1985) *Sex and Germs: The Politics of AIDS*, Boston: South End Press.

Patton, Cindy (1996) *Fatal Advice: How Safe-Sex Education Went Wrong*, Durham, NC: Duke University Press.

Pearl, Monica (1990) Heterosexual women and AIDS, in the ACTUP/NY Women and AIDS Book Group (eds), *Women AIDS and Activism*, Boston: South End Press, 187–90.

Penley, Constance (1992) Feminism, psychoanalysis and the study of popular culture, in L. Grossberg, C. Nelson and P. Treichler (eds) *Cultural Studies*, London: Routledge, 470–500.

Percy, W. and Warner, A. (1990) Sexual liberty and the law, in W. Dynes, W. Johansson and W. Percy (eds) *Encyclopedia of Homosexuality*, Chicago and London: St James Press, 1183–6.

Petchesky, R. (1984) *Abortion and Women's Choice*, London: Longman.

Petersen, A. (1998) *Unmasking the Masculine: 'Men' and 'Identity' in a Sceptical Age*, London: Sage.

Phelan, Shane (1989) *Identity Politics: Lesbian Feminism and the Limits of Community*, Philadelphia: Temple University Press.

Phelan, Shane (1994) *Getting Specific: Postmodern Lesbian Politics*, Minneapolis: University of Minnesota Press.

Phelan, Shane (1998) Public discourse and the closeting of butch lesbians, in Sally Munt (ed.) *Butch/femme: Inside Lesbian Gender*, London: Cassell, 191–9.

Pheterson, Gail (1989) *A Vindication of the Rights of Whores*, Seattle: Seal Press.

Pheterson, Gail (1993) The whore stigma: female dishonor and male unworthiness. *Social Text* 37: 39–64.

Phoenix, Joanna (1999) *Making Sense of Prostitution*, New York: Palgrave.

Pickles (1986) *Queens*, London: Quartet.

Pile, Steve (1996) *The Body and the City: Psychoanalysis, Subjectivity and Space*. London: Routledge.

Pineau, Lois (1996) Date rape: a feminist analysis and a response to my critics, in Leslie Francis (ed.) *Date Rape: Feminism, Philosophy and the Law*, Pennsylvania: Pennsylvania State University Press, 1–26 and 63–107.

Plachy, Sylvia and Ridgeway, James (1996) *Red Light: Inside the Sex Industry*, New York: PowerHouse.

Plummer, Ken (1995) *Telling Sexual Stories: Power, Change and Social Worlds*, London: Routledge.

Plummer, David (1999) *One of the Boys: Masculinity, Homophobia, and Modern Manhood*, New York: Haworth.

Polchin, James (1997) Having something to wear: the landscape of identity on Christopher Street, in Gordon Brent Ingram, Anne-Marie Bouthillette and Yolanda Retter (eds) *Queers in Space: Communities/ Public Places/Sites of Resistance*, Seattle: Bay Press, 381–90.

Pollock, S. and Vaughan, J. (1987) *Politics of the Heart: A Lesbian Parenting Anthology*, New York: Firebrand Books.

Porter, Roy and Hall, Lesley (1995) *The Facts of Life: The Creation of Sexual Knowledge in Britain, 1650–1950*, New Haven: Yale University Press.

Potts, Annie (2002) *The Science/Fiction of Sex: Feminist Deconstruction and the Vocabularies Of Heterosex*, London: Routledge.

Pramaggiore, Maria (1996) BI-ntroduction I: epistemologies of the fence, in Donald E. Hall and Maria Pramaggiore (eds) *RePresenting Bisexualities: Subjects and Cultures of Fluid Desire*, New York: New York University Press, 1–7.

Pranzarone, G. F. (2001) 'Glossary of sexual slang', http://www.sexuality.org/l/sex/slang.html.

Preves, Sharon (2003) *Intersex and Identity*, New Brunswick, NJ: Rutgers University Press.

Price, Sally (1984) *Co-Wives and Calabashes*, Ann Arbor: University of Michigan Press.

Pronger, Brian (1998) On your knees: carnal knowledge, masculine dissolution, doing feminism, in Tom Digby (ed.) *Men Doing Feminism*, London: Routledge, 60–80.

Prosser, J. (1998) *Second Skins: The Body Narratives of Transsexuality*, New York: Columbia University Press.

Queen, Carol, and Schimel, Lawrence (eds) (1997) *Pomosexuals: Challenging Assumptions about Gender and Sexuality*, San Francisco: Cleis Press.

Radicalesbians [Karla Jay, Artemis March, Ellen Bedoz, Cynthia Funk, Rita Mae Brown, Lois Hart, Barbara Gladstone, and others.] (1970) The woman-identified woman, http://scriptorium.lib.duke.edu/wlm/womid

Ragone, H. (1998) Incontestable motivations, in H. Ragone and S. Franklin (eds) *Reproducing Reproduction: Kinship, Power and Technological Innovation*, Philadelphia: University of Pennsylvania Press, 118–31.

Rahman, Momin (2000) *Sexuality and Democracy: Identities and Strategies in Lesbian and Gay Politics*, Edinburgh: Edinburgh University Press.

Rainbow Icon Archive (2003) Icons and information, http://www.enqueue.com/ria.

Raphael, Mitchel (1998) Fetish chic. *The Toronto Star* (August 30):1.

Rawson, Hugh (1995) *Dictionary of Euphemisms and Other Doubletalk*, New York: Crown.

Raymond, Janice (1979) *The Transsexual Empire: The Making of the She-Male*, New York: Teachers College Press.

Reich, June L. (1999) Genderfuck: the law of the dildo, in Fabio Cleto (ed.) *Camp: A Reader*, Edinburgh: Edinburgh University Press, 254–65.

Reich, Wilhem (1972) *Sex-Pol: Essays, 1929–1934*, New York: Random House.

Reynolds, Paul (2002) Rape, law and consent: the scope and limits to sexual regulation by law. *Contemporary Issues in Law: Special Edition on Rape and Sexual Consent* 6(1): 92–102.

Rheingold, Howard (1992) *Virtual Reality*, London: Mandarin.

Rich, Adrienne (1986 [1980]) Compulsory heterosexuality and lesbian existence, in *Blood, Bread, and Poetry, Selected Prose 1979–1985*, New York: Norton, 24–75.

Richardson, D. (2000) *Rethinking Sexuality*, London, Sage Publications.

Riddle, J.M. (1997) *Eve's Herbs: A History of Contraception and Abortion in the West*, Cambridge, MA: Harvard University Press.

Ridley, M. (1993) *The Red Queen: Sex and the Evolution of Human Nature*, London: Viking.

Riveira, Diana M. and Hart, Angela L. (2000) Date rape drugs, *Prosecutor: Journal of the National District Attorneys Association* 34 (1): 33.

Riviere, Joan (1986 [1929]) Womanliness as a masquerade, in Victor Burgin, James Donald, and Cora Kaplan (eds) *Formations of Fantasy*, London and New York: Methuen, 35–44.

Rixecker, Stefanie S. (2000) Exposing queer biotechnology via queer archaeology: the quest to (re)construct the human body from the inside out. *World Archaeology* 32(2): 263–74.

Rixecker, Stefanie S. (2002) Genetic engineering and queer biotechnology: the eugenics of the twenty-first century?, *Journal of Genocide Research* 4(1): 109–26.

Roberts, Celia, Kippax, Susan, Spongberg, Mary and Crawford, June (1996) 'Going down': oral sex, imaginary bodies, and HIV. *Body and Society* 2(3): 107–24.

Rosario, Vernon A. (2002) *Homosexuality and Science. A Guide to the Debates*, Santa Barbara, Denver and Oxford: ABC-CLIO.

Roscoe, Will (1998) *Changing Ones: Third and Fourth Genders in Native North America*, New York: St Martin's Press.

Rose, Jacqueline (1986) *Sexuality in the Field of Vision*, London: Verso.

Rose, Steven, Kamin, Leon J. and Lewontin, R.C. (1984) *Not in our Genes: Biology, Ideology and Human Nature*, London: Penguin.

Rowland, R. (1992) *Living Laboratories. Women and Reproductive Technology*, London: Lime Tree.

Rubin, Gayle (1975) The traffic in women: notes on the 'political economy' of sex, in R. R. Reiter (ed.) *Toward an Anthropology of Women*, New York: Monthly Review Press, 157–210.

Rubin, Gayle (1984) Thinking sex: notes for a radical theory of the politics of sexuality, in Carole Vance (ed.) *Pleasure and Danger: Exploring Female Sexuality*, London: Pandora, 267–319.

Rubin, Gayle (1992) Of catamites and kings: reflections on butch, gender, and boundaries, in Joan Nestle (ed.) *The Persistent Desire: A Femme-Butch Reader*, Boston and London: Alyson Press, 466–82.

Rubin, Henry S. (1998) Reading like a (transsexual) man, in Tom Digby (ed.) *Men Doing Feminism*, London: Routledge, 305–24.

Russell, Diana E.H. (2000) Pornography and rape: a causal model, in Drucilla Cornell (ed.) *Feminism and Pornography*, Oxford: Oxford University Press, 48–93.

Rust, Paula C. (2000) Sexual identity and bisexual identities: the struggle for self-description in a changing sexual landscape, in Tracy E. Ore (ed.) *The Social Construction of Difference and Inequality: Race, Class, Gender, and Sexuality*, Mountain View, CA: Mayfield Publishing Company, 153–70.

Rutledge, Leigh. (1996) *The New Gay Book of Lists*, Boston: Alyson.

Ryan, Chris and Hall, Mike (eds) (2001) *Sex Tourism: Marginal People and Liminalities*, London: Routledge.

Sacher-Masoch, Leopold von (2000 [1870]) *Venus in Furs*, tr. Joachim Neugroschel, Harmondsworth: Penguin.

Saffron, L. (1994) *Challenging Conceptions: Planning a Family by Self-Insemination*, London: Cassell.

Sahlins, Marshall (1976) *The Use and Abuse of Biology*, London: Tavistock.

Salisbury, Joyce E. (1996) Gendered sexuality, in Vern L Bullough. and James A. Brundage (eds) (1996) *Handbook of Medieval Sexuality*, London: Garland Publishing, 81–102.

Sánchez, María Carla and Schlossberg, Linda (eds) (2001) *Passing: Identity and Interpretation in Sexuality, Race and Religion*, New York and London: New York University Press.

Saunders, Penelope (1998) Presentation at a journalists' seminar, http://www.walnet.org/csis/papers/saunders-childpro.html

Savage, Dan (2001) We Have a Winner, http://www.thestranger.com/2001-06-21/savage.html

Schalet, Amy T. (2000) Raging hormones, regulated love: adolescent sexuality and the constitution of the modern individual in the United States and the Netherlands. *Body and Society* 6(1): 75–105.

Scheide, R.V. (2002) Post gay, http://www.newsreview.com/issues/sacto/2002-02-21/cover.asp

Schmidt, M. and Moore, L. J. (1998) Constructing a 'good catch', picking a winner: the development of technosemen and the deconstruction of the monolithic male, in R. Davis-Floyd and J. Dumit (eds) *Cyborg Babies: from Techno-Sex to Techno-Tots*, London: Routledge, 21–39.

Schmidtlein, Jill (1998) Rohypnol. Fact sheet. Drug Policy Information Clearinghouse. Executive Office of the [U.S.] President. Office of National Drug Control Policy. http://www.whitehousedrugpolicy.gov/publications/pdf/rohypnol.pdf

Schor, Naomi and Weed, Elizabeth (eds) (1994) *The Essential Difference*, Bloomington: Indiana University Press.

Schulhofer, Stephen J (1998) *Unwanted Sex: The Culture of Intimidation and the Failure of Law*, Cambridge: Harvard University Press.

Schulman, Sarah (1994) *My American History: Lesbian and Gay Life During the Reagan/Bush Years*, New York: Routledge.

Schwartz, R.H. and Weaver, A.B. (1998) Rohypnol, the date rape drug. *Clinical Pediatrics* 37 (5): 321.

Scott, G.R. (1996) *The History of Corporal Punishment*, London: Senate.

Scott, Meghan (2003) Second Sex #1: Outlaw, http://www.sexuality.org/l/mscott/ssex01.html

Scott, Peter, Cokon, Tony, Kirk, Martin and Pinson, David (1998) *Cottaging and Cruising in Barnet, Brent and Harrow*, London: Barnet AIDS Education Unit and Brent and Harrow Health Promotion.

Scott, Sue and Jackson, Stevi (2000) Sexuality, in Geoff Payne (ed.) *Social Divisions*, London: Macmillan, 168–84.

Searles, Patricia and Berger, Ronald (eds) (1995) *Rape and Society: Readings on the Problem of Sexual Assault*, Boulder, CA: Westview Press.

Sedgwick, Eve Kosofsky (1985) *Between Men: English Literature and Male Homosocial Desire*, New York: Columbia University Press.

Sedgwick, Eve Kosofsky (1991) *Epistemology of the Closet*, Hemel Hempstead: Harvester Wheatsheaf.

Sedgwick, Eve Kosofksy (1994) *Tendencies,* London: Routledge.

Segal, Lynne (1990) *Slow Motion: Changing Masculinities, Changing Men*, London: Virago.

Segal, Lynne (1992) Sweet sorrows, painful pleasures: pornography and the perils of heterosexual desire, in L. Segal and M. McIntosh (eds), *Sex Exposed: Sexuality and the Pornography Debate*, London: Virago, 65–91.

Segal, Lynne (1994) *Straight Sex: The Politics of Pleasure*, London: Virago.

Segal, Lynne (1997) Feminist sexual politics and the heterosexual predicament, in L. Segal (ed.) *New Sexual Agendas*, London: Macmillan Press, 77–88.

Seidler, Victor J. (1991) *Recreating Sexual Politics: Men, Feminism And Politics,* London And New York: Routledge.

Seidman, Steven (1993) Identity and politics in 'postmodern' gay culture: some historical and conceptual notes, in Michael Warner (ed.) *Fear of a Queer Planet*, Minneapolis and London: University of Minnesota Press, 105–42.

Seidman, Steven (ed.) (1996) *Queer Theory/Sociology*, Oxford: Blackwell.

Seidman, Steven (1997) *Difference Troubles: Queering Social Theory and Sexual Politics*, Cambridge: Cambridge University Press.

Servicemembers Legal Defense Network (2002) *Conduct Unbecoming: The 8th Annual Report on 'Don't Ask, Don't Tell, Don't Pursue, Don't Harass'*, Washington, DC: Servicemembers Legal Defense Network Press.

Sexuality.Org (2002) The official watersports training manual, http://www.sexuality.org/l/fetish/ws.html.

SFAF (2001) HIV vaccine: how close are we?, San Francisco AIDS Foundation Out Reach, http://www.thebody.com/sfaf/outreach/nov01/vaccine.html.

Shapiro, Judith (1991) Gender and the mutability of sex, in Julia Epstein and Kristina Straub (eds) *Body Guards: The Cultural Politics of Gender Ambiguity*, London: Routledge, 248–79.

Shaw, C. and McKay, H. (1969) *Juvenile Delinquency and Urban Area*, Chicago: Chicago University Press.

Sherfey, Mary Jane (1972) *The Nature and Evolution of Female Sexuality*, New York: Random House.

Showalter, Elaine (1997) *Hystories: Hysterical Epidemics and Modern Culture*, New York: Columbia University Press.

Shilts, Randy (1988) *And the Band Played On: Politics, People, and the AIDS Epidemic*, New York: Penguin.

Signorile, Michelangelo (1994) *Queer in America: Sex, the Media and the Closets of Power*, London: Abacus.

Simons, G.L. (1975) A *Place For Pleasure: The History of the Brothel*, London: Harwood-Smart Publishing.

Simpson, Mark (ed.) (1996) *Anti-Gay*, London: Cassell.

Sinfield, Alan (1994) *The Wilde Century: Effeminacy, Oscar Wilde and the Queer Moment*, London: Cassell.

Sinfield, Alan (1998) *Gay and After*, London: Serpent's Tail.

Singer, Linda (1993) *Erotic Welfare: Sexual Theory and Politics in the Age of the Epidemic*, London: Routledge.

Sisley, Emily L. and Harris, Bertha (1977) *The Joy of Lesbian Sex*, New York: Simon and Schuster.

Slater, Amy and Tiggemann, Marika (2002) A test of objectification theory in adolescent girls. *Sex Roles: A Journal Of Research* 46 (9–10): 343–9.

Smith, Barbara and Smith, Beverly (1983) Across the kitchen table: a sister-to-sister dialogue, in Cherrie Moraga and Gloria Anzaldua (eds) *This Bridge Called My Back: Writings by Radical Women of Color*, New York: Kitchen Table Women of Color Press, 113–27.

Smith, Bruce R, (1994) *Homosexual Desire in Shakespeare's England*, Chicago: University of Chicago Press.

Smyth, Cherry (1994) Beyond queer cinema: it's in her kiss, in Liz Gibbs (ed.) *Daring to Dissent*, London: Cassell, 194–213.

Sontag, Susan (1990) *AIDS and Its Metaphors*, London: Penguin Books.

Sontag, Susan (1999 [1964]) Notes on camp, in Fabio Cleto (ed.) *Camp: A Reader*, Edinburgh: Edinburgh University Press, 53–65.

Sourbut, E. (1996) Gynogenesis: a lesbian appropriation of reproductive technologies, in N. Lykke and R. Braidotti (eds) *Between Monsters, Goddesses and Cyborgs: Feminist Confrontations with Science, Medicine and Cyberspace*, London: Zed Books, 227–41.

Spurlock, John C. (1988) *Free Love: Marriage and Middle-Class Radicalism in America, 1825–1860*, New York: New York University Press.

Stallybrass, Peter and White, Allon (1986) *The Poetics and Politics of Transgression*, London: Methuen.

Stanley, Julia P. (1977) Gender marking in American English: usage and reference, in Alleen Pace Nilsen, Haig Bosmajian, H. Lee Gershuny, and Julia P. Stanley (eds) *Sexism and Language*, Urbana, IL: NCTE, 43–77.

Steffen, M. (2000) The normalisation of AIDS policies in Europe: patterns, path dependency and innovation, in J-P. Moatti, Y.Souteyrand, A. Prieur, T. Sandfort, and P. Aggleton (eds) *AIDS in Europe: New Challenges for the Social Sciences*, London: Routledge, 207–22.

Stein, Arlene (1992) Sisters and queers: the decentering of lesbian feminism. *Socialist Review* 22(1): 33–55.

Stekel, Wilhelm (1950 [1922]) *Bi-Sexual Love*, tr. J.S. van Teslaar, New York: Emerson Books.

Stekel, Wilhelm (1952[1922]) *Patterns of Psychosexual Infantilism*, New York: Liveright.

Stewart, Gary K. (1998) Intrauterine devices (IUDs), in Robert A. Hatcher (ed.) *Contraceptive Technology*, New York: Ardent Media, 511–44.

Stewart, William (1995) *Cassell's Queer Companion: A Directory of Lesbian and Gay Life and Culture*, London and New York: Cassell.

Stoller, R.J. (1977) Sexual deviations, in F. Beach (ed.) *Human Sexuality in Four Perspectives*, Baltimore: John Hopkins University Press, 190–214.

Stoltenberg, John (1989) *Refusing to be a Man*, London: Fontana.

Stone, Sandy (1991) The empire strikes back: a posttranssexual manifesto, in Julie Epstein, and Kristina Straub (eds) *Body Guards: The Cultural Politics of Gender Ambiguity*, New York: Routledge, 280–304.

Storms, Michael (1980) Theories of sexual orientation. *Journal of Personality and Social Psychology* 38 (5): 738–92.

Strossen, Nadine (1995) *Defending Pornography: Free Speech, Sex, and the Fight for Women's Rights*, New York and London: Scribner.

Stryker, Susan (1998) The transgender issue: an introduction. *GLQ* 4(2): 145–8.

Stryker, Susan (2001) *Queer Pulp: Perverted Passions from the Golden Age of the Paperback*, Landover, MD: Atomic Books.

Stuard, Susan Mosher (ed.) (1987) *Women in Medieval History and Historiography*, Philadelphia: University of Pennsylvania Press.

Sullivan, Nikki (2003) *A Critical Introduction to Queer Theory*, Edinburgh: Edinburgh University Press.

Tan, Cecilia (1995) Bisexuality and S/M: the bi switch revolution, in Naomi Tucker (ed.) *Bisexual Politics: Theories, Queries, and Visions*, New York: Harrington Park Press, 167–70.

Tannahill, Reay (1989) *Sex in History*, London: Abacus Press.

Thompson, B. (1994) *Sadomasochism: Painful Perversion or Pleasurable Play?* London: Cassell.

Thompson, Mark (ed.) (1991) *Leatherfolk: Radical Sex, People, Politics and Practice,* Boston: Alyson.

Thompson, Mark (ed.) (1994) *Long Road to Freedom: The Advocate History of the Gay and Lesbian Movement,* New York: St Martin's Press.

Tiefer, Leonore (1995) *Sex Is Not A Natural Act And Other Essays,* Boulder: Westview Press.

Tomkins, Silvan (1995 [1963]) Shame-humiliation and contempt-disgust, in Eve Sedgwick and Adam Frank (eds) *Shame and Its Sisters: A Silvan Tomkins Reader,* Durham, NC, and London: Duke University Press, 133–78.

Tomlinson, J. (ed.) (1999) *ABC of Sexual Health,* London, BMJ Books.

Torok, Maria (1992 [1962]) The meaning of 'penis envy' in women, tr. David Travis, *Differences* 4(1): 1–39.

Traub, Valerie (1995) The psychomorphology of the clitoris. *GLQ* 2(1–2): 81–113.

Travers, Andrew (1993) 'An essay on self and camp' *Theory, Culture and Society* 10(1): 127–43.

Treichler, Paula A. (1988) AIDS, homophobia, and biomedical discourse: an epidemic of signification, in Douglas Crimp (ed.) *AIDS: Cultural Analysis, Cultural Activism,* Cambridge, MA: MIT Press, 31–70.

Trumbach, Randolph (1994) London's sapphists: from three sexes to four genders in the making of modern culture, in Gilbert Herdt (ed.) *Third Sex, Third Gender: Beyond Sexual Dimorphism in Culture and History,* New York: Zone, 111–36.

Tucker, Naomi (ed.) (1995) *Bisexual Politics: Theories, Queries and Visions,* New York: Harington Park Press.

Turkle, Sherry (1995) *Life on Screen: Identity in the Age of the Internet,* New York: Simon and Schuster.

Turner, Bryan (1996) *The Body and Society,* second edition, London: Sage.

Turner, William (2000) *A Genealogy of Queer Theory,* Philadelphia: Temple University Press.

Udis-Kessler, Amanda (1992) Notes on the Kinsey scale and other measures of sexuality, in Elizabeth Reba Weise (ed.) *Closer to Home: Bisexuality and Feminism,* Seattle: Seal Press, 311–18.

Ultra Violet (1988) *Famous for 15 Minutes: My Years with Andy Warhol,* San Diego: Harcourt Brace Jovanovich.

Underwood, D. (2003) *Gay Men And Anal Eroticism: Tops, Bottoms And Versatiles,* New York: Haworth Press.

Ussher, J. and Baker, C. (1993) *Psychological Perspectives on Sexual Problems: New Directions in Theory and Practice,* London: Routledge.

Valentine, David (2000) 'I know what I am': transgender ethnography, unpublished dissertation, New York University Anthropology Department.

Valentine, David (2002) We're 'not about gender': the uses of 'transgender', in Ellen Lewin and William L. Leap (eds) *Out in Theory: The Emergence of Lesbian and Gay Anthropology*, Urbana and Chicago: University of Illinois Press, 2002, 222–45.

Van De Walle, Etienne, and Renne, Elisha P. (2001) *Regulating Menstruation: Beliefs, Practices, Interpretations*, Chicago: University of Chicago Press.

Van Gulik, Robert Hans (1961) *Sexual Life in Ancient China: A Preliminary Survey of Chinese Sex and Society from ca. 1500 BC till 1644 AD*, Leiden, The Netherlands: E. J. Brill.

Vance, Carole (ed.) (1984) *Pleasure and Danger: Exploring Female Sexuality*, London: Pandora.

Volcano, Del La Grace with Halberstam, Judith (1999) *The Drag King Book*, London: Serpent's Tail.

Walker, Alice (1984) *In Search of Our Mother's Gardens: Womanist Prose*, London: Women's Press.

Walker, Alice and Parmar, Pratibha (1993) *Warrior Marks: Female Genital Mutilation and the Sexual Blinding of Women*, New York, San Diego and London: Harcourt Brace and Co.

Walker, Lisa (1993) How to recognize a lesbian: the cultural politics of looking like what you are. *Signs: Journal of Women in Culture and Society* 18(4): 866–91.

Walkowitz, Rebecca (1993) Reproducing reality: Murphy Brown and illegitimate politics, in Marjorie Garber, Jann Matlock, and Rebecca Walkowitz (eds) *Media Spectacles*, New York: Routledge, 40–56.

Walton, P. and Young, J. (eds) (1998) *The New Criminology Revisited*, London: Macmillan.

Warner, Michael (ed.) (1993) *Fear of a Queer Planet: Queer Politics and Social Theory*, Minneapolis: University of Minnesota Press.

Warner, Michael (1995) Why gay men are having risky sex. *The Village Voice*, January 31: 33–6.

Warner, Michael (1999) *The Trouble with Normal: Sex, Politics, and the Ethics of Queer Life*, Cambridge, MA: Harvard University Press.

Watkins, Elizabeth Siegel (1998) *On The Pill: A Social History of Oral Contraceptives*, London and Baltimore: Johns Hopkins University Press.

Watney, Simon (1988) The spectacle of AIDS, in Douglas Crimp (ed.) *AIDS: Cultural Analysis, Cultural Activism*, Cambridge, MA: MIT Press, 71–86.

Watney, Simon (1994) *Practices of Freedom: Selected Writings on HIV/AIDS*, London: Rivers Oram Press.

Watney, Simon (2001) *Imagine Hope: AIDS and Gay Identity*, London: Routledge.

Weatherford, J. M. (1986) *Porn Row*, New York: Arbor House.

Weedon, Chris (1997) *Feminist Practice and Poststructuralist Theory*, Oxford: Blackwell.

Weeks, Jeffrey (1985) *Sexuality and its Discontents*, London, Boston and Henley: Routledge and Kegan Paul.

Weeks, Jeffrey (1990) *Coming Out: Homosexual Politics in Britain from the Nineteenth Century to the Present*, revised edition. London: Quartet.

Weeks, Jeffrey (1991a) *Between the Acts: Lives of Homosexual Men 1885–1967*, London: Routledge.

Weeks, Jeffrey (1991b) Inverts, perverts and mary-annes: male prostitution and the regulation of homosexuality in England in the nineteenth and early twentieth centuries, in Martin Duberman, Martha Vicinius and George Chauncy, Jr (eds) *Hidden From History: Reclaiming the Gay and Lesbian Past*, Harmondsworth: Penguin, 195–211.

Weeks, Jeffrey Heaphy, Brian and Donovan, Catherine (2000) *Same Sex Intimacies: Families of Choice and other Life Experiments*, London: Routledge.

Wegesin, M.L., Elwood, W.N., and Bowen, A.M. (2000) Top/bottom self-label, anal sex practices, HIV risk and gender role identity in gay men in New York City. *Journal Of Psychology And Human Sexuality* 12 (3): 43–62.

Weinberg, T.S. (ed.) (1995) *S & M: Studies In Dominance And Submission*, Amherst: Prometheus Books.

Weise, Elizabeth Reba (ed.) (1992) *Closer to Home: Bisexuality and Feminism*, Seattle: Seal Press.

Westermarck, Edward (1921[1891]) *History of Human Marriage*, 3 vols, London: Macmillan.

Weston, K. (1991) *Families We Choose: Lesbians, Gays, Kinship*, New York: Columbia University Press.

Whitehead, Stephen, and Barrett, Frank (eds) (2001) *The Masculinities Reader*, Cambridge: Polity.

Whitford, Margaret (1991) *Luce Irigaray: Philosophy in the Feminine*, London: Routledge.

Whittle, Stephen. (2000) *The Transgender Debate: The Crisis Surrounding Gender Identities*, Reading: South Street Press.

Whittle, Stephen (2002) *Respect and Equality: Transsexual and Transgender Rights* London, Sydney, and Portland: Cavendish Publishing.

Wiesner-Hanks, Merry E. (2000) *Christianity and Sexuality in the Early Modern World*, New York and London: Routledge.

Wikholm, Andrew (1999) Biography: Karl Heinrich Ulrichs, http://www.gayhistory.com/rev2/events/ulrichs.htm

Wilchins, Riki Anne (1997) *Read My Lips: Sexual Subversion and the End of Gender*, New York: Routledge.

Wilchins, Riki Anne (ed.) (2002) *Genderqueer: Voices from Beyond the Sexual Binary*, Los Angeles: Alyson Publications.

Wilkinson, Sue (1996) Bisexuality 'à la Mode'. *Women's Studies International Forum* 19(3): 293–301.

Williams, Linda (1990) *Hard Core: Power, Pleasure and the 'Frenzy of the Visible'.* Glasgow: Pandora.

Williams, Walter L. (1986) *The Spirit and the Flesh: Sexual Diversity in American Indian Culture*, Boston: Beacon Press.

Wilson, Elizabeth (1993) Is transgression transgressive?, in Joseph Bristow and Angelia Wilson (eds) *Activating Theory: Lesbian, Gay and Bisexual Politics*, London: Lawrence and Wishart, 107–17.

Winks, Cathy and Semans, Anne (2002) *The Good Vibrations Guide to Sex*, San Francisco: Cleis Press.

Wintemute, R. (1995) *Sexual Orientation and Human Rights: the United States Constitution, the European Convention, and the Canadian Charter*, Oxford: Clarendon Press.

Winter, Bronwyn (1998), Radical feminism, women's studies list file collection, http://research.umbc.edu/~korenman/wmst/radfem1.html

Wiseman, J. (2002) The medical realities of breath control play, http://www.sexuality.org/l/fetish/aspydang.html.

Wittig, Monique (1992) *The Straight Mind*, London: Harvester Wheatsheaf.

Wittman, Carl (1992 [1970]) A Gay Manifesto, in Karla Jay and Allen Young (eds) *Out of the Closets: Voices of Gay Liberation*, London: Gay Men's Press, 330–42.

Wolf, Naomi (1993) *The Beauty Myth*, London: Vintage.

Wolfson, Nicholas (1997) *Hate Speech, Sex Speech, Free Speech*, Westport, CT, and London: Praeger.

Woods, Greg (1987) *Articulate Flesh: Male Homoeroticism and Modern Poetry*, New Haven and London: Yale University Press.

Woodward, Kathryn (ed.) (1997) *Identity and Difference*, London: Sage.

Wright, C. and Jagger, G. (1999) *Changing Family Values: Difference, Diversity and the Decline of Male Order*, London: Routledge.

Wright, J.M. (1998) *Lesbian Step Families: An Ethnography of Love*, New York: Haworth Press.

Wyatt, Nancy (2000) Information on sexual harassment: international perspectives, http://www.de.psu.edu/harassment/generalinfo/international.html

Wylde Wear (2002) Paraphilia, http://www.wylde.com/paraphilia.html

Yalom, Marilyn (1997) *A History of the Breast*, New York: Knopf.

Yalom, Marilyn (2001) *A History of the Wife*, London: Pandora.

Yang, Suzanne (2001) Speaking of the surface: the texts of Kaposi's sarcoma, in Tim Dean and Christopher Lane (eds) *Homosexuality and Psychoanalysis*, Chicago: University of Chicago Press, 322–48.

Young, Iris Marion (1990) *Justice and the Politics of Difference*, Princeton: Princeton University Press.

Young, Iris Marion (1984) Pregnant embodiment: subjectivity and alienation. *Journal of Medicine and Philosophy* 9: 45–62.

Young, R.J.C. (1995) *Colonial Desire: Hybridity in Theory, Culture and Race*, London: Routledge.

Zaviacic, Milan (1999) *The Female Prostate*, Bratislava: Slovak Academic Press.

Zita, Jacqueline (1998) Male lesbians and the postmodernist body, in *Body Talk: Philosophical Reflections on Sex and Gender*, New York: Columbia University Press, 85–108.